Urological Surgery: Current Techniques

Urological Surgery: Current Techniques

Editor: Holly Penn

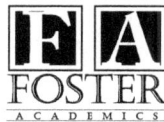

FOSTER
ACADEMICS

www.fosteracademics.com

www.fosteracademics.com

FA
FOSTER
ACADEMICS

Cataloging-in-Publication Data

Urological surgery : current techniques / edited by Holly Penn.
    p. cm.
Includes bibliographical references and index.
ISBN 978-1-63242-965-0
1. Genitourinary organs--Surgery. 2. Urinary organs--Surgery. 3. Surgery. 4. Urology. I. Penn, Holly.
RD571 .U76 2020
617461--dc23

Foster Academics,
118-35 Queens Blvd., Suite 400,
Forest Hills, NY 11375, USA

ISBN 978-1-63242-965-0 (Hardback)

Contents

Preface IX

Chapter 1 **Traumatic penile amputation** 1
Tushar Patial, Girish Sharma and Pamposh Raina

Chapter 2 **Hyaluronic acid-carboxymethylcellulose reduced postoperative bowel
adhesions following laparoscopic urologic pelvic surgery** 5
U-Syn Ha, Jun Sung Koh, Kang Jun Cho, Byung Il Yoon, Kyu Won Lee,
Sung Hoo Hong and Ji Youl Lee

Chapter 3 **Virtual reality suturing task as an objective test for robotic
experience assessment** 11
Michael A. Liss, Christopher J. Kane, Tony Chen, Joel Baumgartner and
Ithaar H. Derweesh

Chapter 4 **Heavy hematuria requiring cystectomy in a patient with hemophilia A** 18
Satoshi Washino, Masaru Hirai, Yutaka Kobayashi, Kimitoshi Saito and
Tomoaki Miyagawa

Chapter 5 **Rethinking of ureteral stent removal using an extraction string; what patients
feel and what is patients' preference?** 22
Dae Ji Kim, Jeong Hwan Son, Seok Heun Jang, Jae Won Lee, Dae Sung Cho and
Chae Hong Lim

Chapter 6 **Effects of tadalafil treatment after bilateral nerve-sparing radical prostatectomy:
quality of life, psychosocial outcomes, and treatment satisfaction results** 29
Hitendra R Patel, Dapo Ilo, Nimish Shah, Béatrice Cuzin, David Chadwick,
Robert Andrianne, Carsten Henneges, Jane Barry, Katja Hell-Momeni,
Julia Branicka and Hartwig Büttner

Chapter 7 **MMP9 overexpression is associated with good surgical outcome in children
with UPJO** 39
Sabrina Thalita Reis, Kátia R. M. Leite, Nayara Izabel Viana, Roberto Iglesias Lopes,
Caio Martins Moura, Renato F. Ivanovic, Marcos Machado, Francisco Tibor Denes,
Amilcar Giron, William Carlos Nahas, Miguel Srougi and Carlo C. Passerotti

Chapter 8 **A pilot randomized trial of conventional versus advanced pelvic floor exercises
to treat urinary incontinence after radical prostatectomy** 44
Daniel Santa Mina, Darren Au, Shabbir M. H. Alibhai, Leah Jamnicky,
Nelly Faghani, William J. Hilton, Leslie E. Stefanyk, Paul Ritvo, Jennifer Jones,
Dean Elterman, Neil E. Fleshner, Antonio Finelli, Rajiv K. Singal,
John Trachtenberg and Andrew G. Matthew

Chapter 9   **Physical activity before radical prostatectomy reduces sick leave after surgery** 54
E. Angenete, U. Angerås, M. Börjesson, J. Ekelund, M. Gellerstedt,
T. Thorsteinsdottir, G. Steineck and E. Haglind

Chapter 10   **Comparison of patient-reported quality of life outcome questionnaire response rates between patients treated surgically for renal cell carcinoma and prostate carcinoma** 63
David D. Thiel, Andrew J. Davidiuk, Gregory A. Broderick, Michelle Arnold,
Nancy Diehl, Andrea Tavlarides, Kaitlynn Custer and Alexander S. Parker

Chapter 11   **3D vs 2D laparoscopic radical prostatectomy in organ-confined prostate cancer: comparison of operative data and pentafecta rates** 69
Pierluigi Bove, Valerio Iacovelli, Francesco Celestino, Francesco De Carlo,
Giuseppe Vespasiani and Enrico Finazzi Agrò

Chapter 12   **Comparison of continence outcomes of early catheter removal on postoperative day 2 and 4 after laparoscopic radical prostatectomy** 77
Masashi Matsushima, Akira Miyajima, Seiya Hattori, Toshikazu Takeda,
Ryuichi Mizuno, Eiji Kikuchi and Mototsugu Oya

Chapter 13   **Risk factors for biochemical recurrence after robotic assisted radical prostatectomy** 85
Ryuta Tanimoto, Yomi Fashola, Kymora B Scotland, Anne E Calvaresi,
Leonard G Gomella, Edouard J Trabulsi and Costas D Lallas

Chapter 14   **A novel stepwise micro-TESE approach in non obstructive azoospermia** 92
Giorgio Franco, Filomena Scarselli, Valentina Casciani, Cosimo De Nunzio,
Donato Dente, Costantino Leonardo, Pier Francesco Greco, Alessia Greco,
Maria Giulia Minasi and Ermanno Greco

Chapter 15   **Sensitivity of initial biopsy or transurethral resection of bladder tumor(s) for detecting histological variants on radical cystectomy** 100
Peng Ge, Zi-Cheng Wang, Xi Yu, Jian Lin and Qun He

Chapter 16   **Diagnostic and treatment factors associated with poor survival from prostate cancer are differentially distributed between regional and metropolitan Victoria** 106
Rasa Ruseckaite, Fanny Sampurno, Jeremy Millar, Mark Frydenberg and
Sue Evans

Chapter 17   **Predicting 90-day and long-term mortality in octogenarians undergoing radical cystectomy** 116
Michael Froehner, Rainer Koch, Matthias Hübler, Ulrike Heberling,
Vladimir Novotny, Stefan Zastrow, Oliver W. Hakenberg and
Manfred P. Wirth

Chapter 18   **Multi-tract percutaneous nephrolithotomy combined with EMS lithotripsy for bilateral complex renal stones**..123
Taisheng Liang, Chenming Zhao, Gang Wu, Botao Tang, Xiangdong Luo,
Shangguang Lu, Yu Dong and Huan Yang

Chapter 19   **Application and analysis of retroperitoneal laparoscopic partial nephrectomy with sequential segmental renal artery clamping for patients with multiple renal tumor**..128
Jundong Zhu, Fan Jiang, Pu Li, Pengfei Shao, Chao Liang, Aiming Xu,
Chenkui Miao, Chao Qin, Zengjun Wang and Changjun Yin

Chapter 20   **Single-stage laparoscopic surgery for bilateral organ tumors using a transumbilical approach with a zigzag incision**..133
Yoichiro Kato, Renpei Kato, Misato Takayama, Daiki Ikarashi, Mitsutaka Onoda,
Tomohiko Matsuura, Mitsugu Kanehira, Ryo Takata, Shigeaki Baba,
Toshimoto Kimura, Koki Otsuka, Jun Sugimura, So Omori, Akira Sasaki and
Wataru Obara

Chapter 21   **Circumcision-related tragedies seen in children at the Komfo Anokye Teaching Hospital**...138
Kwaku Addai Arhin Appiah, Christian Kofi Gyasi-Sarpong, Roland Azorliade,
Ken Aboah, Dennis Odai Laryea, Kwaku Otu-Boateng, Kofi Baah-Nyamekye,
Patrick Opoku Manu Maison, Douglas Arthur, Isaac Opoku Antwi,
Benjamin Frimpong-Twumasi, Edwin Mwintiereh Yenli, Samuel Kodzo Togbe
and George Amoah

Chapter 22   **Continuous saline bladder irrigation for two hours following transurethral resection of bladder tumors in patients with non-muscle invasive bladder cancer does not prevent recurrence or progression compared with intravesical Mitomycin-C**...146
Andrew T. Lenis, Kian Asanad, Maher Blaibel, Nicholas M. Donin and
Karim Chamie

Chapter 23   **Acceptability of dietary and physical activity lifestyle modification for men following radiotherapy or radical prostatectomy for localised prostate cancer**...........155
Lucy E. Hackshaw-McGeagh, Eileen Sutton, Raj Persad, Jonathan Aning,
Amit Bahl, Anthony Koupparis, Chris Millett, Richard M. Martin and
J. Athene Lane

Chapter 24   **Pattern of varicocele vein blood gases in patients undergoing microsurgical Varicocelectomy**..166
Khaleeq ur Rehman, Hafsa Zaneb, Abdul Basit Qureshi, Ahsan Numan,
Muhammad Shahbaz Yousaf, Imtiaz Rabbani and Habib Rehman

Chapter 25   **Evaluation and treatment for ovotesticular disorder of sex development (OT-DSD)**...172
Yu Mao, Shaoji Chen, Ru Wang, Xuejun Wang, Daorui Qin and Yunman Tang

Chapter 26   **Systematic review and meta-analysis of randomised trials of perioperative outcomes comparing robot-assisted versus open radical cystectomy**..................179
Zhiyuan Shen and Zhongquan Sun

Chapter 27   **Laparoscopic radical cystectomy with pelvic re-peritonealization: the technique and initial clinical outcomes** 188
Qiang Cao, Pengchao Li, Xiao Yang, Jian Qian, Zengjun Wang, Qiang Lu and Min Gu

Chapter 28   **Transperineal ultrasound-guided prostate biopsy is safe even when patients are on combination antiplatelet and/or anticoagulation therapy** 194
Kimitoshi Saito, Satoshi Washino, Yuhki Nakamura, Tsuzumi Konishi, Masashi Ohshima, Yoshiaki Arai and Tomoaki Miyagawa

Chapter 29   **Bilateral benign renal oncocytomas and the role of renal biopsy** 200
Andrew R. Leone, Laura C. Kidd, Gregory J. Diorio, Kamran Zargar-Shoshtari, Pranav Sharma, Wade J. Sexton and Philippe E. Spiess

Chapter 30   **Surgical management of large adrenal tumors: impact of different laparoscopic approaches and resection methods on perioperative and long-term outcomes** 206
Wei Chen, Yong Liang, Wei Lin, Guang-Qing Fu and Zhi-Wei Ma

Chapter 31   **Preoperative lipiodol marking and its role on survival and complication rates of CT-guided cryoablation for small renal masses** 214
Fumiya Hongo, Yasuhiro Yamada, Takashi Ueda, Terukazu Nakmura, Yoshio Naya, Kazumi Kamoi, Koji Okihara, Yusuke Ichijo, Tsuneharu Miki, Kei Yamada and Osamu Ukimura

Permissions

List of Contributors

Index

Preface

This book has been a concerted effort by a group of academicians, researchers and scientists, who have contributed their research works for the realization of the book. This book has materialized in the wake of emerging advancements and innovations in this field. Therefore, the need of the hour was to compile all the required researches and disseminate the knowledge to a broad spectrum of people comprising of students, researchers and specialists of the field.

The field of urological surgery deals with kidney structure abnormalities and urinary tract defects. The management of cancers, kidney stones, ureteral stones, renal cysts and urinary tract obstruction is under the scope of this field. Modern urological surgery involves a wide use of technology. Minimally invasive surgical procedures, such as laser-assisted surgeries, as well as laparoscopic and robotic surgeries are performed with the aid of fiber-optic endoscopic equipment, real-time ultrasound guidance and lasers. The field of transplant surgery, which deals with the transplantation of ureters, kidneys, bladder tissue and penis, is an important area of urological surgery. This book elucidates new procedures of urological surgery in a comprehensive manner. It strives to provide a fair idea about urological disorders and to help develop a better understanding of the latest advances within urology. As this field is emerging at a rapid pace, the contents of this book will help the readers understand the modern concepts and applications of the subject.

At the end of the preface, I would like to thank the authors for their brilliant chapters and the publisher for guiding us all-through the making of the book till its final stage. Also, I would like to thank my family for providing the support and encouragement throughout my academic career and research projects.

Editor

Traumatic penile amputation

Tushar Patial[1]* ⓘ, Girish Sharma[2] and Pamposh Raina[3]

Abstract

Background: Traumatic amputation of the penis is a rare surgical emergency. Although repair techniques have been well described in literature, failure of replantation and its causes are poorly understood and reported. Herein, we report the case of a 9 year old boy who underwent replantation of his amputated penis with delayed failure of the surgery, along with a discussion of recent advances in the management of this condition.

Case Presentation: A 9-year-old boy was referred to our hospital for traumatic amputation of the penis. Papaverine aided microsurgical replantation of the severed part was performed, but by 48 h, the glans became discoloured and necrosis set in by 4 days. Unfortunately, by day 12 two thirds of the re-implanted penis was lost along with overlying skin.

Conclusion: Replantation of an amputated penis in a pediatric patient is a daunting task even for experienced surgeons. The vasodilatory effect of papaverine for vascular anastomosis is well described, but the use of a paediatric cannula for identification and instillation of papaverine into penile vasculature, has not been described for the repair of penile amputation. Despite its apparent failure, we believe this technique may be valuable to surgeons who might encounter this rare event in their surgical practice, especially in resource limited settings like ours.

Keywords: Case report, Microsurgery, Penile injury, Replantation, Traumatic amputation

Background

Traumatic amputation of the penis is a rare surgical emergency. A systematic review of 80 cases from 1996 to 2007 reported only 37.5% of cases undergoing a successful replantation [1]. The main etiologies for penile amputation are self-mutilation, accidents, circumcision, assault and animal attacks. Back in the 1970's, an epidemic of penile amputations was reported from Thailand, where women amputated their husbands' genitalia for infidelity. That case series of 18 patients remains the largest till date [2].

We report the case of a 9 year old boy who underwent unsuccessful microsurgical repair for traumatic penile amputation.

Case report

A 9-year-old boy was referred to our hospital after his sister amputated his penis with a sickle. The sister was being treated for a mental illness, and the incident occurred after the two of them got into an argument while playing. After initial evaluation at a primary health center, the patient arrived at our hospital approximately 12 h after the injury. The amputated part of the penis was brought to us in a polythene bag immersed in muddied tap water. On examination of the genital area, the amputation had divided the penis into two halves. (Fig. 1).

After resuscitation, the patient was started on broad spectrum antibiotics and given tetanus toxoid for prophylaxis. Prior to replantation, the part was cleaned with normal saline and placed in an ice box for temporary storage. After carefully preparing the genital area, a 12 Fr Foley's catheter was inserted through the amputated part and passed into the urinary bladder via the urethra at the amputated stump. The integrity of the corpus, urethra and dorsal vessels was verified. After orientation and alignment of the two ends an end-to-end anastomosis of the urethra was done using Vicryl 7–0. Next, the corporal bodies, were reattached using interrupted sutures of Vicryl 5–0, with special care taken near the dorsal aspect, to avoid injury to blood vessels. After carefully re-assessing the dorsal vein and artery,

---
* Correspondence: drtusharpatial@gmail.com
[1]Department of General Surgery, Indira Gandhi Medical College & Hospital, Shimla, Himachal Pradesh 171001, India
Full list of author information is available at the end of the article

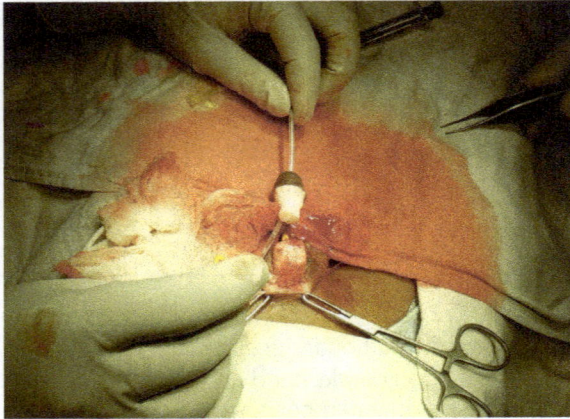

Fig. 1 Photograph of amputated penis with stump remnant

both vessels were cannulated with a 24 G cannula in succession and papaverine was injected to aid anastomosis. (Figure 2) Under loupe magnification, anastomosis of the dorsal vein and one dorsal artery was established using Prolene 9–0. Adequacy of the vascular anastomosis was confirmed by visible demonstration of the return of capillary refill at the glans and sustained bleeding from a deliberate needle puncture over the

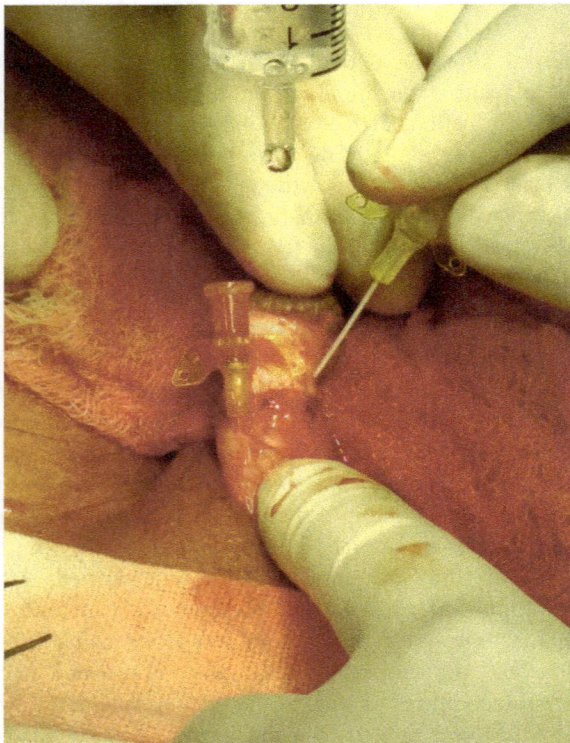

Fig. 2 Cannulation of dorsal artery and delivery of papaverine

same area. Finally, the skin was closed with Prolene 3–0 sutures. (Figure 3) A corrugated drain was brought through just below the surgical site. No evidence of necrosis was seen during or immediately after the surgery. The wound was dressed with paraffin gauze and bacitracin ointment and the total duration of the surgery was just over 8 h. Post operatively, the patient was started on intravenous heparin. Monitoring was done with aPTT (activated partial thromboplastin time) and clinical examination performed every 8 h. By 48 h, the glans had become discoloured, with prolonged refill time as evidenced at the glans. The skin had also darkened, and necrosis set in by 4 days. No vascularity was found on Doppler examination. The patient was observed for 12 days. During this time, a Psychiatric consultation was done for both the victim and his sister. Despite best efforts, two thirds of the implanted penis was lost along with its overlying skin. The patients' family refused further investigations and hence the necrotic tissue could not be sent for histopathological examination.

Discussion

The first case of macroscopic penile replantation was reported in 1926 by Ehrich without repair of neurovascular structures. This fallacy was repudiated by the year 1977 due to the advancement of microsurgical techniques [1]. Regardless of technique, the two primary objectives for the treatment of any penile amputation are, preservation of penile length and maintenance of erectile as well as voiding functions [2].

Replantation of the penis is dependent on the condition of the stump and the amputated segment. If wound conditions at the amputation site are not favourable, debridement and closure of stump, followed by secondary reconstruction is preferable [3].

Successful replantation entails the following principles; removal of debris, debridement of necrotic tissue,

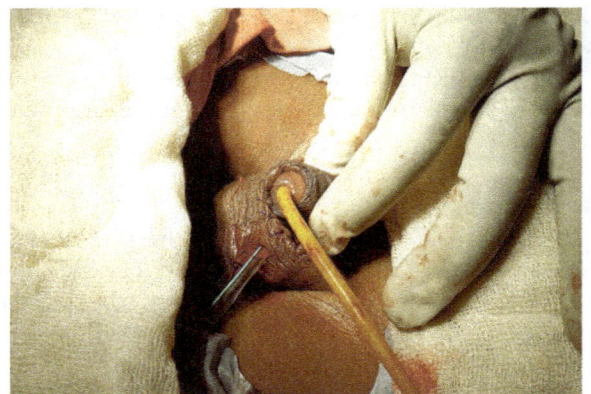

Fig. 3 Replantation complete, with Foley's catheter in situ and corrugated drain

anastomosis of the severed urethra, repair of corporal bodies and tunica, and microsurgical repair of the dorsal neurovascular plexus. When repaired without the use of a microscope there is a higher rate of erectile dysfunction and urethral strictures [4].

All patients presenting as cases of assault should be resuscitated and stabilized, before considering repair. A secondary survey should be mandatory to rule out other injuries.

In all cases an attempt to salvage the severed penis should be made [4]. The penis should be washed clean of all debris and placed in normal saline, and then placed in ice. Care should be taken to avoid the severed part being in direct contact with ice. Hypothermia increases the ischemia time and successful replantation has been reported as late as 16 h [2].

The opioid alkaloid Papaverine is well known for its vasodilatory effects and is commonly used during microsurgical repair. As a topical agent, it primarily acts as a phosphodiesterase inhibitor inhibiting the myosin light chain kinase [5]. A secondary mechanism of calcium antagonism has also been proposed for the agent [6]. The drug takes between 1 to 5 min to take effect and is known to reverse as well as prevent vasospasm [5].

Common complications of penile replantation include penile deformation, erectile dysfunction, hematoma formation, abscess, urethral fistula, urethral stenosis, delayed/ absent penile sensation and failure of replantation [4]. Since mental illness is often associated with these cases, a thorough psychiatric evaluation is a must for all patients, including those with failed implantation for possible future issues with body image and sexuality [2].

There are many causes for a failed anastomosis. These include, hematoma formation, intimal fibrosis, arterial spasm, destruction of the intima from trauma and bleeding in the media. The factors responsible for failed microvascular anastomosis can be classified as, surgical factors (e.g experience, fatigue, technique), the diameter of vessels and pre-existing vessel damage [7].

Due to the lack of histopathological evaluation of the necrosed part, any attempt at trying to identify the potential cause for anastomotic failure would be pure speculation. However, in our opinion, the presence of soil debris, the small diameter of vessels to be anastomosed, physical manipulation by the child and the time from injury till completion of repair, approximately 20 h, were major factors precluding successful anastomosis.

Post anastomosis monitoring, has been traditionally done by visual assessment. However, this was considered unreliable because of factors such as ambient temperature, vasospasm and positioning. To provide an objective evaluation, newer methods like transcutaneous oxygen measurement, Doppler flowmeters, implantable venous Doppler monitoring and transit-time flow

monitoring have been proposed. Traditional intraoperative methods for anastomosis monitoring have been, clinical evaluation, optical visualization and in some centres Doppler examination. An upcoming real time method is the phase-resolved Doppler optical coherence tomography, which has already undergone animal trials at the Johns Hopkins University [8].

Conclusion

Traumatic penile amputation is a rare emergency and despite being well described in literature, it is poorly understood. The use of papaverine as a vasodilator for vascular anastomosis is well described. But the use of a paediatric cannula for instillation of the drug into the penile vasculature, has not been described for repair of penile amputation. An operative microscope may not be available at many centres due to limited resources. Despite its limitations, a loupe based repair can provide acceptable results. We believe, this technique may be valuable to surgeons who might encounter this rare event in their surgical practice.

Abbreviations
aPTT: Activated partial thromboplastin time; Fr: French; G: Gauge

Acknowledgements
None.

Funding
None.

Authors' contributions
TP: Concept, Design, Literature search, Manuscript preparation. GS: Literature search, manuscript preparation, manuscript editing and review. PR: Literature search, manuscript preparation, manuscript editing and review. All authors have read and approved the final manuscript.

Competing interests
The authors declare that they have no competing interests.

Author details
[1]Department of General Surgery, Indira Gandhi Medical College & Hospital, Shimla, Himachal Pradesh 171001, India. [2]Department of Urology, Indira Gandhi Medical College & Hospital, Shimla, Himachal Pradesh 171001, India. [3]Department of Urology, Indira Gandhi Medical College & Hospital, Shimla, Himachal Pradesh 171001, India.

References
1. Babaei AR, Safarinejad MR. Penile replantation, science or myth? A systematic review. Urol J. 2009;4(2):62–5.
2. Jezior JR, Brady JD, Schlossberg SM. Management of penile amputation injuries. World J Surg. 2001;25(12):1602–9.
3. Yeniyol CÖ, Yener H, Keçeci Y, Ayder AR. Microvascular replantation of a self amputated penis. Int Urol Nephrol. 2002;33(1):117–9.

4. Biswas G. Technical Considerations and Outcomes in Penile Replantation. Seminars in Plastic Surgery. 2013;27(4):205–210. doi:10.1055/s-0033-1360588.
5. Ricci JA, Koolen PG, Shah J, Tobias AM, Lee BT, Lin SJ. Comparing the outcomes of different agents to treat vasospasm at microsurgical anastomosis during the papaverine shortage. Plast Reconstr Surg. 2016; 138(3):401e–8e.
6. Kerschner JE, Futran ND. The effect of topical vasodilating agents on microvascular vessel diameter in the rat model. Laryngoscope. 1996;106(11): 1429–33.
7. Lidman D, Daniel RK. Evaluation of clinical microvascular Anastomoses-reasons for failure. Ann Plast Surg. 1981;6(3):215–23.
8. Huang Y, Tong D, Zhu S, Wu L, Mao Q, Ibrahim Z, et al. Evaluation of microvascular anastomosis using real-time ultrahigh resolution Fourier domain Doppler optical coherence tomography. Plast Reconstr Surg. 2015; 135(4):711e.

Hyaluronic acid-carboxymethylcellulose reduced postoperative bowel adhesions following laparoscopic urologic pelvic surgery

U-Syn Ha[1], Jun Sung Koh[2,5*], Kang Jun Cho[2], Byung Il Yoon[3], Kyu Won Lee[4], Sung Hoo Hong[1] and Ji Youl Lee[1]

Abstract

Background: To assess the anti-adhesive effect of treatment with hyaluronic acid-carboxymethylcellulose following laparoscopic radical prostatectomy.

Methods: This was a randomized, controlled, single-blind, parallel-group study using hyaluronic acid-carboxymethylcellulose in patients who underwent laparoscopic radical prostatectomy. Sixty patients were enrolled in the study. All patients were randomly assigned to either the hyaluronic acid-carboxymethylcellulose treatment group ($n = 30$) or the control group ($n = 30$). Viscera slide ultrasounds and plain X-rays were obtained at enrollment (V0), postoperative week 12 (V1), and 24 (V2). The primary end point was the difference in the excursion distance in the viscera slide ultrasound between V0 and V2.

Results: A total of 50 patients completed this study. The average excursion distance at V2 in the experimental group ($n = 25$) was significantly longer than in the control group ($n = 25$, 2.7 ± 1.2 vs. 1.3 ± 1.0 cm, respectively; $p < 0.001$). The differences in the V0 and V2 excursion distances were significantly higher in the control group than in the experimental group (1.48 ± 1.5 vs. 2.9 ± 1.2 cm, respectively; $p < 0.001$). None of patients showed adverse events associated with the use of hyaluronic acid-carboxymethylcellulose.

Conclusion: This randomized study demonstrated that hyaluronic acid-carboxymethylcellulose treatment resulted in a reduction in bowel adhesion to the abdominal wall after laparoscopic pelvic surgery and had good clinical safety.

Keywords: Postoperative adhesion, Laparoscopy, Adhesion barrier

* Correspondence: gostraight@catholic.ac.kr
[2]Department of Urology, Bucheon St. Mary's Hospital, College of Medicine, The Catholic University of Korea, Seoul, Republic of Korea
[5]Department of Urology, Bucheon St. Mary's Hospital, College of Medicine, The Catholic University of Korea, 327, Sosa-ro, Wonmi-gu, Bucheon-si, Gyeonggi-do 14647, Republic of Korea
Full list of author information is available at the end of the article

Background

Postoperative adhesions frequently occur following abdominal surgery [1, 2]. Peritoneal adhesions are a consequence of surgical trauma such as dissection, cutting, and coagulation, and can result in adhesion-related complications that can increase health care costs. To date, there no effective treatments for adhesions have been developed. Thus, the prevention and reduction of adhesions is the best management strategy [3].

Many researchers have been trying to find effective methods to prevent adhesions, and various barrier materials have been developed and studied. Individual studies with barrier materials have reported positive results in the prevention of postoperative adhesions [4, 5]. However, another study on barriers did not demonstrate efficacy in reducing adhesions [6]. A meta-analysis from 28 trials (5191 patients) reported that oxidized regenerated cellulose and Hyaluronic acid-carboxymethylcellulose (HA/CMC) can safely reduce the clinically relevant consequences of adhesions [7]. Most of the trial agents evaluated in the above studies were based on open bowel surgery. Recently, laparoscopic surgery has been expanding rapidly and has gained acceptance as a viable alternative to traditional open surgery [8]. A certain degree of peritoneum loss should be also inevitable during laparoscopic pelvic surgery (i.e., laparoscopic radical prostatectomy and cystectomy), although the loss of peritoneum should be smaller than open surgery.

There are a few studies based on patients who have undergone laparoscopic surgery [5, 9, 10], but no study has targeted laparoscopic urologic surgery. In addition, these studies did not directly assess the presence of adhesions. The purpose of this study was to assess the presence of adhesions as determined by viscera slide ultrasound after treatment with HA/CMC following laparoscopic radical prostatectomy.

Methods

This was a prospective, randomized, controlled, single-blind, parallel-group study using HA/CMC (marketed as Guardix-sol®, Hanmi Medicare, Seoul, Korea) in patients who underwent laparoscopic radical prostatectomy between November 2011 and June 2014. All the patients were informed in detail about the aims and the procedures of the study and they signed a written informed consent prior inclusion into the study. The protocol and the written informed consent were approved by the local ethical committee (Catholic Medical Center, Clinical Research Coordinator Center; approval number XC11DIMI10098H).

Subjects

Men who were 50–75 years old and diagnosed with prostate cancer were eligible if they were scheduled to undergo laparoscopic radical prostatectomy. Exclusion criteria included any history of abdominal or pelvic surgery, hypersensitivity or an allergic reaction to the study material, pelvic lymph node dissection at the same time as prostatectomy, the presence of surgical site infection or contamination, a history of a medical disease causing bowel adhesion, or a history of severe drug allergies.

Study design and protocol

The laparoscopic radical prostatectomy was performed in same surgical procedures and steps by two surgeons (USH and JSK) who have experienced over 150 cases of laparoscopic radical prostatectomy. The laparoscopic radical prostatectomy was performed using the five-port fan-shaped transperitoneal approach. After the introducing the peritoneal cavity, incising the parietal peritoneum between the medial umbilical ligaments are incised and dissection is carried through the fatty alveolar tissue to develop the space of Retzius. After that, the surgical steps are following order (1) incision of the endopelvic fascia; (2) ligation of the dorsal vein complex; (3) division of the bladder neck; (4) dissection of the seminal vesicles; (5) incision of the Denonvillier fascia and control of the lateral pedicles with antegrade neurovascular bundle dissection; (8) apical dissection and division of the dorsal vein and the urethra; (9) urethrovesical anastomosis.

Considering about 30 % of dropout rate (under the assumption of 40 % difference between HA/CMC treatment group and the control group based on previous similar study[10]), by which the target enrollment for this trial was 60 subjects (30 subjects per group). The sample size was determined assuming a level of significance of $\alpha = 0.05$ (two-side) and a 80 % statistical power of test. All patients were randomly assigned to either the HA/CMC treatment group ($n = 30$) or the control group ($n = 30$) using a computer-generated randomization table. The surgeon was blinded to treatment assignments before randomization. Patients were also blinded to their treatment group throughout the study. HA/CMC was applied in all port sites and the peritoneal incision line of the medial umbilical ligament with a single-use applicator attached to a sprayer that allowed for the precise application to the required sites (Fig. 1). The amount of HA/CMC applied was 5 ml. Information regarding the duration of illness and medical history were collected at the time of enrollment (V0). Viscera slide ultrasound and plain X-ray were recorded at the time of the operation (V0) and 12 (V1) and 24 week (V2) after the operation.

The primary end point was the difference in excursion distance on viscera slide ultrasound between V0 and V2. The secondary end point was excursion distance on

Hyaluronic acid-carboxymethylcellulose reduced postoperative bowel adhesions following laparoscopic urologic...

7

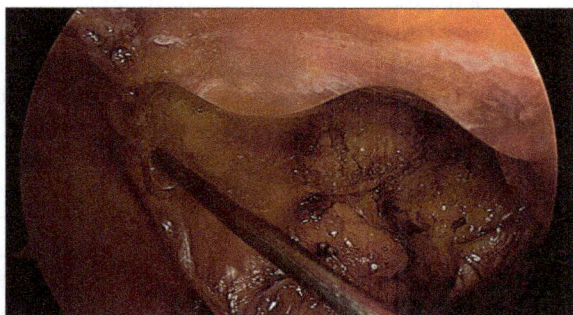

Fig. 1 A view of HA/CMC application: HA/CMC was applied to the port site and peritoneal incision line of the medial umbilical ligament with a single-use applicator

viscera slide ultrasound at V2 and the presence of restriction of viscera slide on ultrasound at V2.

Assessment of efficacy and safety

Twelve and 24 weeks after the operation, bowel adhesion to the abdominal wall was evaluated by ultrasound and plain X-rays. We performed viscera slide ultrasound according to a technique that has been previously described [11]. By dividing the abdomen into 5 segments and examining the viscera slide in each segment, a prediction of the extent of the adhesions was made for each patient. Figure 2 shows the division of the abdomen into 5 segments and their numbering. At the time of the viscera slide ultrasound, data were also collected on the location of the scars on the abdomen. The main point of interest was the distance of the longitudinal

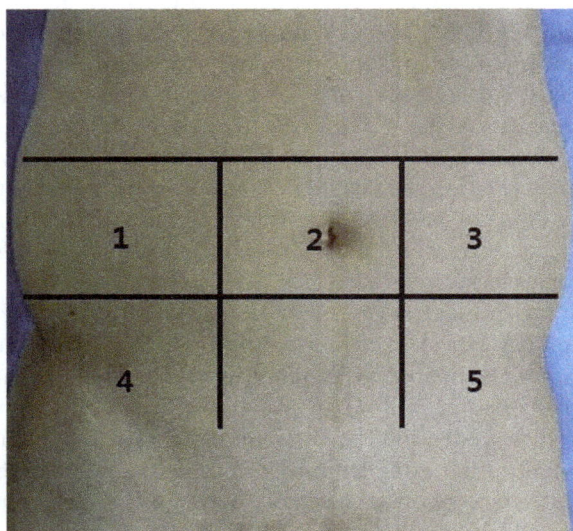

Fig. 2 Map of the abdomen divided into 5 segments by bilateral, vertical, and proximal one-third clavicular lines, a transverse line across the supraumbilical region, and a transverse line across the anterior superior iliac spines

excursion of the selected area in relation to the fixed abdominal wall. Normal viscera sliding movement was defined as equal to or greater than 1 cm of longitudinal movement. Restricted viscera slide was defined as less than 1 cm of longitudinal movement during both normal and exaggerated respiration. The ultrasound was performed by two sonographers who had been well instructed for study assessment. The assessment by ultrasound was double-checked. The sonographer, radiologist and all accessor was blind to the randomization during the all study period.

Statistical analysis

The data for this study are expressed as mean ± standard deviation of the mean. The comparisons of the 2 groups were made using a χ^2 test, an independent Student's t test, or repeated measure ANOVA. P-values <0.05 were considered significant. Statistical calculations were carried out with IBM SPSS statistics, Version 21 (IBM Corp, Armonk, NY).

Results

A total of 60 patients who diagnosed with prostate cancer were enrolled and 50 patients completed this study. In the HA/CMC group, two patients were lost to follow-up, two patients dropped out because they don't want to undergo a sonography test and one patient was switched to open radical prostatectomy. In the control group, two patients were lost to follow-up and three patient dropped out because they don't want to undergo a sonography test. The characteristics of the patients who completed the study are summarized in Table 1. There were no statistically significant differences in the baseline characteristics between groups. There were also no differences in the perioperative findings between groups (Table 2), nor were there any differences in the number of ports used for each patient (5 ports), the size of the ports (1.1 cm), or the site of insertion. None of the patients enrolled in this study showed postoperative complications such as wound infections, bladder urethral anastomosis leakage, post-operative ileus, or adverse events (e.g. hypersensitivity or an allergic reaction) associated with the use of HA/CMC.

Table 3 shows the results of the adhesion characteristics in the experimental and control groups. The average post-operative excursion distance in the experimental group (2.7 ± 1.2 cm) was significantly longer than that of the control group (1.3 ± 1.0 cm; $p < 0.001$). The differences in the V0 and V2 excursion distances were significantly higher in the control group (2.9 ± 1.2 cm) than in the experimental group (1.48 ± 1.5 cm; $p < 0.001$).

According to the restriction criteria, a total of 43 sites showed visceral slide restriction in the experimental group, while a total of 74 sites in the control group

Table 1 Demographic data of the Hyaluronic acid-carboxymethylcellulose (HA/CMC) group and the control group

	HA/CMC group (n = 25)	Control group (n = 25)	p- value
Age (years), mean ± SD	67.5 ± 9.3	65.4 ± 10.5	0.542
BMI (kg/m²), mean ± SD	24.7 ± 2.9	25.1 ± 2.6	0.453
Combined disease, n (%)			
DM	6	4	0.480
Cardiovascular dis.	8	7	0.758
Gastrointestinal dis., hepatitis	12	10	0.569
Smoking history			
Current smoker	10	12	0.569
Non-smoker	15	13	
ASA physical status classification			
1	14	17	0.382
2	11	8	
3–6	0	0	

BMI body mass index, *DM* diabetes mellitus, *ASA* American Society of Anesthesiologists

showed restriction, which was a significant difference. Plain X-rays showed an ileus gas pattern in patients in both groups (experimental group: 8 % [2/25], control group: 16 % [4/25]), but none of the participants complained of abdominal pain.

Discussion

The main findings of this study are that HA/CMC treatment increased bowel excursion distance in patients after laparoscopic pelvic surgery, suggesting that it reduced and prevented bowel adhesion to the damaged layer between anterior abdominal wall and peritoneum including port site. Furthermore, there were no reports of complications associated with the use of HA/CMC.

The key sites of adhesion formation are the port sites and damaged surface lining of the peritoneum between the medial umbilical ligaments. The peritoneal injury between anterior abdominal wall and anterior peritoneum,

Table 2 Operative and post-operative clinical data in the Hyaluronic acid-carboxymethylcellulose (HA/CMC) group and the control group

	HA/CMC group (n = 25)	Control group (n = 25)	p-value
Pathological stage			
II	21	18	0.306
III	4	7	
IV	0	0	
Total operative surgical time (min), mean ± SD	214.7 ± 82.5	202.1 ± 92.6	0.212
Estimated blood loss (ml)	158.8 ± 120.7	173.9 ± 113.5	0.382

which is inevitable, can cause a local inflammatory reaction with fibrous exudate and fibrin formation. Various factors can lead to postoperative adhesions, including the type and technique of surgery, individual predisposing factors, thermal injury, trauma, and a history of previous surgery. The balance between fibrin deposition and degradation is crucial in determining whether normal peritoneal healing or adhesion formation occurs, with peritoneal injury promoting an imbalance in fibrin kinetics which may serve as a scaffold for fibroblasts and capillary in-growth that form peritoneal adhesions [12]. Keeping peritoneal surfaces separate for peritoneal re-epithelialization is critical for preventing and decreasing adhesion.

Adhesive strength that can withstand gravity is considered to be an important factor for measuring success because the target site in this study is the abdominal wall. Park et al. conducted a study using Seprafilm® (a hyaluronate/carboxycellulose-based membrane) and found that this membrane type was brittle and difficult to apply, with liquid devices likely to be more useful in this setting [13]. Another animal study showed that a liquid device appeared to be superior to Seprafilm® [14]. The idea of using HA/CMC gel to reduce bowel adhesions to the abdominal wall was based on its relatively high adhesive strength, and previous studies have demonstrated a significant reduction of post-surgical adhesions after the instillation of HA/CMC solutions as tissue barriers during the healing process [15–17]. HA/CMC, which is a liquid-type synthetic physical sol–gel barrier with a viscosity ranging from 2500 to 3500 cP, is an anionic polysaccharide that is composed of D-glucuronic acid and N-acetyl-D-glucosamine [15]. Thus, HA/CMC is sticky and coats the peritoneum for a sufficient period and make up damage when it is sprayed on the tissue [18]. In addition to physical barrier to maintain a space, HA/CMC can reduce inflammation by preventing the migration of leukocyte and fibroblasts to the operation site. Sohn et al showed in his experimental study that HA/CMC treatment significantly decrease average degrees of polymorphonuclear leukocyte and myofibroblasts infiltration [19].

In the present study, our results showed significantly increased bowel excursion distance in the treatment group as compared to the control group. The fact that patients treated with HA/CMC had reduced postoperative bowel adhesions to the abdominal wall can be attributed to the extended presence of the barrier and the maintenance of coating activity between the abdominal wall and bowel.

One distinctive feature of this study is its examination of the prevention of adhesions in laparoscopic pelvic surgery in the urologic field. This study is the first clinical report to evaluate the efficacy of strategies to

Table 3 Adhesion characteristics in the Hyaluronic acid-carboxymethylcellulose (HA/CMC) group and the control group

	HA/CMC group (n = 25)			Control group (n = 25)			p-value
	V0 (0 week)	V2 (24 weeks)	p-value	V0 (0 week)	V2 (24 weeks)	p-value	
Ultrasound findings							
Average excursion distance of the viscera slide	4.2 ± 0.6	2.7 ± 1.2	<0.001[a]	4.1 ± 0.7	1.3 ± 1.0	<0.001[a]	
Difference in V0 and V2	1.48 ± 1.5			2.9 ± 1.2			<0.001[b]
% of restricted viscera slide sites	0	34.4 (43/125)		0	59.2 (74/125)		<0.001[c]

[a]independent t-test, [b]repeated measure ANOVA, [c]χ^2 test

prevent adhesions to the abdominal wall, such as at the port site and the incision line of the medial umbilical ligament, in patients who have undergone laparoscopic radical prostatectomy. Most previous studies evaluating the use of HA/CMC have been conducted with open surgery. The fact that minimally invasive surgeries such as laparoscopic or robot-assisted laparoscopic surgery have become more popular in pelvic surgery without bowel resection and manipulation could affect the efficacy of HA/CMC as compared to previous studies. Thus, we conducted a study targeting patients who have undergone laparoscopic radical prostatectomy.

Another unique feature of this study is that we used ultrasonic detection and mapping of abdominal wall adhesions as an evaluation method, which was developed by Sigel B et al [11]. Although adhesions are the main cause of small bowel obstruction and ileus, postoperative adhesions do not always result in bowel obstruction, especially when pelvic surgery is performed without bowel resection or manipulation. Bowel adhesion to the abdominal wall is expected to be one of the most frequent sites of adhesion in patients who have undergone surgery without bowel resection or manipulation. This means that the presence of adhesions cannot be fully assessed by plain x-ray or by clinical history in patients who have undergone surgery without bowel resection or manipulation. Ultrasound examination is a specific and reliable method to identify and detect adhesion-free areas [20, 21]. Previous studies have relied on second-look operations for the evaluation of post-operative adhesions, which is invasive and cannot be used to evaluate all patients who have had surgery. We selected ultrasound as an evaluation method to specifically evaluate adhesions between the abdominal wall and bowel.

This study had a relatively small sample size, resulting in limitation of its statistical power. Another initial concern was a lack of interest among patients to be enrolled in the control group because many wanted to be treated with HA/CMC. These data and results must be considered as a preliminary report, although the fact that these findings were statistically significant should be noted.

Conclusions

This randomized study provided preliminary data demonstrating that HA/CMC treatment resulted in a reduction in bowel adhesion to the abdominal wall after laparoscopic pelvic surgery with good clinical safety.

Abbreviation
HA/CMC, hyaluronic acid-carboxymethylcellulos

Acknowledgements
We would like to acknowledge the support provided by all the staff of the Department of Urology, The Catholic University of Korea, Seoul, Korea. We also thank the Hanmi Medicare for providing HA/CMC.

Funding
The study was funded by Hanmi Medicare, Seoul, Korea. The funding sources had no role in study design; in the collection, analysis and interpretation of data; in the writing of the report; and in the decision to submit the article for publication.

Authors' contributions
USH and JSK participated in the study design. KJC, BIY, SHH, KWL and JYL acquired the data. JSK analysed and interpreted the data. USH and KJC drafted the manuscript. JSK and JYL critically revised the manuscript for important intellectual content. All authors read and approved the final manuscript.

Competing interests
The authors declare that they have no competing interests.

Consent for publication
The informed consent included the agreement of publication of any pictures in anonymity of the patient.

Author details
[1]Department of Urology, Seoul St. Mary's Hospital, College of Medicine, The Catholic University of Korea, Seoul, Republic of Korea. [2]Department of Urology, Bucheon St. Mary's Hospital, College of Medicine, The Catholic University of Korea, Seoul, Republic of Korea. [3]Department of Urology, Catholic Kwandong University, International St. Mary's Hospital, Incheon, Republic of Korea. [4]Department of Urology, St. Paul's Hospital, College of Medicine, The Catholic University of Korea, Seoul, Republic of Korea. [5]Department of Urology, Bucheon St. Mary's Hospital, College of Medicine, The Catholic University of Korea, 327, Sosa-ro, Wonmi-gu, Bucheon-si, Gyeonggi-do 14647, Republic of Korea.

References

1. Becker JM, Dayton MT, Fazio VW, Beck DE, Stryker SJ, Wexner SD, et al. Prevention of postoperative abdominal adhesions by a sodium hyaluronate-based bioresorbable membrane: a prospective, randomized, double-blind multicenter study. J Am Coll Surg. 1996;183:297–306.

2. Menzies D, Ellis H. Intestinal obstruction from adhesions–how big is the problem? Ann R Coll Surg Engl. 1990;72:60–3.

3. Diamond MP, Wexner SD, diZereg GS, Korell M, Zmora O, Van Goor H, et al. Adhesion prevention and reduction: current status and future recommendations of a multinational interdisciplinary consensus conference. Surg Innov. 2010;17:183–8.

4. Larsson B, Lalos O, Marsk L, Tronstad SE, Bygdeman M, Pehrson S, et al. Effect of intraperitoneal instillation of 32 % dextran 70 on postoperative adhesion formation after tubal surgery. Acta Obstet Gynecol Scand. 1985;64:437–41.

5. Takeuchi H, Kitade M, Kikuchi I, Shimanuki H, Kumakiri J, Kinoshita K. Adhesion-prevention effects of fibrin sealants after laparoscopic myomectomy as determined by second-look laparoscopy: a prospective, randomized, controlled study. J Reprod Med. 2005;50:571–7.

6. Tang CL, Jayne DG, Seow-Choen F, Ng YY, Eu KW, Mustapha N. A randomized controlled trial of 0.5 % ferric hyaluronate gel (Intergel) in the prevention of adhesions following abdominal surgery. Ann Surg. 2006;243:449–55.

7. ten Broek RP, Stommel MW, Strik C, van Laarhoven CJ, Keus F, van Goor H. Benefits and harms of adhesion barriers for abdominal surgery: a systematic review and meta-analysis. Lancet. 2014;383:48–59.

8. Mettler L. Pelvic adhesions: laparoscopic approach. Ann N Y Acad Sci. 2003; 997:255–68.

9. Fossum GT, Silverberg KM, Miller CE, Diamond MP, Holmdahl L. Gynecologic use of Sepraspray Adhesion Barrier for reduction of adhesion development after laparoscopic myomectomy: a pilot study. Fertil Steril. 2011;96:487–91.

10. Tchartchian G, Hackethal A, Herrmann A, Bojahr B, Wallwiener C, Ohlinger R, et al. Evaluation of SprayShield™ Adhesion Barrier in a single center: randomized controlled study in 15 women undergoing reconstructive surgery after laparoscopic myomectomy. Arch Gynecol Obstet. 2014;290:697–704.

11. Sigel B, Golub RM, Loiacono LA, Parsons RE, Kodama I, Machi J, et al. Technique of ultrasonic detection and mapping of abdominal wall adhesions. Surg Endosc. 1991;5:161–5.

12. Arung W, Meurisse M, Detry O. Pathophysiology and prevention of postoperative peritoneal adhesions. World J Gastroenterol. 2011;17:4545–53.

13. Park CM, Lee WY, Cho YB, Yun HR, Lee WS, Yun SH, et al. Sodium hyaluronate-based bioresorbable membrane (Seprafilm) reduced early postoperative intestinal obstruction after lower abdominal surgery for colorectal cancer: the preliminary report. Int J Colorectal Dis. 2009;24:305–10.

14. Oncel M, Remzi FH, Senagore AJ, Connor JT, Fazio VW. Comparison of a novel liquid (Adcon-P) and a sodium hyaluronate and carboxymethylcellulose membrane (Seprafilm) in postsurgical adhesion formation in a murine model. Dis Colon Rectum. 2003;46:187–91.

15. Hong JH, Choe JW, Kwon GY, Cho DY, Sohn DS, Kim SW, et al. The effects of barrier materials on reduction of pericardial adhesion formation in rabbits: a comparative study of a hyaluronan-based solution and a temperature sensitive poloxamer solution/gel material. J Surg Res. 2011;166:206–13.

16. Leach RE, Burns JW, Dawe EJ, SmithBarbour MD, Diamond MP. Reduction of postsurgical adhesion formation in the rabbit uterine horn model with use of hyaluronate/carboxymethylcellulose gel. Fertil Steril. 1998;69:415–8.

17. Lee JM, Baek S. Antiadhesive effect of mixed solution of sodium hyaluronate and sodium carboxymethylcellulose after blow-out fracture repair. J Craniofac Surg. 2012;23:1878–83.

18. Kimmelman CP, Edelstein DR, Cheng HJ. Sepragel sinus (hylan B) as a postsurgical dressing for endoscopic sinus surgery. Otolaryngol Head Neck Surg. 2001;125:603–8.

19. Sohn EJ, Ahn HB, Roh MS, Ryu WY, Kwon YH. Efficacy of temperature-sensitive Guardix-SG for adhesiolysis in experimentally induced eyelid adhesion in rabbits. Ophthal Plast Reconstr Surg. 2013;29:458–63.

20. Zinther NB, Zeuten A, Marinovskij E, Haislund M, Friis-Andersen H. Detection of abdominal wall adhesions using visceral slide. Surg Endosc. 2010;24:3161–6.

21. Kolecki RV, Golub RM, Sigel B, Machi J, Kitamura H, Hosokawa T, et al. Accuracy of viscera slide detection of abdominal wall adhesions by ultrasound. Surg Endosc. 1994;8:871–4.

3

Virtual reality suturing task as an objective test for robotic experience assessment

Michael A. Liss[1], Christopher J. Kane[1], Tony Chen[2], Joel Baumgartner[3] and Ithaar H. Derweesh[1,4*]

Abstract

Background: We performed a pilot study using a single virtual-simulation suturing module as an objective measurement to determine functional use of the robotic system. This study will assist in designing a study for an objective, adjunctive test for use by a surgical proctor.

Methods: After IRB approval, subjects were recruited at a robotic renal surgery course to perform two attempts of the "Tubes" module without warm-up using the Da Vinci® Surgical Skills Simulator™. The overall MScore (%) from the simulator was compared among various skill levels to provide construct validity. Correlation with MScore and number of robotic cases was performed and pre-determined skill groups were tested. Nine metrics that make up the overall score were also tested via paired t test and subsequent logistic regression to determine which skills differed among experienced and novice robotic surgeons.

Results: We enrolled 38 subjects with experience ranging from 0- < 200 robotic cases. Median time to complete both tasks was less than 10 min. The MScore on the first attempt was correlated to the number of previous robotic cases ($R^2 = 0.465$; $p = 0.003$). MScore was different between novice and more experienced robotic surgeons on the first (44.7 vs. 63.9; $p = 0.005$) and second attempt (56.0 vs. 69.9; $p = 0.037$).

Conclusion: A single virtual simulator exercise can provide objective information in determining proficient use of the robotic surgical system.

Keywords: Education, Robotics, Simulation, Virtual reality

Background

Surgical training has met immense challenges from the rapid growth of minimally invasive surgery (MIS) across all surgical specialties, compounded by limitations in training hours [1, 2]. In particular, robotic surgery has expanding indications in many surgical specialties [3]. As with diffusion of any new technology, early adoption of robotic surgery was associated with adverse patient outcomes [4, 5]. Robotic simulation may improve the learning curve and may also improve the operative characteristics of surgeons with simulation training [6–9].

Robotic surgery encompasses new challenges in assessing skill, proctoring, and credentialing of surgeons [10]. Proctoring is an essential patient safety component of surgeon privileging for specific operations, including the

use of new technology. However, the proctor has limited guidelines, assessment parameters, or objective tools to assess other surgeons and their comfort level with new technology [11].

Objective testing of the adequate use of a robotic surgical system may provide added information for institutions and proctors regarding specific surgeons' comfort level and competency with the robotic equipment prior to live patient operative experience. We investigate whether the overall score calculated from one advanced module ("Tubes") on the Da Vinci® Surgical Skills Simulator™ (DVSSS, Intuitive Surgical, Inc., Sunnyvale, CA, USA) is associated with a number of previous robotic cases and assumed comfort with using the robotic system safely.

Methods
Participants and setting

University of California San Diego Institutional Review Board reviewed and approved the ethical conduct of the study (IRB#: 130298). After IRB approval and informed

* Correspondence: iderweesh@ucsd.edu
[1]Department of Urology, UC San Diego Health System, San Diego, CA, USA
[4]UC San Diego Moores Cancer Center, 3855 Health Sciences Drive #0987, La Jolla, CA 92093-0987, USA
Full list of author information is available at the end of the article

consent, participants enrolled in an American Urological Association-sponsored "Hands on Robotic Renal Surgery" course on May 3, 2013 were asked to perform the "Tubes" training module on the DVSSS twice at one sitting. Each participant was given a number for confidentiality in analysis and was asked to record the number of previous robotic cases performed as primary surgeon. This identification number was entered into the simulator as their user name. After watching the instructional video at the beginning of the module, the participant was not given any other direction. The results from the individual components and the overall score were recorded within the software and retrieved after all participants completed the task.

Simulator

We used the DVSSS, which incorporates the Mimic software program (Mimic Technologies, Inc. Seattle, WA, USA) to provide an MScore™ developed from individual skill metrics (Table 1, Fig. 1a and b). The MScore™ and metric percentages were developed from the mean and standard deviation of 100 robotic surgeons who have completed at least 75 robotic cases (similar to the Fundamentals of Laparoscopic Surgery FLS™ protocol) to facilitate credentialing and privileging (http://www.mimic simulation.com/products/dv-trainer/mscore-evaluation). The DVSSS uses the actual Da Vinci Si° surgical robotic console (Intuitive Surgical, Inc., Sunnyvale, CA, USA) with the video cable to the simulation pack that fits on the posterior aspect of the console (Fig. 1a). The "Tubes" module is a virtual simulation of a suturing task mimicking an anastomosis of two tubular structures and has been validated in previous studies [12]. The simulator and software have been evaluated favorably for face, content, construct, and concurrent validity, though were found to be limited on predictive validity [6, 13–15].

Study design and data collection

We performed a construct validity observational study of urologic surgeons and residents at the AUA course described above. The one-day course consisted of didactic learning regarding technique, simulation of robotic tasks, and hands-on robotic porcine laboratory experience. Data was collected from the DVSS in Microsoft Excel format including all metrics for the first and second attempt at the Tubes module. The database was expanded to include the number of previous robotic cases. We categorized participants into two groups. The first group included novice robotic surgeons (0–10 cases) and intermediate/experienced robotic surgeons (>10 cases) based on previous studies [16]. The second group for sub-analysis included residents (0 cases), novice robotic surgeon (0 cases), intermediate (1–49 cases), experienced (50–200) and expert (>200) [17, 18].

Outcomes

We hypothesized that the overall score on the virtual simulation module "Tubes" without warm up is able to distinguish novice surgeons from intermediate and experienced surgeons. Our primary outcome was the overall score on the advanced suturing virtual simulation "Tubes" module as a continuous variable. A secondary outcome was the difference in the scores between the first and second attempt, which we hypothesized would be more distinct in novice surgeons. We then examined the individual metrics to determine any trends that categorize common mistakes between novice and experienced robotic surgeons.

Statistical analysis

We investigated the correlation of the number of robotic cases and the individual overall performance MScore on the first attempt. Subsequently, we compared the mean overall MScore on the first attempt comparing novice robotic surgeons (<10 cases) to more experienced robotic surgeons (>10 cases) using the t-test. Each subgroup's (resident, novice, intermediate, and experienced) achievement of overall MScore was compared to the "expert" group scores using the Wilcoxon Rank test with Benjamini and Hochberg adjustment. In order to

Table 1 Metric definitions

Metric		Definitions
Overall score	-	The weighted average of metric scores
Economy of motion	1	Total distance (measured in centimeters) traveled by all instruments
Time to complete	2	Total time (measured in seconds) the user spends on the exercise
Instrument collisions	3	Total number of instrument-on-instrument collisions exceeding a minimum force threshold
Master workspace range	4	Diameter (measured in centimeters) of user's working volume on master grips
Critical errors	5	Number of metrics whose % score is zero
Instruments out of view	6	Total distance (measured in centimeters) traveled by instruments outside the user's field of view
Excessive force	7	Total time (measured in seconds) an excessive instrument force is applied above a prescribed threshold
Missed targets	8	Number of missed targets
Drops	9	Number of times an object or objects are dropped in an inappropriate region of the scene

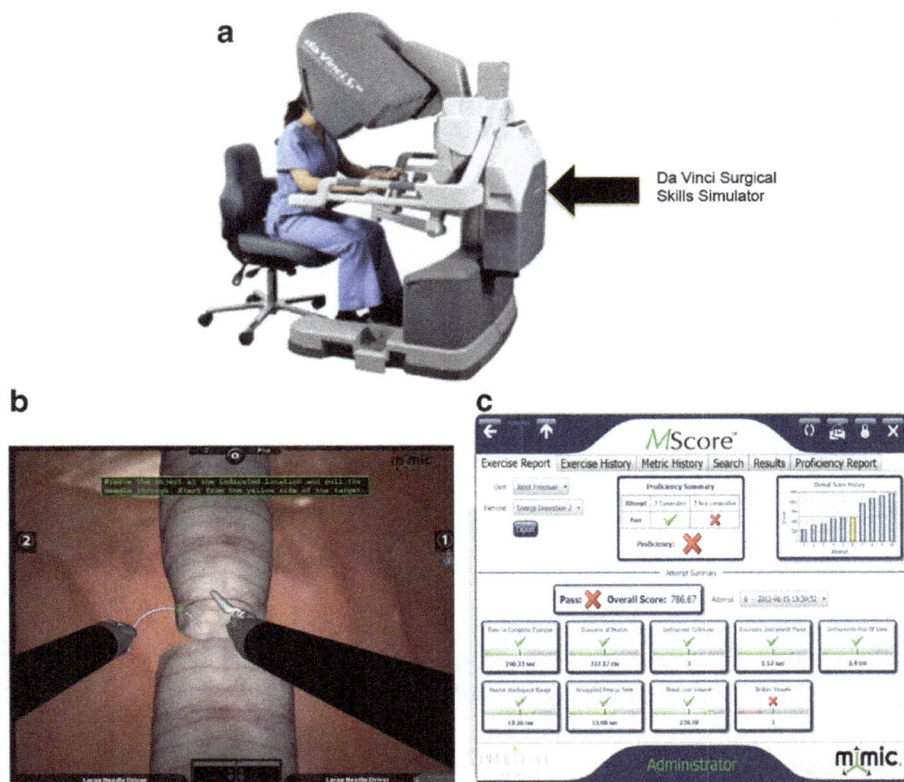

Fig. 1 a: Da Vinci® Surgical Skills Simulator™. **b**: Tubes module. **c**: MScore evaluation score sheet

investigate the amount of improvement from the first attempt to the second, a paired t-test was utilized and is displayed using a bar bell graph for each group. Secondarily, we compared each individual component metric that makes up the Mscore from the first and second attempt using the Students t test to determine differences in specific areas. We investigated the correlation of the number of robotics cases compared to the overall Mscore on the first and second attempts at the "Tubes" task on the simulator using Spearman's rho. Univariate and multivariate analyses were performed using logistic regression for individual components of the overall score to determine in which areas the novice robotic surgeons perform poorly. Subsequently, we performed bidirectional stepwise multiple logistic regression to find the most significant of these metrics compared to overall score. Finally, we attempted to determine a cut point between 50 % and 80 % that could be used as the MScore percent, which would maintain a difference between novice and more experienced robotic surgeons while maximizing the number of surgeons who would qualify as proficient to use the robot. All p values <0.05 are considered significant. Statistical analysis was performed using the R statistical package.

Results and discussion

We enrolled 38 subjects in the study with a previous experience range from 0–2,000 robotic cases. All participants completed the "Tubes" module twice, in which raw and percentage values were obtained for the overall score and the 9 individual metrics included raw and software calculated percent (%) score. The median time to complete the task was 4.5 (2.5–13.6) min on the first attempt and 3.9 (1.9–14.2) min on the second attempt. In addition to the overall score, the individual metrics that improved from the first attempt to the second were: use of the workspace, economy of motion, missed targets, and time to complete the task (Table 2).

Educational experience consisted of residents (n = 9), novice robotic surgeons (n = 7), intermediate (n = 9), experienced (n = 7), and expert robotic surgeons (n = 6). Compared to expert surgeons, residents in training and novice robotic surgeons showed significantly lower overall MScores on the Tubes module on both attempts (first attempt p = 0.039 and second attempt p = 0.023) (Table 3). The median overall MScore on the first attempt was 47.5 (range 0–95) and the second attempt was 62.5 (range 2–98). The MScore on the first attempt was correlated to the number of previous robotic cases (Spearman Correlation

Table 2 MScores

Metrics	N	1st attempt Median/Mean (SD)	2nd attempt Median/Mean (SD)	P value Paired student's t test
Overall MScore	38	47.5/53.76 (22.11)	62.5/62.58 (20.73)	0.012
Workspace	38	9/9.08 (1.88)	8/8.16 (1.26)	0.015
Collisions	38	5.5/8.32 (7.73)	5/7.24 (8.06)	0.474
Economy of Motion	38	478/510.4 (196.7)	385/440.11 (207.38)	0.043
Excessive For	38	0.0/0.68 (1.65)	0.0/ 2.58 (12.81)	0.376
Instruments Out of View	38	0.0/1.52 (2.73)	0.5/1.45 (2.14)	0.865
Missed Targets	38	7/9.08 (7.57)	4/5.71 (6.24)	0.029
Time to complete task	38	272/325.7 (150.6)	236/260.42 (122.66)	0.011

Overall MScores obtained by subjects based on experience group in the first and second attempt to complete the "Tubes" simulator module

0.465 (p = 0.003) (Fig. 2a). The second attempt was no longer correlative (Spearman 0.200; p = 0.228) (Fig. 2b). Significant differences in the mean MScores were noted comparing the novice robotic surgeons and surgeons with some robotic experience on the first (44.7 vs. 63.9; p = 0.005) and second attempt (56.0 vs. 69.9; p = 0.037). The overall scores did improve on the second attempt by 8.82 %, in which the novice group improved to a greater extent than the experienced group (11.4 % vs. 6 %; p = 0.012). We graphed each individual subject's 1st and 2nd attempts and connected each score with a line to display trends of improvement within each sub-group of experience level (Fig. 3). In this figure, novice and residents without attending level experience on the robot nearly unanimously improved on the second attempt. The other levels of robotic experience seem to be less predictable, possibly due to their particular robotic expertise or experience with this particular simulator.

In order to identify metrics most influential to the overall MScore, we performed logistic regression and identified that experienced surgeons had more out of view penalties if adjusting for missed targets (p = 0.014)

on the first attempt despite having higher overall scores. On the second attempt, time (p = 0.014) and missed targets (p = 0.004) were the most significant factors between the novice and experienced groups (Table 4).

Therefore, the "Tubes" simulator module within the DVSSS does have construct validity to determine if the subject has performed more than 10 cases previously. The virtual simulation task, therefore, may be useful as an objective assessment of proficient use of the robotic console defined as basic functional use of the robot system (not surgical proficiency). Limiting the test to only one difficult virtual reality simulation may limit the amount of information obtained, however, the test can be performed quickly (approximately 5 min) and efficiently.

A previous study has suggested that the use of virtual reality robotic simulation may serve as an assessment tool in a variety of settings [19]. We tested a wide range of robotic surgical experience to determine if one task or module ("Tubes") could have the ability to provide assessment value in proctoring in a future study. Proctoring requires another surgeon to assess the new surgeon's ability to perform a particular surgery and report to the

Table 3 Overall MScores based on experience level

Overall MScore			Median/Mean overall Mscore (SD)					
Experience level	N	Number of robotic cases	1st attempt	P value*	2nd attempt	P value*	Mean difference (SD)	P value*
Resident	9	0	42/45.22 (21.94)	0.039	61/62.56 (13.70)	0.97	17.33 (14.99)	0.023
Novice	7	0	34/39.57 (7.48)	0.039	61/59.29 (11.86)	0.97	19.71 12.75)	0.023
Intermediate	9	1-49	57/60.67 (21.42)	0.28	74/61.56 (32.35)	0.97	0.89 (29.32)	0.555
Experienced	7	50 - 200	42/49.86 (22.12)	0.149	55/60.71 (23.23)	0.97	10.86 (16.50)	0.305
Expert	6	>200	80/77.33 (16.52)	-	72/70.17 (17.28)	-	-7.17 (11.43)	-
				P Value**		P Value**		P Value**
Novice	20	≤10	42.5/44.65 (16.91)	0.006	60/56.00 (19.83)	0.037	11.4 (23.2)	0.429
Experienced	18	>10	68/63.89 (23.21)		72.5/69.8 (19.70)		5.9 (17.3)	

*Compared to Expert (Wilcoxin Rank with Benjamini and Hochberg adjustment)
**Student t test

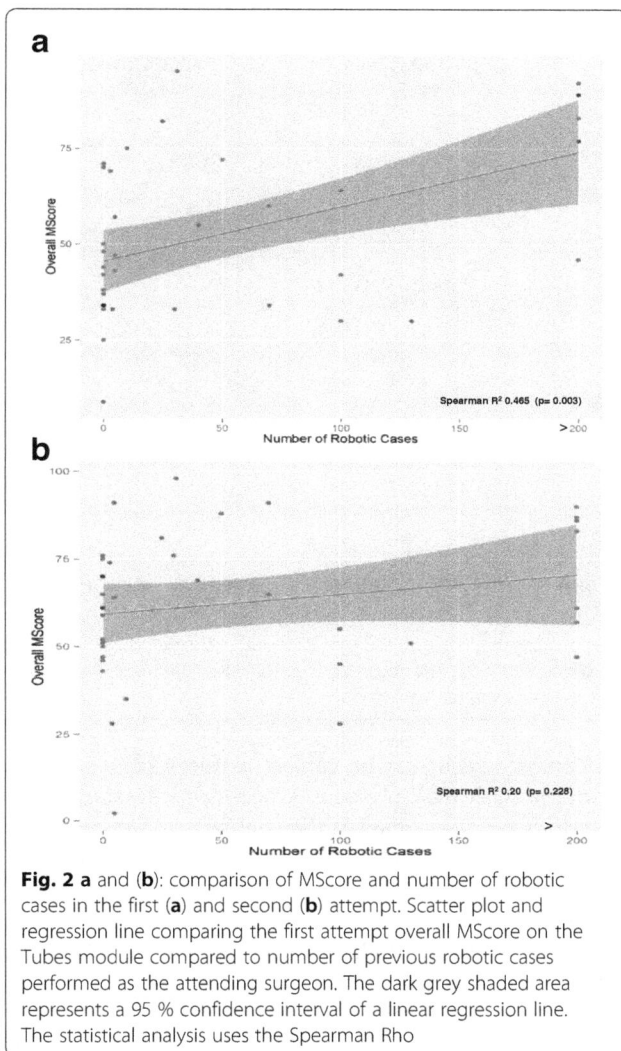

Fig. 2 a and (**b**): comparison of MScore and number of robotic cases in the first (**a**) and second (**b**) attempt. Scatter plot and regression line comparing the first attempt overall MScore on the Tubes module compared to number of previous robotic cases performed as the attending surgeon. The dark grey shaded area represents a 95 % confidence interval of a linear regression line. The statistical analysis uses the Spearman Rho

moving robotic arms out of the field, potentially causing safety concerns to which a common reaction would be: "I know where the arm is." Even experienced surgeons should use the simulation as an opportunity for improvement. Another scenario would be if a novice scored exceptionally well on the MScore tasks. The surgeon would still go through the usual proctoring and prove the ability to troubleshoot the robotic system, but may not need additional mentored robotic console training.

The simulator can provide these metrics; however, in order to incorporate them into proctoring, a benchmark needs to be set to provide assessment. Many proficiency based surgical curricula and training programs are based on pass rates of 80 %–91 % to progress to the next level [9, 21]. We then identified that an overall MScore of 75 % would serve as the lowest possible score that could still distinguish surgeon experience even if the surgeon is granted a second attempt. On first attempt only 1 of 20 (5 %) novice surgeons were able to pass compared to 8 of 18 (44 %) surgeons with >10 robotic cases (p = 0.001). When given a second attempt, 2 additional novices (15 %) and 1 additional surgeon with some robotic experience (50 %) were able to pass with maintenance of statistically significant difference between the groups (p = 0.020). Overall, 23 failed both attempts and 6 passed both attempts, 3 passed on the first but not second and 6 failed on first and passed on second attempt. We emphasize the contrast in distinguishing familiarity with the robotic console and basic operation, not surgical proficiency. The cutoff values are arbitrary but should be consistent to compare surgeons to their peers and provide baseline proficiency.

If a surgeon "fails" their first attempt, the natural inclination is to try again. Therefore, we had the subjects perform the task a second time to determine improvement levels, as described above. We found that both the novice and experienced groups were able to improve their overall MScore on the second attempt, with the novice group able to improve to a greater extent. The improvement provides suggestive information that the simulator does have a learning curve and repeated measures may improve their virtual reality score, which may in turn provide improved operative efficiency [9]. Thus, turning the proctoring experience into an opportunity for improvement with specific recommendations on areas of focus. Based on the simulator results, the learner can be directed to a surgeon-specific training curriculum if needed.

The culture regarding operative safety has drastically improved in the last few decades with the use of safety checklists, pathways, and guidelines [22]. One component of safety that has not been investigated sufficiently is the incorporation of new technology and the surgeon. Previous studies suggest a reduction in errors may be

credentialing authority [20]. The proctor's prior training, experience and ability to judge competency may be highly variable; however, the proctor does have the authority and responsibility to recommend further training prior to a surgeon being given unrestricted privileges to perform robotic surgery [10, 20]. Therefore, introducing an objective measure to assess the surgeon's comfort with the robotic system may be helpful to identify those surgeons who may need to take part in a standardized robotic curriculum prior to robotic privileging.

The simulator can identify particular tasks the user may need additional practice or training on, making the test a learning opportunity (Fig. 1). Metrics such as workspace utilization, economy of motion, missed targets and time all play important factors in the overall MScore and can provide an opportunity for self-reflection and improvement. No to be understated, the more experienced group of robotic surgeons had more "out of view" errors. More experienced surgeons may be

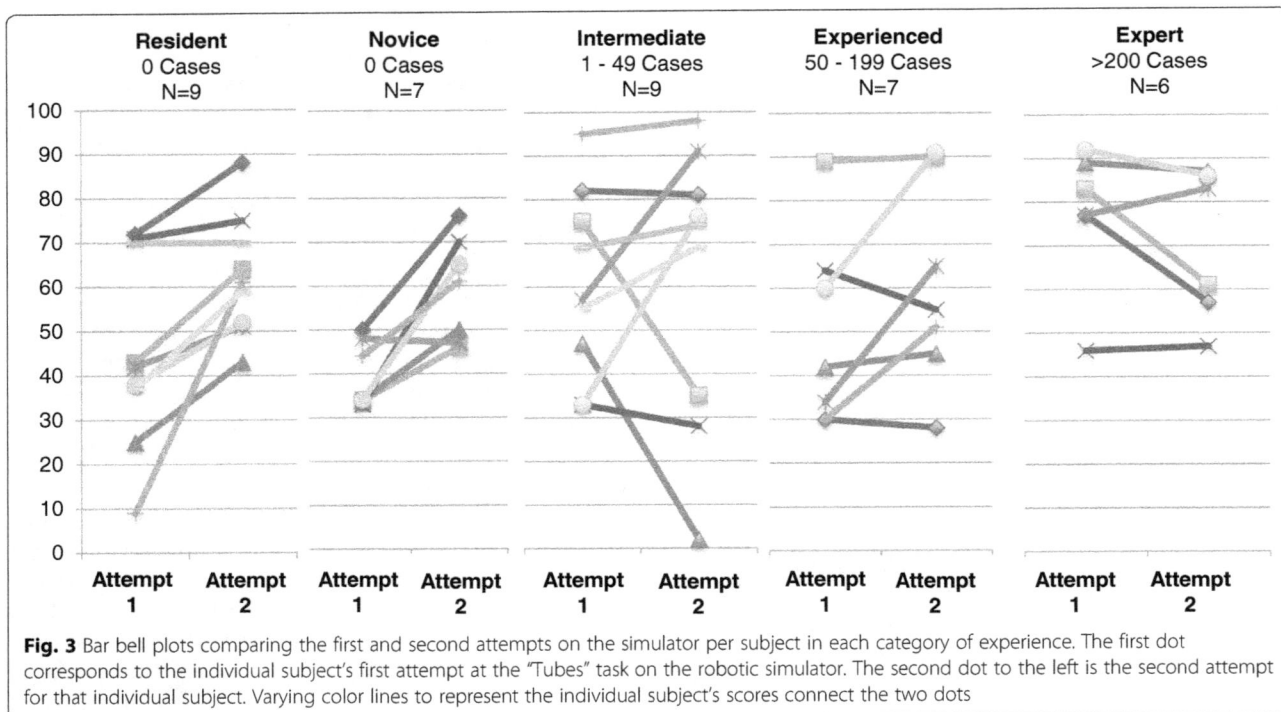

Fig. 3 Bar bell plots comparing the first and second attempts on the simulator per subject in each category of experience. The first dot corresponds to the individual subject's first attempt at the "Tubes" task on the robotic simulator. The second dot to the left is the second attempt for that individual subject. Varying color lines to represent the individual subject's scores connect the two dots

achieved with the use of surgical simulation similar to flight simulation in the aviation industry [23]. Currently, simulators for surgical training, practice and warm-up are not widely utilized [24]. Barriers of cost, validation, and optimal specific simulators and tasks have hampered widespread adoption.

Our study is limited by the sample size and number of repeated measures. In addition, we relied on the surgeons to remember the number of robotic cases they have

Table 4 Experience and individual metrics of the overall MScore

Univariate	Attempt 1	Attempt 2
	P value	P value
Workspace	0.943	0.586
Collisions	0.136	0.081
Economy of Motion	0.104	0.121
Excessive Force	0.101	0.3
Out of View	0.025	0.546
Missed Targets	0.083	0.91
Overall Time	0.021	0.13
Multivariate[a]		
Excessive Force	0.078	
Out of View	0.014	
Missed Targets	0.127	0.014
Overall Time		0.004

Metrics obtained by subjects based on experience group (novice ≤10 cases, experienced >10 cases) in the first and second attempt to complete the "Tubes" simulator module
[a]Using Akaike Info Criterion Model Selection

performed, which may be subject to recall bias. Of note, we did not ask their previous experience with simulators. The study was developed in the context of a robotic training course, which interjects some bias regarding the participants. The novice surgeons and residents are not yet at the point of requiring robotic surgical privileges, although a range of skill was needed for the purposes of the study. Additionally, the use of surgical simulators have limitations in that the DVSSS is attached to the actual console and can only be performed when not in use for patient care. Similar software has been used in the Da Vinci Trainer (Mimic Technologies, Seattle, WA, USA) as a tabletop simulator that may be more mobile though may have less working space [12]. The simulator's virtual reality environment is improving but continues to have low fidelity compared to actual human surgery. Therefore, simulator based testing can only offer an assessment regarding operation of the robotic equipment and not surgical decision-making. We stress that this single simulator test is helpful, but may not be ready for widespread use and standardization. Subjects may not be familiar with the simulator and may need to perform practice sessions first; due to time constraints of the study, we selected one tool and performed it twice. The use of simulators prior to incorporating them into credentialing should be rigorously studied and tested, such as the Fundamentals of Laparoscopic Surgery examination for general surgeons [25, 26]. Proctors with robotic experience would be needed to evaluate actual robotic surgical proficiency. With the help of telemedicine, these opportunities may be offered to hospitals that do not have experienced robotic surgeons available [27].

Conclusions

A single virtual simulator exercise can provide objective information to assist surgical proctors in assessing the use of the surgical robot in addition to the usual proctoring process. This study supports further research regarding the proctoring process for robotic privileges and further incorporation of simulation into robotic skills testing. The results from the virtual simulation process may be used as a learning tool and guideline for individualized robotic curriculum to improve the surgeon's efficiency on the robotic console.

Competing interests
Dr. Christopher J. Kane is a consultant for Intuitive Surgical, Inc. Dr. Ithaar H. Derweesh is an investigator in a study sponsored by GlaxoSmithKline. Michael A. Liss, Tony Chen and Joel Baumgartner have no conflicts of interest or financial ties to disclose.

Authors' contributions
ML conceived and designed the study along with data collection, statistical analysis, and writing the manuscript. CK provided support for the study, assisted with data collection, and edited the manuscript. TC performed data collection and formation of tables. JB performed statistical analysis. ID performed oversight of the project and manuscript editing. All authors read and approved the final manuscript.

Acknowledgements
We would like to acknowledge Intuitive Surgical, Inc. for assistance in obtaining the data from the surgical simulators that were provided for the robotic surgical course.

Author details
[1]Department of Urology, UC San Diego Health System, San Diego, CA, USA.
[2]University of California, San Diego School of Medicine, La Jolla, CA, USA.
[3]Department of Surgery, UC San Diego Health System, San Diego, CA, USA.
[4]UC San Diego Moores Cancer Center, 3855 Health Sciences Drive #0987, La Jolla, CA 92093-0987, USA.

References
1. Chung RS, Ahmed N. The impact of minimally invasive surgery on residents' open operative experience: analysis of two decades of national data. Ann Surg. 2010;251:205–12.
2. Antiel RM, Reed DA, Van Arendonk KJ, Wightman SC, Hall DE, Porterfield JR, Horvath KD, Terhune KP, Tarpley JL, Farley DR. Effects of duty hour restrictions on core competencies, education, quality of life, and burnout among general surgery interns. JAMA Surg. 2013;148:448–55.
3. Anderson JE, Chang DC, Parsons JK, Talamini MA. The first national examination of outcomes and trends in robotic surgery in the United States. J Am Coll Surg. 2012;215:107–14. discussion 114-106.
4. Mirheydar HS, Parsons JK. Diffusion of robotics into clinical practice in the United States: process, patient safety, learning curves, and the public health. World J Urology. 2013;31:455–61.
5. Ellison EC, Carey LC. Lessons learned from the evolution of the laparoscopic revolution. Surg Clin North Am. 2008;88:927–41.
6. Lendvay TS, Brand TC, White L, Kowalewski T, Jonnadula S, Mercer LD, Khorsand D, Andros J, Hannaford B, Satava RM. Virtual reality robotic surgery warm-up improves task performance in a dry laboratory environment: a prospective randomized controlled study. J Am Coll Surg. 2013;216:1181–92.
7. Seymour NE, Gallagher AG, Roman SA, O'Brien MK, Bansal VK, Andersen DK, Satava RM. Virtual reality training improves operating room performance:

8. results of a randomized, double-blinded study. Ann Surg. 2002;236:458–63. discussion 463-454.
8. Lerner MA, Ayalew M, Peine WJ, Sundaram CP. Does training on a virtual reality robotic simulator improve performance on the da Vinci surgical system? J Endourol. 2010;24:467–72.
9. Ahlberg G, Enochsson L, Gallagher AG, Hedman L, Hogman C, McClusky 3rd DA, Ramel S, Smith CD, Arvidsson D. Proficiency-based virtual reality training significantly reduces the error rate for residents during their first 10 laparoscopic cholecystectomies. Am J Surg. 2007;193:797–804.
10. Zorn KC, Gautam G, Shalhav AL, Clayman RV, Ahlering TE, Albala DM, Lee DI, Sundaram CP, Matin SF, Castle EP, et al. Training, credentialing, proctoring and medicolegal risks of robotic urological surgery: recommendations of the society of urologic robotic surgeons. J Urol. 2009;182:1126–32.
11. Sachdeva AK, Russell TR. Safe introduction of new procedures and emerging technologies in surgery: education, credentialing, and privileging. Surg Clin North Am. 2007;87:853–66.
12. Liss MA, Abdelshehid C, Quach S, Lusch A, Graversen J, Landman J, McDougall EM. Validation, correlation, and comparison of the da Vinci trainer() and the daVinci surgical skills simulator() using the Mimic() software for urologic robotic surgical education. J Endourol. 2012;26:1629–34.
13. Finnegan KT, Meraney AM, Staff I, Shichman SJ. da Vinci Skills Simulator construct validation study: correlation of prior robotic experience with overall score and time score simulator performance. Urology. 2012;80:330–5.
14. Kenney PA, Wszolek MF, Gould JJ, Libertino JA, Moinzadeh A. Face, content, and construct validity of dV-trainer, a novel virtual reality simulator for robotic surgery. Urology. 2009;73:1288–92.
15. Lendvay TS, Casale P, Sweet R, Peters C. VR robotic surgery: randomized blinded study of the dV-Trainer robotic simulator. Stud Health Technol Inform. 2008;132:242–4.
16. Perrenot C, Perez M, Tran N, Jehl JP, Felblinger J, Bresler L, Hubert J. The virtual reality simulator dV-Trainer((R)) is a valid assessment tool for robotic surgical skills. Surg Endosc. 2012;26:2587–93.
17. Seixas-Mikelus SA, Kesavadas T, Srimathveeravalli G, Chandrasekhar R, Wilding GE, Guru KA. Face validation of a novel robotic surgical simulator. Urology. 2010;76:357–60.
18. van der Meijden OA, Broeders IA, Schijven MP. The SEP "robot": a valid virtual reality robotic simulator for the Da Vinci Surgical System? Surg Technol Int. 2010;19:51–8.
19. Lee JY, Mucksavage P, Kerbl DC, Huynh VB, Etafy M, McDougall EM. Validation study of a virtual reality robotic simulator–role as an assessment tool? J Urology. 2012;187:998–1002.
20. Livingston EH, Harwell JD. The medicolegal aspects of proctoring. Am J Surg. 2002;184:26–30.
21. Zhang N, Sumer BD. Transoral robotic surgery: simulation-based standardized training. JAMA Otolaryngol. 2013;139:1111–7.
22. de Vries EN, Prins HA, Crolla RM, den Outer AJ, van Andel G, van Helden SH, Schlack WS, van Putten MA. Effect of a comprehensive surgical safety system on patient outcomes. New England J Med. 2010;363:1928–37.
23. Henriksen K, Battles JB, Marks ES, et al. Advances in Patient Safety: From Research to Implementation (Volume 4: Programs, Tools, and Products). Rockville (MD): Agency for Healthcare Research and Quality (US); 2005.
24. Liss MA, McDougall EM. Robotic surgical simulation. Cancer. 2013;19:124–9.
25. Derossis AM, Fried GM, Abrahamowicz M, Sigman HH, Barkun JS, Meakins JL. Development of a model for training and evaluation of laparoscopic skills. Am J Surg. 1998;175:482–7.
26. Vassiliou MC, Dunkin BJ, Marks JM, Fried GM. FLS and FES: comprehensive models of training and assessment. Surg Clin North Am. 2010;90:535–58.
27. Ereso AQ, Garcia P, Tseng E, Dua MM, Victorino GP, Guy LT. Usability of robotic platforms for remote surgical teleproctoring. Telemed J and E-health. 2009;15:445–53.

4

Heavy hematuria requiring cystectomy in a patient with hemophilia A

Satoshi Washino*, Masaru Hirai, Yutaka Kobayashi, Kimitoshi Saito and Tomoaki Miyagawa

Abstract

Background: Hemophilia A is an X-linked recessive disorder caused by a deficiency in factor VIII. Hemophilia A affects 1 in 5,000–10,000 males. Hematuria is frequent in hemophilia. Hematuria in hemophilia is generally considered benign and manageable with conservative therapy; however, severe hematuria requiring surgical therapy has rarely been reported.

Case presentation: A 60-year-old male with hemophilia A presented with persistent gross hematuria of unknown cause. He was treated with recombinant factor VIII products, followed by several conservative therapies as follows: clot evacuation by vesicoclysis, continuous bladder irrigation with normal saline, and intravesical instillation of aluminum hydroxide/magnesium hydroxide (Maalox); however, these failed to resolve the hemorrhaging. The patient was offered and consented to cystectomy with an ileal conduit. Intraoperative clotting was normal with the infusion of adequate recombinant factor VIII products and transfusion of fresh-frozen plasma, and the procedure was performed safely. After surgery, the patient had blood in his stool several times. No bleeding site was demonstrated in the colon by colonoscopy and ^{99m}Technetium-human serum albumin-diethylenetriaminepenta-acetic acid scintigraphy demonstrated that the extravasation of radioactive isotope was detected at the anal side of terminal ileum but not at the oral side. These findings were suspected to be bleeding from the ileoileal anastomosis. However, the bleeding was managed with recombinant factor VIII products.

Conclusions: Cystectomy in hemophilia may be safe, if monitored appropriately. Urinary diversion using the intestine may be avoided because anastomotic hemorrhage may become a problem.

Background

Hemophilia A and B are X-linked recessive disorders caused by deficiencies in factors VIII and IX, respectively. Hemophilia A affects 1 in 5,000–10,000 males, whereas hemophilia B affects 1 in 25,000–30,000 males [1]. Hematuria is a frequent manifestation of hemophilia. Historically, hematuria in hemophilia has generally been considered benign and manageable with conservative therapy [1]. However, severe hematuria in hemophilia has rarely been reported [2, 3]. Here, we present a case of severe hematuria requiring surgical therapy. This is the first case report to date of cystectomy with an ileal conduit urinary diversion in a patient with hemophilia A.

---
* Correspondence: suwajiisan@jichi.ac.jp
The Department of Urology, Saitama Medical Center Jichi Medical University, 1-847, Amanuma-cho, Omiya-ku, Saitama city, Saitama, Japan

Case presentation

A 60-year-old male with a mild factor VIII deficiency presented to the hematology clinic at our hospital with a 1-week history of asymptomatic gross hematuria. He had suffered a hemorrhagic gastric ulcer at the age of 48 and was diagnosed with mild hemophilia A (his factor VIII levels were 6 % of normal) at that time. He had suffered a cerebral hemorrhage at the age of 59. For several years beginning at the age of 50, the patient had experienced mild hematuria, and he had experienced one episode of intramuscular and subcutaneous hemorrhage; both conditions were managed with recombinant factor VIII products.

A physical examination revealed no abnormal signs. Laboratory tests revealed that the patient's activated partial thromboplastin time (aPTT) was prolonged to 74.6 s (normal range, 28.5–40.9 s), but his prothrombin time-international normalized ratio, platelet count, serum creatinine level, and prostate-specific antigen level were unremarkable. The patient's urinalysis results were normal, except for the gross hematuria, and urine cytology revealed no cancer cells. The patient was treated with a third-generation recombinant factor VIII product (Advate). However, he had persistent hematuria, followed by clot retention. Thus, he was referred to the Department of Urology. Computed tomography demonstrated that his bladder was filled with a blood clot (Fig. 1), but his prostate and upper urinary tract were apparently normal.

He was admitted to our hospital and received the following therapy: clot evacuation by vesicoclysis, continuous bladder irrigation with normal saline, and intravesical instillation of aluminum hydroxide/magnesium hydroxide (Maalox) concurrent with the administration of Advate, which failed to resolve the hemorrhage. Consequently, the patient had repeated transfusions of packed red cells. Although the patient also underwent transurethral coagulation of the bladder mucosa under anesthesia, the bleeding presented with oozing throughout the mucosa and was not controlled. Subsequently, the patient developed pyelonephritis in his left kidney with a severe reduction (<50 mL) in his bladder capacity. Conservative management for 2 months failed to resolve the patient's symptoms, so he was offered a cystectomy with ileal conduit and consented to it after a detailed discussion.

The quality of intraoperative clotting seemed to be normal with the use of sufficient Advate to raise the levels of factor VIII to 100 % (3000 U, IV bolus) and the transfusion of 3 U of fresh-frozen plasma. His aPTT was 54 s during surgery. The cystectomy was performed safely without severe bleeding events. A 15-cm length of ileal segment at 15 cm from the ileocecal valve was used for the ileal conduit. The technique of side-to-side stapled anastomosis was used for the ileoileal anastomosis, and the Bricker anastomosis technique was used for ureteroileal anastomosis. The total operating time was 220 min and the estimated blood loss was 800 mL.

The resected specimen revealed multiple erosions and ulcers in the bladder mucosa, and sclerosis of the bladder wall. Histological examinations demonstrated inflammatory cell infiltration and fibrous changes in the bladder wall without malignant figures. The cause of the hematuria was unclear.

Postoperatively, Advate (3000 U, q12 h) was administered to maintain 100 % levels of factor VIII for 2 days with no bleeding complications. After removal of the ureteral catheters on postoperative day 13, the patient had urinary leakage from the ureteroileal anastomosis, which induced a pelvic abscess followed by septic shock and acute respiratory distress syndrome. Blood cultures were positive for *Candida tropicalis*. Several antibiotics and surgical drainage of the abscess were needed.

At 4 months after the cystectomy, the patient had blood in his stool requiring a transfusion of packed red cells. No bleeding site was demonstrated in the colon by colonoscopy and [99m]Technetium-human serum albumin-diethylenetriaminepenta-acetic acid scintigraphy demonstrated that the extravasation of radioactive isotope was detected at terminal ileum, cecum, ascending and transverse colon but not at the oral side of terminal ileum (Fig. 2). These findings were suspected to be bleeding from the ileoileal anastomosis. The patient was given Advate (2000–4000 U) three times per week for 6 months, and the

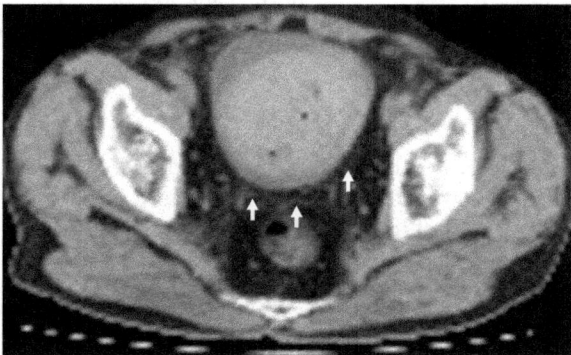

Fig. 1 Computed tomography demonstrated that the bladder was filled with a blood clot (arrow)

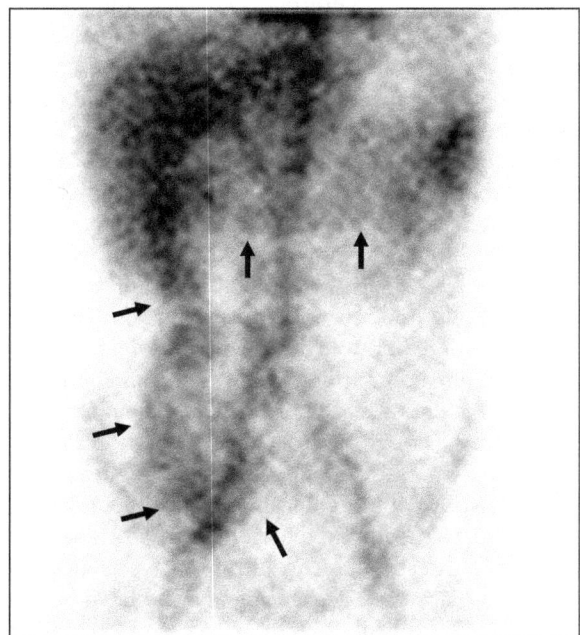

Fig. 2 [99m]Technetium-human serum albumin-diethylenetriaminepenta-acetic acid scintigraphy demonstrated that the extravasation of radioactive isotope was detected at terminal ileum, cecum, ascending and transverse colon (arrow), but not at the oral side of terminal ileum

blood in his stool resolved. His condition recovered gradually and he was discharged at 8 months after admission.

After discharge, he had mild gastrointestinal bleeding and mild hematuria several times a year; however, this was controlled by Advate. The patient had been doing well, other than the bleeding tendency, until he suffered a malignant lymphoma at the age of 66 and was transferred to another clinic for treatment.

Discussion

Hemophilia A and B are rare X-linked recessive disorders caused by deficiencies in factors VIII and IX, respectively. They exhibit a range of clinical severity that correlates well with assayed factor VIII and IX levels. Severe disease is defined as < 1 % factor activity, whereas 1–5 % and > 5 % of normal are deemed moderate and mild disease, respectively [4]. Hematuria is a frequent manifestation of hemophilia. In two studies of hemophiliacs, 66 % had a history of hematuria [5, 6]. The etiology of hematuria is broad, ranging from benign causes to potentially life-threatening malignancies, including bladder cancer, renal cell cancer, and prostate cancer [7]. However, the etiology of hematuria in hemophilia is often unclear, and it may be attributable to the underlying coagulation deficiency [1]. Historically, hematuria in hemophiliacs is generally considered benign in nature and usually responds to conservative therapies, including hydration, bed rest, and infusions of factor concentrate [1]. However, severe hematuria in classic or acquired hemophilia has rarely been reported [2, 3]. In our case, severe hematuria occurred without any obvious cause except the hemophilia, and persisted despite several conservative therapies. After failure of several conservative therapies we next chose a surgical treatment, cystectomy, because he had not only severe hematuria but also pyelonephritis with a severe reduction in his bladder capacity although selective embolization of any major bleeding vessels prior to cystectomy may also be one of treatment options. Histological analyses, which indicated non-specific inflammatory cell infiltration in the bladder, also failed to demonstrate the cause of the hemorrhage.

Performing a surgical procedure in hemophiliac patients is a demanding challenge for the surgeon and hematologist. Various open abdominal operations, including appendectomy, cholecystectomy, splenectomy, and gastric/intestinal procedures, in patients with hemophilia of varying degrees of severity have been reported [8]. In the urology field, successful prostatectomies for prostate cancer in hemophiliac patients have been reported [9, 10]. However, cystectomy in a hemophiliac patient has not been reported before. In our case, with adequate intraoperative factor replacement therapy and the transfusion of fresh-frozen plasma, the quality of intraoperative clotting seemed to be normal and the cystectomy was performed safely.

Our patient experienced urinary leakage from the ureteroileal anastomosis after removal of the ureteral stent, leading to abscess formation and sepsis. The time to stent removal on postoperative day 13 was supposed to be sufficient. The rate of urinary leakage from an anastomosis has been reported to be ~2 % with the routine use of soft plastic stents placed across the ureteroenteric anastomosis [11]. However, it has been reported that wound healing is impaired in hemophilia but that normal healing can be obtained with adequate hemostatic replacement therapy for 7 days [12, 13]. It is possible that tissue healing at an anastomosis is also impaired in hemophilia. Adequate factor VIII concentrate for an extended period of time and the delay of stent removal at an anastomotic site may be required in hemophiliac patients. Stentogram before removal of ureteric stent after ileal conduit construction may also be required to detect leakage of urine at the ureteroenteric anastomosis in hemophiliac patients although routine postoperative stentogram is not recommended in patients with a normal postoperative course [14].

Our patient also had intestinal bleeding, probably from the ileoileal anastomosis. Generally, anastomotic hemorrhage is considered a rare entity. To our knowledge, there is no previous report on an ileoileal anastomotic hemorrhage. The incidence of colorectal anastomotic hemorrhage is reported to be as high as 5 % [15]. There is one report of a severe anastomotic hemorrhage in a hemophiliac patient after total gastrectomy with a Roux-en-Y reconstruction [16]. The intestinal bleeding in our case was likely attributable to his bleeding tendency. Because anastomotic bleeding may be serious in hemophilia, urinary diversion using the intestine should be avoided if possible.

Conclusion

To our knowledge, this is the first case report of cystectomy in a patient with hemophilia A. In our case, the procedure was performed safely with normal intraoperative clotting, but ureteroileal anastomotic leakage and intestinal bleeding were problematic.

Consent

Written informed consent was obtained from the patient for publication of this case report and any accompanying images. A copy of the written consent is available for review by the Editor of this journal.

Abbreviation
aPTT: Activated partial thromboplastin time.

Competing interests
The authors declare that they have no competing interests.

Authors' contributions

SW, MH, and YK were responsible for all the medical and surgical treatment of this case, including the cystectomy. SW drafted the manuscript. SW provided imaging description and figures. MH, YK, and KS assisted with manuscript preparation and literatures collection. TM revised the manuscript. All authors have read and approved the final manuscript.

Acknowledgements

We thank Hitoshi Sugawara and Akira Ishii for patient care and medical advice. The authors received no funding for this study.

References

1. Quon DV, Konkle BA. How we treat: Haematuria in adults with haemophilia. Haemophilia. 2010;16(4):683–5.
2. Kawamura J, Sawanishi K, Takayama H, Ueyama H, Yasunaga K. "Hemophilia A" presenting unusual vesical bleeding; report of a case. Hinyokika kiyo Acta urologica Japonica. 1969;15(12):827–46.
3. Kannan MS, Raj Kumar TR, Subramanian S. Acquired factor VIII inhibitor syndrome: A rare cause of hematuria. Indian J Urol. 2015;31(1):73–4.
4. White GC, Rosendaal F, Aledort LM, Lusher JM, Rothschild C, Ingerslev J, et al. Definitions in hemophilia - Recommendation of the Scientific Subcommittee on factor VIII and factor IX of the Scientific and Standardization Committee of the International Society on Thrombosis and Haemostasis. Thromb Haemost. 2001;85(3):560.
5. Beck P, Evans KT. Renal abnormalities in patients with haemophilia and Christmas disease. Clin Radiol. 1972;23(3):349–54.
6. Prentice CR, Lindsay RM, Barr RD, Forbes CD, Kennedy AC, McNicol GP, et al. Renal complications in haemophilia and Christmas disease. Q J Med. 1971;40(157):47–61.
7. Cohen RA, Brown RS. Microscopic hematuria. N Engl J Med. 2003;348(23):2330–8.
8. Ingram GIC. Haemophilia and the forbidden abdomen. Haemophilia. 2000;6(6):719–22.
9. Lavery HJ, Senaratne P, Gainsburg DM, Samadi DB. Robotic Prostatectomy in a Patient with Hemophilia. JSLS. 2010;14(3):439–41.
10. Petros S, Siegemund T, Stolzenburg JU, Siegemund A, Engelmann L. Coagulation monitoring with thrombin generation test during endoscopic extraperitoneal radical prostatectomy for prostate cancer in a patient with severe haemophilia B. Haemophilia. 2007;13(5):677–9.
11. Farnham SB, Cookson MS. Surgical complications of urinary diversion. World J Urol. 2004;22(3):157–67.
12. Hoffman M, Harger A, Lenkowski A, Hedner U, Roberts HR, Monroe DM. Cutaneous wound healing is impaired in hemophilia B. Blood. 2006;108(9):3053–60.
13. Hoffman M, Monroe DM. Wound healing in haemophilia - breaking the vicious cycle. Haemophilia. 2010;16:13–8.
14. Touma N, Spodek J, Kuan J, Shepherd RR, Hayman WP, Chin JL. Confirming routine stentograms after cystectomy is unnecessary. Can Urol Assoc J. 2007;1(2):103–5.
15. Tang S-J, Rivas H, Tang L, Lara LF, Sreenarasimhaiah J, Rockey DC. Endoscopic hemostasis using endoclip in early gastrointestinal hemorrhage after gastric bypass surgery. Obes Surg. 2007;17(9):1261–7.
16. Onda M, Urazumi K, Abe R, Matsuo K. Obstructive ileus caused by blood clot after emergency total gastrectomy in a patient with hemophilia A: Report of a case. Surg Today. 1998;28(12):1266–9.

Rethinking of ureteral stent removal using an extraction string; what patients feel and what is patients' preference?

Dae Ji Kim, Jeong Hwan Son*, Seok Heun Jang, Jae Won Lee, Dae Sung Cho and Chae Hong Lim

Abstract

Background: Ureteral stent removal using an extraction string is advantageous because it can obviate an invasive cystoscopy, but there is a paucity of data on how patients feel about it, and how bothersome or beneficial it is. We performed this study to evaluate patients' preference for stent removal using an extraction string and which parameters could affect it.

Methods: In total, 114 consecutive patients undergoing ureteral stent insertion after ureteroscopic stone removal (URS) for unilateral recurrent ureter stones were enrolled. Patients were randomized to a string group or a no string group.
Stent removal was performed on the first visit within 7 days postoperatively. All patients were asked to complete the ureteral stent symptom questionnaire, to rate the degree of pain during stent removal using a visual analog scale (VAS) and to answer to questions regarding their preference.

Results: No significant differences were found in domain total scores including urinary symptoms (p = 0.17), pain (p = 0.62), general health (p = 0.37), work performance (p = 0.41). However, regarding separate questions for 'dysuria' and 'difficulties with heavy physical activity', there were significant intergroup differences (p = 0.03 and p = 0.04, respectively). Particular, a significantly higher proportion of patients in the string group checked 'stoppage of sexual intercourse due to stent-related problems' than in the no string group (p = 0.03).
VAS score on stent removal was significantly higher in the no string group than the string group (p = 0.005). Among the patients who remember the experience of an indwelling ureteral stent in the past, 85 % (17/20) of the no string group answered 'No' to the question of 'difference between the methods used in this time and in the past'. On the contrary, 84.2 % (16/19) answered 'Yes' to the same question in the string group. And, all 16 patients of the string group who noted differences between the methods preferred ureteral stent removal using an extraction string to the past method.

Conclusions: Despite of minor increased morbidity related to the extraction string, patients preferred ureteral stent removal using the extraction string after URS. The patients with the extraction string felt less pain on stent removal than flexible cystoscopic stent removal.

Keywords: Urolithiasis, Ureteral stent, Stent removal, Pain, Preference

* Correspondence: sjhwany@dmc.or.kr
Department of Urology, Bundang Jesaeng Hospital, 180 Seohyeon-rho
Bundang-gu, Seongnam 463-774, Republic of Korea

Background

Removing a ureteral stent using an extraction string was first described by Siegel et al. in 1986 as a simple method to avoid general anesthesia and unnecessary urethral instrumentation for pediatric patients [1]. Subsequently, several descriptions of a method to remove ureteral stents using an extraction string have been published [2–6].

The method is advantageous because it can obviate an invasive cystoscopic procedure, but there is wide variability in its clinical application and a paucity of data on how many urological surgeons use extraction strings, how patients feel about them, and how bothersome or beneficial they are.

The ureteral stent is an integral armamentarium in the urologic surgical field. However, urologists must understand the morbidities related to removing a ureteral stent and the patients' perception of stent removal as well as ureteral stent *in situ*-related morbidities.

The primary objective of this study was to evaluate patients' preference for removing a ureteral stents using an extraction string. A secondary objective was to evaluate parameters that could affect patients' preference using a visual analog scale (VAS) for pain during ureteral stent removal and the Ureteral Stent Symptom Questionnaire (USSQ) with respect to their ureteral stent *in situ*.

Methods

In total, 114 consecutive patients undergoing insertion of ureteral stent after ureteroscopic stone removal (URS) between July 2012 and November 2014 were enrolled. This study was approved by Bundang Jesaeng General Hospital Institutional Review Board. Consent was obtained from all patients after providing with verbal and written information about the study.

Inclusion criteria were patients who had a double J ureteral stent inserted after URS for unilateral recurrent ureteral stones. Exclusion criteria were coexisting non-calculous disease (e.g., malignant obstruction, renal insufficiency, or congenital anomaly of urinary tract), solitary kidney, ureteral stricture, pregnancy, or complicated URS requiring long-term stent placement (>7 days). Patients who were taking an alpha-blocker or anti-cholinergic agent to treat lower urinary tract symptoms or who were taking analgesics for chronic pain were also excluded to rule out any influence of the drugs on the symptom questionnaire results.

After completing the URS, patients who met the inclusion criteria were randomized into the string-stent group or the no string-stent group (Fig. 1). Group allocation was performed using the random-number generator in Excel 2010 on an operating room computer before stent insertion.

All stents (6-F Percuflex plus; Boston Scientific, Natick, MA, USA) were inserted via a retrograde approach under cystoscopic guidance. Stent lengths were determined based on patient height. The stent string was manipulated to leave a new air knot 1 cm from the stent end, as described by Bockholt et al. [3]. The distal end of the string (4–5 cm long) was left protruding from the urethral meatus without securing it to the skin.

All patients were discharged the day following the operation with prescriptions for prophylactic antibiotics and non-steroidal anti-inflammatory drugs for several days until the first visit. Alpha-blockers and anti-cholinergics were not administered. The string-stent group patients were reminded to be cautious regarding the string to prevent inadvertent extraction.

Stents were removed in the outpatient department on the first visit within 7 days postoperatively. All patients were asked to complete the validated Korean version of the USSQ [7] immediately before the stent was removed. Urology residents removed the string-stents by pulling the string out without use of lidocaine jelly or an analgesic before the procedure. The no string-stents were removed by urology residents through flexible cystoscopic procedures in which 2 % lidocaine jelly was applied in the urethra without an analgesic. The patient was asked to rate the degree of pain during stent removal on a 10-cm VAS (Fig. 1).

We asked the following four questions regarding their preference:

"Have you ever had an operation to treat urolithiasis?"

"Do you remember your experience with a ureteral indwelling stent?"

"Was there a difference between the method used this time and the one used in the past regarding ureteral stent maintenance and removal?"

"Which method do you prefer?" (Figs. 1 and 2)

Sample size was calculated based on the results of previous ureteral stent studies. A sample size of 50 patients in each group was sufficient for 80 % power to detect a 20 % difference in each USSQ domain score.

Statistical analyses were performed using SPSS ver. 19.0 software (SPSS Inc., Chicago, IL, USA). Numerical data were compared using Student's t-test. Categorical data were analyzed using the χ^2 test. Statistical significance was set at $P < 0.05$.

Results

In total, 114 patients were randomized into 58 patients in the string-stent and 56 in the no string-stent groups. No differences were observed for age, stone size, laterality, stone location, or *in situ* ureteral stent duration between the groups (Table 1).

The USSQ was completed by 89 of 114 patients; 43 in the string group and 46 in the no string group. The VAS and the preference questions were completed by all patients except three patients who had suffered inadvertent

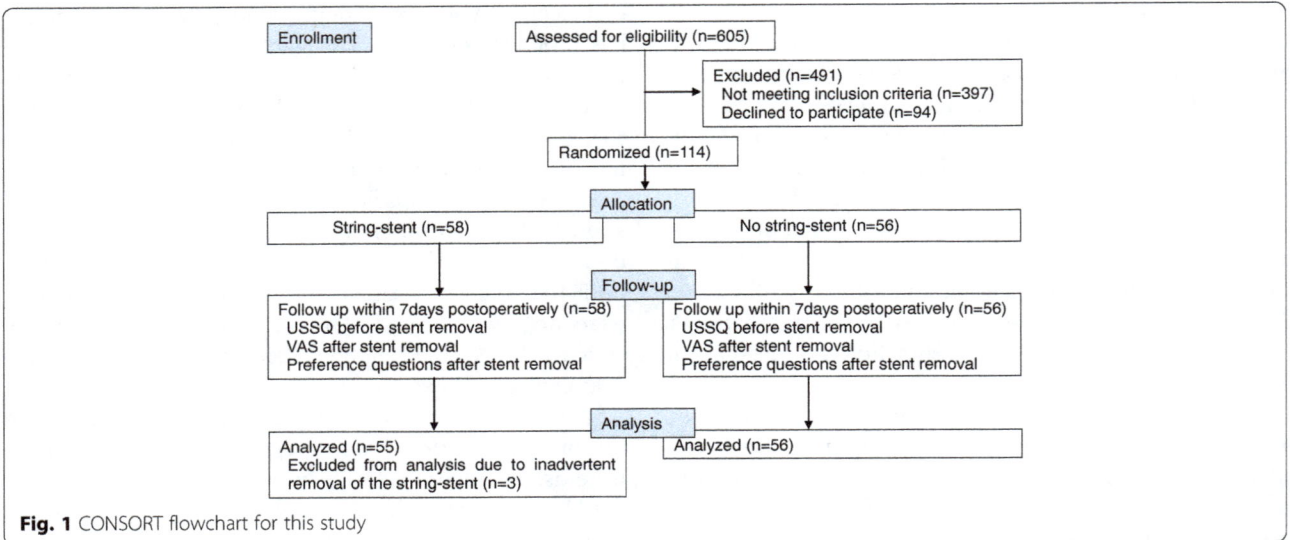

Fig. 1 CONSORT flowchart for this study

removal of the string-stent before the first outpatient clinic visit.

Overall ureteral stent *in situ*-related symptoms are shown in Table 2. No significant differences were found in domain total scores, including urinary symptoms, pain, general health, or work performance. However, significant differences were observed between the groups for separate questions on "dysuria" and "difficulties with heavy physical activity" (2.96 vs. 2.36, p = 0.03, and 2.77 vs. 2.18, p = 0.04, respectively). In particular, all patients who completed the USSQ, except one in the string group, answered "no active sexual life". Among them, 22 patients checked "stopped sexual intercourse after insertion of stent ", which was "due to a stent-related problem" in 17 patients and was significantly higher than that in the no string group (77 % vs. 44.4 %, p = 0.03).

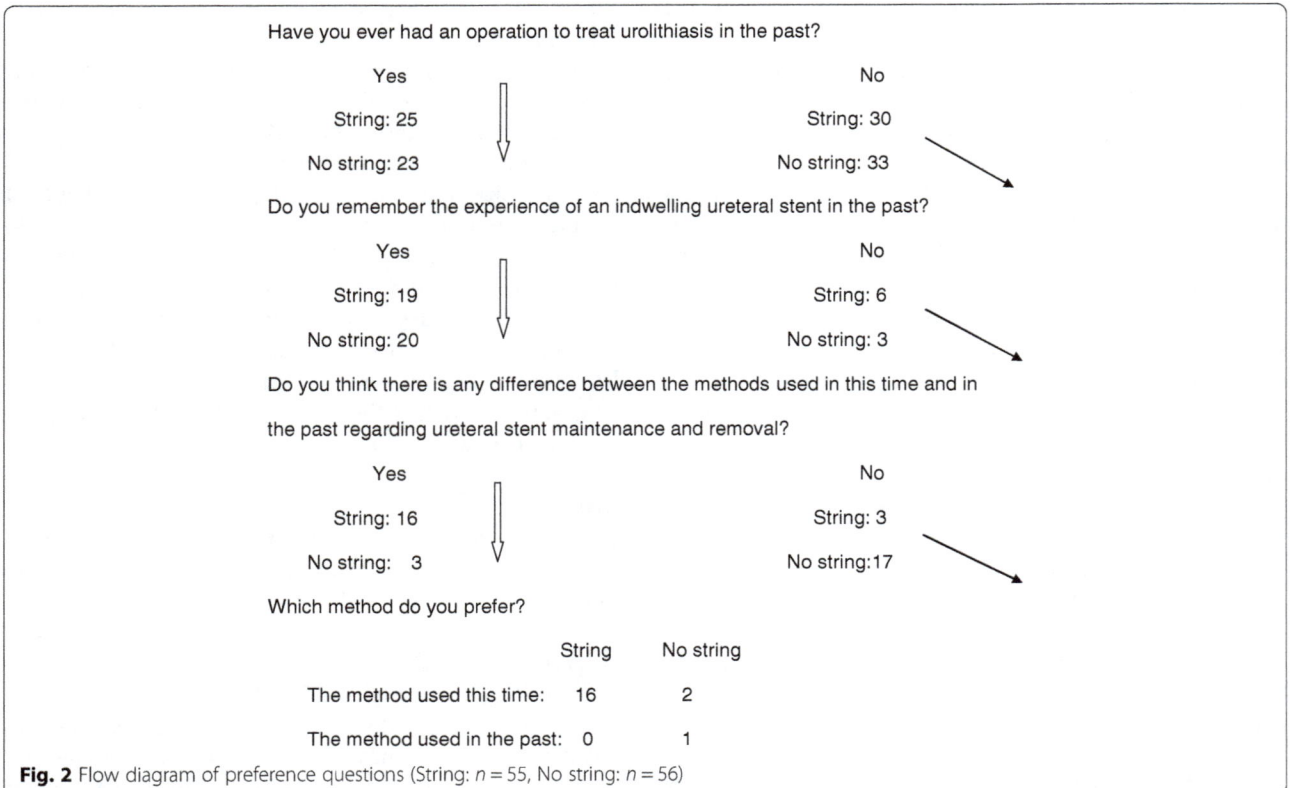

Fig. 2 Flow diagram of preference questions (String: *n* = 55, No string: *n* = 56)

Table 1 Patient characteristics

Characteristic	String	No string	P-value
Patients(n)	58	56	
Male:Female	42:16	36:20	0.34
Age(years)	50.97±12.20	50.54±14.28	0.86
Stone size(mm)	6.83±2.04	7.64±1.68	0.32
Laterality (n) Right:Left	28:30	27:29	0.85
Stone location(n) upper: mid: lower	4:12:42	7:12:37	0.53
Stent duration(days)	5.97	6.28	0.12

Male patients in the string and no string groups showed significant higher urinary symptom scores (33.14 vs. 25.87, p = 0.006, and 29.69 vs. 26.26, p = 0.012). No differences were found between the two sex subgroups in the other domains of pain, general health, or work performance (Table 3).

The VAS scores are presented in Table 4. Overall, the mean pain score was 2.94 in those with string-stents and 4.23 in those with no string-stents who underwent the flexible cystoscopic removal procedure (p = 0.005).

As shown in Fig. 2, among patients who remembered their experience with an indwelling ureteral stent in the past, 85 % (17/20) in the no string group answered "No" to the question of a "difference between the method used this time and the one used in the past". In contrast, 84.2 % (16/19) answered "Yes" to the same question in the string group. All 16 patients in the string group who noted a difference between the methods preferred removal of their ureteral stent using an extraction string compared to the method used previously.

No significant complications were noted, except three cases of inadvertent removal of the string-stent before the first outpatient clinic visit, none of which required replacement. No patient suffered from a febrile urinary tract infection requiring additional antibiotic treatment or a therapeutic procedure (Table 2).

Discussion

The ureteral stent has long been an integral part of urology, as it reduces postoperative complications, such as stricture, urine leakage, and renal colic due to edema of the ureter [8]. However, various *in situ*-related ureteral stent problems, such as flank pain, hematuria, and lower urinary tract symptoms, can develop [9, 10]. Many studies have assessed how *in situ*-related stent discomfort can be alleviated, how long ureteral stents should be in-place, and the possibility of eliminating use of a ureteral stent after a ureteroscopic procedure. These studies consistently show that medications, such as alpha-blocker and anticholinergic agents, only alleviate some *in situ*-related

ureteral stent symptoms. [11–16] Moreover, ureteral stent indwelling durations have been shortened [17, 18] and an indwelling ureteral stent is not required under certain conditions [19–21].

In addition to *in situ*-related ureteral stent problems, urologists must pay more attention to ureteral stent removal procedures, which are troublesome for patients. However, few studies have investigated alleviating *in situ*-related ureteral stent discomfort. Several reports have described endoscopic and non-endoscopic methods intended to reduce pain during cystoscopic stent removal or provide a substitute for the cystoscopic procedure. The ureteral stent extraction string is an alternative that can obviate the need for a cystoscopic procedure [1–6, 22, 23].

Most ureteral stents from various manufacturers have a string connected to the stent, which is used for removing or intraoperative repositioning of a stent. Some surgeons believe the string is useful to avoid an invasive cystoscopic procedure to remove a stent and reduce cost. However, others hesitate to use a string-stent due to possible inadvertent removal or increased stent-related discomfort or complications. Our result that 84.2 % of the string group found a difference between methods used this time and previously and 85 % of the no string group did not find any difference suggests that the extraction string had not been used popularly in our study cohort.

In a recent study on ureteral stent extraction strings, Barnes et al. [4] reported that the index scores for the USSQ domains of urinary symptoms, pain, general health, and work performance were not different between the groups and that use of a stent extraction string after URS for stone disease did not increase stent-related urinary symptoms, complications, or morbidity during removal.

In addition to such parameters, our study focused on evaluating patients' preference for ureteral stent removal using an extraction string. As results, we noted that most patients preferred removal of the ureteral stent using an extraction string, although there were concerns about the impact on their sex life and minor increases in stent-related urinary symptoms, such as dysuria and difficulties with heavy physical activity. The general domain scores on the USSQ were not different between the two groups, except for the questions on "dysuria" and "difficulties with heavy physical activity", suggesting that the stent extraction string only slightly increased *in situ*-related stent urinary symptoms or complications.

Male patients showed significantly higher urinary symptom scores in both groups, suggesting that males tend to suffer more from urinary symptoms related to a ureteral stent *in situ*. This may also result from anatomic differences between males and females, for example with respect to the prostate gland and a longer urethra.

Table 2 Overall ureteral stent in situ-related symptoms

Domains	Items	Scores		Standard deviation		P
		String	No string	String	No string	
Urinary symptoms	Domain total	30.6	28.2	8.54	7.25	0.17*
	Daytime frequency	3.02	3.37	1.14	1.25	0.17*
	Nocturia	2.58	2.40	1.07	1.30	0.48*
	Urgency	2.21	1.97	1.01	1.11	0.31*
	Urge incontinence	1.42	1.33	0.63	0.82	0.59*
	Non urge incontinence	1.37	1.16	0.72	0.63	0.14*
	Residual urine sensation	3.02	2.60	1.18	1.29	0.11*
	Dysuria	2.95	2.36	1.53	1.05	0.03*
	Hematuria frequency	3.12	2.80	1.61	1.27	0.31*
	Hematuria amount	2.32	2.29	1.06	0.87	0.86*
	Interference in life	2.81	2.44	1.31	1.12	0.16*
	Quality of life impact	5.76	5.51	1.50	1.31	0.40*
Pain	Domain total	21.02	20.40	6.39	5.38	0.62*
	Presence or absence of pain	1.23	1.16	0.43	0.37	0.39*
	VAS	6.27	5.71	2.84	2.90	0.36*
	Pain associated with amount of physical activities	3.20	3.02	1.25	1.32	0.50*
	Sleep disturbance	2.20	2.13	1.10	1.04	0.74*
	Pain at voiding	3.33	3.09	1.24	1.04	0.34*
	Flank pain at voiding	1.37	1.47	0.49	0.50	0.37*
	Frequency of painkiller	2.16	2	1.13	0.93	0.46*
	Overall bother	3.05	2.84	1.31	1.04	0.42*
General health	Domain total	15.12	14.04	5.97	5.09	0.37*
	Difficulties with light physical activity	2.23	1.91	1.36	0.99	0.20*
	Difficulties with heavy physical activity	2.77	2.18	1.46	1.21	0.04*
	Feeling tired	2.33	2.4	1.21	1.18	0.77*
	Feeling calm and peaceful	3.40	3.53	1.43	1.42	0.65*
	Social life enjoyment	2.88	2.62	1.33	1.34	0.36*
	Need extra help	1.51	1.4	0.91	0.86	0.56*
Work performance	Domain total	14.41	15.6	6.32	7.04	0.41*
	Type of employment	2.30	3.31	2.22	2.65	0.06*
	Number of days bed rest all day long	1.79	1.47	2.73	2.30	0.55*
	Number of days reduced more than half daily activity	1.80	2.24	1.80	2.64	0.30*
	Position or role in workplace	1.81	1.75	0.93	0.84	0.74*
	Frequency of rest	1.98	1.08	2.44	1.22	0.06*
	Stent related changes on work	2.28	1.98	1.22	1.05	0.22*
	Changes in work duration	2.51	2.44	1.45	1.27	0.82*
Sexual matters						
	No active sexual life: n (%)	42(97.6)	38(82.6)	-	-	0.02**
	Stop of sexual Intercourse after stent: n (%)	22(52)	18(47.3)	-	-	0.82**
	Stop of sexual intercourse due to stent-related problem: n (%)	17(77)	8(44.4)	-	-	0.03**
Additional problems	Need for additional antibiotics (%)	0	0	-	-	-
	Admission or additional therapeutic procedure(%)	0	0	-	-	-

* Student's t-test, ** χ^2 test.

Table 3 Comparison of ureteral stent in situ-related symptoms between male and female subgroups

Domains		String	No string	P-value[a]
Urinary symptoms	Overall	30.60 ± 8.54	28.20 ± 7.25	0.17
	Male	33.14 ± 7.59	29.69 ± 6.79	0.08
	Female	25.87 ± 8.43	26.26 ± 7.56	0.89
	P-value[b]	0.006	0.012	
Pain	Overall	21.02 ± 6.39	20.40 ± 5.38	0.62
	Male	23.14 ± 6.08	21.58 ± 6.43	0.36
	Female	22.27 ± 7.79	21.16 ± 5.51	0.63
	P-value[b]	0.69	0.82	
General health	Overall	15.12 ± 5.97	14.04 ± 5.09	0.37
	Male	14.93 ± 4.98	13.50 ± 5.42	0.32
	Female	15.47 ± 7.68	14.79 ± 4.64	0.75
	P-value[b]	0.78	0.41	
Work performance	Overall	14.41 ± 6.32	15.60 ± 7.04	0.41
	Male	13.68 ± 6.24	14.50 ± 6.93	0.65
	Female	15.80 ± 6.47	17.11 ± 7.12	0.58
	P-value[b]	0.30	0.22	

[a]between string group and no string group, [b]between male and female

Overall VAS scores were different between the string and no string groups but were more marked in male than female patients. Barnes et al. [4] reported no difference in VAS pain scores of patients during stent removal (2.5 in those with a stent string and 3.1 in those with no string using cystoscopy, p = 0.45). In a small study that used a VAS to evaluate pain during stent removal using rigid cystoscopy, Kuehhas et al. [24] found no difference in pain between patients undergoing cystoscopy and extraction using a stent string. These results differ from our VAS scores and may have been influenced by the conditions of our cystoscopic stent removal procedure, such as use of lidocaine jelly but not an analgesic. In addition, different clinical experiences may have caused these differences, as Kuehhas et al. [24] reported that clinical experience is correlated with pain scores of cystoscopic procedures. In fact, mean VAS scores for cystoscopic stent removal were 1.87–8 in several studies. This broad range is thought to be due to heterogeneous settings, such as type of cystoscope or whether any adjunctive medications or local anesthesia was used [4, 24–26].

A few pain-related studies have reported cystoscopic removal of stents, but the results were obtained under heterogeneous settings. Large, controlled studies on pain related to cystoscopic stent removal are warranted.

Loh-Doyle et al. [26] investigated patient experiences of, and preference for, removing ureteral stents through an anonymous website-based survey that included a large sample size and reported the following results by method : "willingness to undergo the same procedure again"; cystoscopy in clinic in 51 %, doctor's office pulled string in 55 %, cystoscopy in the operating room in 67 %, and pulling the string myself in 60 %. We acknowledge the small sample size of our study and that it was aimed at patients with recurrent ureteral stones. However, our study had a relative strength, as it presented the preferences of a patient cohort that experienced several procedures. The second limitation was that patients only had stents in-place for only 7 days after URS. So, whether this method is useful in cases that require a stent for a longer period, such as URS for complicated pyelonephritis, traumatic URS, ureteroscopic surgery for a ureteral stricture, or periodic stent changes for a malignant ureteral stricture, is unknown. Additional studies are necessary to determine perceptions and related morbidities in patients who have an indwelling ureteral stent and extraction string for a longer period.

Table 4 VAS pain scores on ureteral stent removal

VAS score	String	No string	P-value*
Overall	2.94±1.35	4.23±2.45	0.005
Male	3.19±1.09	4.58±2.23	0.006
Female	2.46±1.71	3.54±2.82	0.25
P-value**	0.22	0.11	

*between string group and no string group, **between male and female

Conclusions

Despite a minor increase in morbidity related to the extraction string, patients preferred removal of their ureteral stent using an extraction string after URS. The patients in the extraction string group felt less pain when the stent was removed than when it was removed with a flexible cystoscope.

However, appropriate counseling for the minor increase in morbidities is needed before applying the method clinically. In particular, concerns related to sexual activity should be considered for patients with an active sexual life.

Abbreviations
VAS: Visual analog scale; USSQ: Ureteral Stent Symptom Questionnaire; URS: Ureteroscopic stone removal.

Competing interests
The authors declare that they have no competing interests.

Authors' contributions
CHL and JHS contributed with the conception and design of the study and drafted the manuscript, SHJ, JWL, DSC, and DJK collected data and performed the analyses. All authors read and approved the final manuscript.

Acknowledgements
No authors received any external funding for the present study.

References
1. Siegel A, Altadonna V, Ellis D, Hulbert W, Elder J, Duckett J. Simplified method of indwelling ureteral stent removal. Urology. 1986;28(5):429. Epub 1986/11/01.
2. Campbell RJ, Griffith DP. Exchange ureteral stent insertion using pullout suture after extracorporeal shock-wave lithotripsy. Urology. 1987;29(6):653–5. Epub 1987/06/01.
3. Bockholt NA, Wild TT, Gupta A, Tracy CR. Ureteric stent placement with extraction string: no strings attached? BJU international. 2012;110(11 Pt C): E1069-73. Epub 2012/05/15.
4. Barnes KT, Bing MT, Tracy CR. Do ureteric stent extraction strings affect stent-related quality of life or complications after ureteroscopy for urolithiasis: a prospective randomised control trial. BJU international. 2014;113(4):605–9. Epub 2014/04/26.
5. Althaus AB, Li K, Pattison E, Eisner B, Pais V, Steinberg P. Rate of dislodgment of ureteral stents when using an extraction string after endoscopic urological surgery. The Journal of urology. 2015;193(6):2011–4. Epub 2014/12/30.
6. Kajbafzadeh AM, Nabavizadeh B, Keihani S, Hosseini Sharifi SH. Revisiting the tethered ureteral stents in children: a novel modification. International urology and nephrology. 2015;47(6):881–5. Epub 2015/04/04.
7. Park J, Shin DW, You C, Chung KJ, Han DH, Joshi HB, et al. Cross-cultural application of the Korean version of Ureteral Stent Symptoms Questionnaire. Journal of endourology / Endourological Society. 2012;26(11): 1518–22. Epub 2012/06/06.
8. Liatsikos E, Kallidonis P, Stolzenburg JU, Karnabatidis D. Ureteral stents: past, present and future. Expert review of medical devices. 2009;6(3):313–24. Epub 2009/05/08.
9. Joshi HB, Okeke A, Newns N, Keeley Jr FX, Timoney AG. Characterization of urinary symptoms in patients with ureteral stents. Urology. 2002;59(4):511–6. Epub 2002/04/03.
10. Damiano R, Autorino R, De Sio M, Cantiello F, Quarto G, Perdona S, et al. Does the size of ureteral stent impact urinary symptoms and quality of life? A prospective randomized study. European urology. 2005;48(4):673–8. Epub 2005/07/26.
11. Wang CJ, Huang SW, Chang CH. Effects of specific alpha-1A/1D blocker on lower urinary tract symptoms due to double-J stent: a prospectively randomized study. Urological research. 2009;37(3):147–52. Epub 2009/03/12.
12. Park SC, Jung SW, Lee JW, Rim JS. The effects of tolterodine extended release and alfuzosin for the treatment of double-j stent-related symptoms. Journal of endourology / Endourological Society. 2009;23(11): 1913–7. Epub 2009/10/10.
13. Lim KT, Kim YT, Lee TY, Park SY. Effects of tamsulosin, solifenacin, and combination therapy for the treatment of ureteral stent related discomforts. Korean journal of urology. 2011;52(7):485–8. Epub 2011/08/24.
14. Lamb AD, Vowler SL, Johnston R, Dunn N, Wiseman OJ. Meta-analysis showing the beneficial effect of alpha-blockers on ureteric stent discomfort. BJU international. 2011;108(11):1894–902. Epub 2011/04/02.
15. Lee YJ, Huang KH, Yang HJ, Chang HC, Chen J, Yang TK. Solifenacin improves double-J stent-related symptoms in both genders following uncomplicated ureteroscopic lithotripsy. Urolithiasis. 2013;41(3):247–52. Epub 2013/03/22.
16. Singh I, Tripathy S, Agrawal V. Efficacy of tamsulosin hydrochloride in relieving "double-J ureteral stent-related morbidity": a randomized placebo controlled clinical study. International urology and nephrology. 2014;46(12): 2279–83. Epub 2014/09/10.
17. Aoyagi T, Hatano T, Tachibana M, Hata M. Short-term ureteral catheter stenting after uncomplicated transurethral uretero-lithotomy. World journal of urology. 2004;22(6):449–51. Epub 2004/11/13.
18. Shigemura K, Yasufuku T, Yamanaka K, Yamahsita M, Arakawa S, Fujisawa M. How long should double J stent be kept in after ureteroscopic lithotripsy? Urological research. 2012;40(4):373–6. Epub 2011/09/20.
19. Keeley Jr FX, Timoney AG. Routine stenting after ureteroscopy: think again. European urology. 2007;52(3):642–4. Epub 2007/02/06.
20. Shao Y, Zhuo J, Sun XW, Wen W, Liu HT, Xia SJ. Nonstented versus routine stented ureteroscopic holmium laser lithotripsy: a prospective randomized trial. Urological research. 2008;36(5):259–63. Epub 2008/09/18.
21. Tang L, Gao X, Xu B, Hou J, Zhang Z, Xu C, et al. Placement of ureteral stent after uncomplicated ureteroscopy: do we really need it? Urology. 2011;78(6): 1248–56. Epub 2011/07/19.
22. Soylemez H, Sancaktutar AA, Bozkurt Y, Atar M, Penbegul N, Yildirim K. A cheap minimally painful and widely usable alternative for retrieving ureteral stents. Urologia internationalis. 2011;87(2):199–204. Epub 2011/08/09.
23. Kawahara T, Ito H, Terao H, Yamashita Y, Tanaka K, Ogawa T, et al. Ureteral stent exchange under fluoroscopic guidance using the crochet hook technique in women. Urologia internationalis. 2012;88(3):322–5. Epub 2012/03/22.
24. Kuehhas FE, Miernik A, Sharma V, Sevcenco S, Javadli E, Herwig R, et al. A prospective evaluation of pain associated with stone passage, stents, and stent removal using a visual analog scale. Urology. 2013;82(3):521–5. Epub 2013/06/19.
25. Kim JH, Park SY, Kim MG, Choi H, Song D, Cho SW, et al. Pain and satisfaction during rigid cystoscopic ureteral stent removal: a preliminary study. BMC urology. 2014;14:90. Epub 2014/11/20.
26. Loh-Doyle JC, Low RK, Monga M, Nguyen MM. Patient experiences and preferences with ureteral stent removal. Journal of endourology / Endourological Society. 2015;29(1):35–40. Epub 2014/07/16.

Effects of tadalafil treatment after bilateral nerve-sparing radical prostatectomy: quality of life, psychosocial outcomes, and treatment satisfaction results

Hitendra R Patel[1*], Dapo Ilo[2], Nimish Shah[3], Béatrice Cuzin[4], David Chadwick[5], Robert Andrianne[6], Carsten Henneges[7], Jane Barry[2], Katja Hell-Momeni[7], Julia Branicka[8] and Hartwig Büttner[7]

Abstract

Background: This multicenter, randomized, double-blind, double-dummy, placebo-controlled trial primarily evaluated the efficacy of tadalafil once-daily (OaD) or on-demand ("pro-re-nata"; PRN) treatment, started early post-nsRP. Secondary outcome-measures on quality-of-life (QoL) and treatment satisfaction are reported.

Methods: Patients, aged <68 yrs, with adenocarcinoma of the prostate (Gleason ≤ 7, normal preoperative erectile function [EF]) were randomized post-nsRP 1:1:1 to 9-month treatment with tadalafil 5 mg OaD, tadalafil 20 mg PRN, or placebo, followed by 6-week drug-free washout and 3-month open-label tadalafil OaD treatment (OLT). The main outcome measures were Changes in Expanded Prostate Cancer Index Composite (EPIC-26), Erectile Dysfunction Inventory of Treatment Satisfaction (EDITS), and Self-Esteem and Relationship (SEAR) questionnaires (mixed-model-for-repeated-measures, including terms for treatment, visit, treatment-by-visit interaction, age-group, country, baseline-score). LS means with 95% confidence interval (CI) are reported.

Results: 423 patients were randomized to 3 treatment-groups: tadalafil OaD (N = 139), PRN (N = 143), or placebo (N = 141). In each group, 57 (41.0%), 58 (40.6%), and 50 (35.5%) patients were aged 61-68 yrs. At the end of double-blind treatment (DBT), patients' EPIC sexual domain-scores improved significantly with tadalafil OaD versus placebo (treatment effect [95% CI]: 9.6 [3.1,16.0]; p = 0.004); comparisons of PRN versus placebo at end of DBT, and comparisons of tadalafil OaD and PRN versus placebo after OLT were not significant. Only in older patients (61-68 yrs; age-by-treatment p ≤ 0.1), EPIC urinary incontinence domain-scores also improved significantly with tadalafil OaD versus placebo (overall treatment effect across all visits, 8.3 [0.4,16.1]; p = 0.040). Treatment satisfaction increased significantly in both tadalafil groups, EDITS total-scores increased significantly with OaD and PRN versus placebo during DBT (p = 0.005 and p = 0.041, respectively). At the end of OLT, improvement was significant for tadalafil OaD versus placebo only (p = 0.035). No significant differences were observed for SEAR.

Conclusions: These results suggest that chronic dosing of tadalafil improves QoL of patients post-nsRP. The improvement of urinary incontinence in elderly patients randomized to tadalafil OaD may contribute to this effect.

Keywords: PDE5 inhibitor, Tadalafil, Erectile dysfunction, Randomized clinical trial, Prostate cancer, Prostatectomy, Quality of life, Urinary incontinence

* Correspondence: urology@hrhpatel.org
[1]Department of Urology, University Hospital North Norway, Sykehusvegen 38, 9038 Tromsø, Norway
Full list of author information is available at the end of the article

Background

Erectile dysfunction (ED) is a common problem after nerve-sparing radical prostatectomy (nsRP) for localized prostate cancer [1,2]. First-line therapy for ED after nsRP is the use of a phosphodiesterase type 5 (PDE5) inhibitor [3]. Alternative treatment options include intracavernosal injections, e.g., of the "trimix" combination of alprostadil, phentolamine, and papaverine, intrautheral alprostadil suppositories, vacuum erection devices, or inflatable penile prosthesis [3]. PDE5 inhibitors are generally well-tolerated and effective treatments of ED after nsRP, although they are less effective in the post-nsRP population than in the general population [1,4,5]. There is still considerable debate as to which patients might benefit most from PDE5 inhibitor treatment after nsRP, and what would be the optimal time for treatment initiation, the optimal duration of treatment, and the most appropriate efficacy endpoints [6].

To date, there have been 4 randomized controlled trials evaluating the impact of the early use of PDE5 inhibitors in men with ED following nsRP. Nightly administration of sildenafil for 36 weeks, starting 4 weeks after surgery, markedly increased the return of normal spontaneous erections; the study was stopped early since it was expected not to meet its primary endpoint [7]. Vardenafil treatment for 9 months, starting within 2 weeks after surgery, was efficacious when used on-demand (pro-re-nata, PRN), but had no significant effect on unassisted erectile function (EF) after drug-free washout [5]. In a recent study, 3 months of treatment with avanafil 100 or 200 mg PRN significantly improved drug-assisted EF after prostatectomy, but a sustained effect on unassisted EF was not assessed [8]. Finally, the REACTT trial has evaluated the effect of the long-acting PDE5 inhibitor tadalafil, showing that tadalafil once daily [OaD] was most effective on drug-assisted EF during 9 months of double-blind treatment (DBT) [9]. The study suggested a potential role of tadalafil OaD provided early after surgery in contributing to EF recovery, and a significant protection from penile length loss, possibly by protecting from penile structural changes. However, also in this trial, unassisted EF was not improved after drug-free washout following DBT [9].

These post-nsRP studies have predominantly looked at standard ED outcomes, including the International Index of Erectile Function (IIEF) domain scores and Sexual Encounter Profile (SEP) questions. However, prostate cancer patients frequently report other associated symptoms, e.g., penile length loss, climacturia, or urinary incontinence, which may have a pronounced impact on their quality of life (QoL).

This manuscript addresses secondary outcome measures on QoL and treatment satisfaction in early post-nsRP patients who participated in the REACTT trial [9]. The QoL questionnaires used evaluate those aspects of QoL which are specifically relevant for prostate cancer patients and patients with ED, for example the Expanded Prostate Cancer Index Composite Short Form (EPIC-26) [10,11]. This questionnaire addressed 4 different domains — sexual, urinary (divided into incontinence and irritation/obstruction subscales), bowel, and hormonal function [10,11]. The sexual and urinary incontinence domain scores are the most relevant to QoL of post-nsRP prostate cancer patients, as ED and urinary incontinence are common sequelae of nsRP [12,13]; other subscales are more pertinent to prostate cancer patients who have had radiation or hormonal deprivation therapy. This study also used the Erectile Dysfunction Inventory of Treatment Satisfaction (EDITS) questionnaire to assess patient and partner satisfaction with ED treatment, and the Self-Esteem and Relationship (SEAR) instrument, which assessed patient and partner sexual relationship confidence and self-esteem [14,15].

Methods

Patients

All enrolled patients were adult men, aged < 68 years at the time of nsRP, with normal preoperative EF (IIEF-EF domain score $\geq$ 22) [9] who underwent nsRP for organ-confined, non-metastatic prostate cancer (Gleason score $\leq$ 7, prostate specific antigen <10 ng/mL). These patients were enrolled between November 2009 and August 2011, in 50 centers in 9 European countries and Canada; detailed trial design and eligibility criteria are available at www.clinicaltrials.gov (NCT01026818) and in [9]. The study was approved by the responsible ethical review boards (Additional file 1: Table S1).

Trial design

This multicenter, Phase IV, randomized, double-blind, 3-arm, placebo-controlled, parallel-group trial was conducted in accordance with the declaration of Helsinki; appropriate ethical review boards approved the study protocol for each country. All patients signed written informed consent. The trial consisted of a screening period (including nsRP), 9 months of randomized, double-blind, double-dummy, treatment with tadalafil 5 mg OaD, tadalafil 20 mg PRN, or placebo, starting within 6 weeks after nsRP (double-blind treatment; DBT), 6 weeks of drug-free washout, and 3 months of open-label treatment with tadalafil 5 mg OaD (OLT, all patients) (Additional file 1: Figure S1). Matching placebo tablets identical to the 5 mg and 20 mg tadalafil tablets were used to ensure that the blinded regimen was identical for all treatment groups. During DBT, patients received tadalafil 5 mg OaD (+ placebo PRN), tadalafil 20 mg PRN (+ placebo OaD) or placebo (OaD + PRN). For PRN dosing, patients were permitted to take up to 3 tablets per week (and no more than 1 per day). During drug-free washout, patients received no study drug. During the open-label period, all patients received tadalafil 5 mg OaD.

Main outcome measures

Patients' EF was assessed using the IIEF-EF domain score at baseline (post-nsRP), the end of DBT, and the end of OLT [16].

EPIC-26 domain scores [10,11], with a special focus on the sexual and urinary incontinence domain scores, were used to assess patients' prostate-specific QoL status at baseline, the end of DBT, and the end of OLT. In addition, partners were asked to complete the EPIC-26P questionnaire. Individual item and EPIC domain scores were standardized to a 0 to 100 scale; higher scores represent better QoL [10,11].

The 11-item EDITS questionnaire was used to assess patients' treatment satisfaction at the end of DBT and OLT [14]. Responses were based on the 4 weeks preceding assessments. Each question was rated from 0 to 4 with higher scores indicating higher satisfaction, and the total score (average of the individual item scores) was reported.

The SEAR questionnaire was used to assess the patients' sexual relationships and self-esteem at baseline, the end of DBT, and the end of OLT [15]. The SEAR questionnaire has 2 domains of sexual relationship (domain score range 8 to 40) and confidence (range 6 to 30), the latter of these domains can be divided into 2 subscales on self-esteem (range 4 to 20) and overall relationship (range 2 to 10) [15]. Higher scores indicate a more favorable response.

Statistical analysis

The planned sample size of 412 patients was based on the primary outcome (proportion of patients achieving IIEF-EF ≥ 22) at the end of drug-free washout period [9]. All analyses were based on the intent-to-treat (ITT)

Table 1 Baseline characteristics

	Tadalafil OaD (N = 139)		Tadalafil PRN (N = 143)[a]		Placebo (N = 141)		Overall (N = 423)[a]	
Age, years								
Mean (SD)	58.6 (5.07)		57.5 (5.91)		57.6 (5.69)		57.9 (5.58)	
<61 years, n (%)	82	(59.0)	85	(59.4)	91	(64.5)	258	(61.0)
61-68 years, n (%)	57	(41.0)	58	(40.6)	50	(35.5)	165	(39.0)
nsRP approach, n (%)								
Open surgery	68	(48.9)	65	(45.5)	56	(39.7)	189	(44.7)
Conventional laparoscopy	29	(20.9)	31	(21.7)	28	(19.9)	88	(20.9)
Robot-assisted laparoscopy	31	(22.3)	41	(28.7)	44	(31.2)	116	(27.4)
Other	11	(7.9)	6	(4.2)	13	(9.2)	30	(7.1)
IIEF-EF at randomization (V4, after prostatectomy)								
N with data	137		140		137		414	
Mean (SD)	6.0	(5.80)	6.7	(5.57)	6.5	(6.08)	6.4	(5.81)
EPIC sexual domain score								
N with data	133		140		137		410	
Mean (SD)	19.8 (19.56)		21.9 (20.16)		20.1 (21.87)		20.6 (20.53)	
EPIC urinary incontinence domain score								
N with data	133		139		137		409	
Mean (SD)	46.7 (30.71)		47.9 (28.89)		49.5 (28.05)		48.0 (29.17)	
EPIC urinary irritative/obstructive domain score								
N with data	131		137		134		402	
Mean (SD)	78.1 (18.92)		81.5 (15.08)		81.3 (16.42)		80.4 (16.88)	
EPIC bowel domain total score								
N with data	129		134		136		399	
Mean (SD)	88.3 (15.32)		91.2 (10.31)		89.9 (13.69)		89.8 (13.27)	
EPIC hormonal domain score								
N with data	130		137		136		403	
Mean (SD)	90.0 (12.71)		92.0 (10.51)		91.4 (10.89)		91.2 (11.39)	

[a]Data presented for all patients randomized. One patient assigned to tadalafil PRN did not receive any study drug and was therefore not included in the ITT population.
Abbreviations: EPIC Expanded Prostate Cancer Index Composite (EPIC-26), *IIEF-EF* International Index of Erectile Function – Erectile Function, *ITT* intent-to-treat, *N* number of patients, *n* number of patients with characteristic, *nsRP* bilateral nerve-sparing prostatectomy, *NSS* Nelson Nerve-Sparing score, *OaD* once daily, *PRN* "pro-re-nata"/on-demand, *SD* standard deviation, *V* visit EPIC scores range from 0–100, higher scores indicate better values.

population, which included all randomized patients with baseline data and at least 1 post-baseline visit. Pre-specified treatment group comparisons were tadalafil OaD versus placebo and tadalafil PRN versus placebo.

Changes from baseline in EPIC and SEAR domain scores, and actual EDITS total scores were assessed using a pre-specified mixed model for repeated measures (MMRM), assuming an unstructured covariance matrix and included terms for baseline domain score, treatment, country, visit, visit-by-treatment interaction, age group, and age-group-by treatment interaction (included only if $p < 0.1$). Least squares means (LS mean) changes from baseline and the associated 95% CIs were provided for the 2 key visits (end of DBT and end of OLT). In case of a significant age-group by treatment interaction ($p < 0.1$), the overall treatment effect (across all visits) by age group was also provided. Agreement between patient- and partner-rated EPIC scores was assessed using unweighted Cohen's kappa statistics, which is adjusted for agreement by chance.

Spearman rank correlation coefficients and the associated 95% CIs were calculated post-hoc to assess correlations at baseline, end of DBT, and end of OLT between: (a) EPIC sexual and urinary incontinence domain scores;

(b) IIEF-EF scores and EPIC sexual and urinary incontinence domain scores.

A 2-sided 5% level of significance was used for p-values for treatment group comparisons; a 10% level of significance was used for p-values for interaction terms. No other adjustments for multiplicity were applied for the analyses reported here. Data were analyzed using SAS 9.2 software (SAS Institute Inc., Cary, USA).

Results

Patient disposition and baseline characteristics

Of 583 patients screened, 423 were randomized to DBT, 422 were included in the ITT population: 139 (32.9%) patients were treated with tadalafil OaD, 142 (33.7%) with tadalafil PRN, and 141 (33.4%) with placebo (Additional file 1: Figure S2). Patient disposition, baseline demographics [12], and relevant disease characteristics were balanced in the 3 treatment groups (Table 1). As per inclusion criteria, all patients had IIEF-EF domain scores ≥22 before nsRP.

EPIC domain scores – patient rating

EPIC sexual and urinary domain scores improved in all 3 treatment groups during DBT and continued to improve during OLT (Table 2). EPIC sexual domain scores improved

Table 2 LS mean changes [95%CI] in EPIC domain scores from baseline

	Tadalafil OaD (N = 139)	Tadalafil PRN (N = 142)	Placebo (N = 141)
EPIC sexual domain (age-group by treatment interaction: p = 0.083)[a]			
End of DBT	+27.5 [21.6, 33.4]**	+20.7 [15.3, 26.1]	+18.0 [12.1, 23.8]
End of OLT	+36.6 [30.0, 43.1]	+32.6 [26.6, 38.6]	+33.4 [27.0, 39.8]
Men ≤60 years	*+30.1 [23.2, 36.9]*	*+31.2 [24.8, 37.6]*	*+24.9 [18.2, 31.6]*
Men 61–68 years	*+34.0 [26.0, 42.0]*	*+22.1 [14.6, 29.5]*	*+26.5 [18.5, 34.4]*
EPIC urinary incontinence domain (age-group by treatment interaction: p = 0.084)[a]			
End of DBT	+34.1 [29.3, 38.9]	+31.1 [26.7, 35.5]	+30.6 [25.9, 35.3]
End of OLT	+37.4 [32.6, 42.3]	+35.5 [31.1, 40.0]	+35.4 [30.7, 40.2]
Men ≤60 years	*+33.0 [27.7, 38.3]*	*+34.6 [29.6, 39.7]*	*+35.8 [30.5, 41.1]*
Men 61–68 years	*+38.5 [32.2, 44.8]**	*+32.0 [26.2, 37.9]*	*+30.2 [24.0, 36.5]*
EPIC urinary irritative/obstructive domain			
End of DBT	+13.8 [11.5, 16.1]	+13.3 [11.2, 15.4]	+12.3 [10.0, 14.5]
End of OLT	+13.9 [11.5, 16.2]	+13.8 [11.7, 15.9]	+12.3 [10.0, 14.6]
EPIC bowel domain			
End of DBT	+5.9 [3.7, 8.2]	+6.3 [4.2, 8.3]	+6.5 [4.3, 8.7]
End of OLT	+6.9 [4.7, 9.1]	+6.5 [4.5, 8.5]	+6.8 [4.6, 8.9]
EPIC hormonal domain			
End of DBT	+1.7 [−0.8, 4.3]	+2.7 [0.4, 5.1]*	−0.2 [−2.7, 2.3]
End of OLT	+2.5 [0.1, 4.9]	+2.9 [0.8, 5.1]	+3.0 [0.7, 5.4]

**p < 0.01, *p < 0.05 versus placebo (MMRM).
[a]Significant at the 10% level.
Abbreviations: CI confidence interval, *DBT* double-blind treatment, *EPIC* Expanded Prostate Cancer Index Composite (EPIC-26), *LS mean* least squares mean, *MMRM* mixed model for repeated measures, *N* number of patients in the ITT population, *OaD* once daily, *OLT* open-label treatment, *PRN* "pro-re-nata"/on-demand.
Data are from MMRM, including baseline domain score, treatment, country, visit, visit-by-treatment interaction, and age group (men ≤60 years, men 61–68 years) (combined sexual/ incontinence score: additionally adjusted for body mass index, smoking status, nerve-sparing score, and type of surgery [open, conventional, robot-assisted, other]). Age-group-by-treatment interaction was included only if significant at the 10% level. For men ≤60 years and 61–68 years (data shown in italics), the overall treatment effect presented includes all visits from baseline to end of OLT.

significantly with tadalafil OaD versus placebo at the end of DBT (Figure 1; treatment group difference [95% CI]: 9.6 [3.1, 16.0]; p = 0.004), but not with tadalafil PRN versus placebo. The difference between groups was no longer significant at the end of OLT, i.e. after all patients had received tadalafil OaD treatment for 3 months (3.2 [−4.3, 10.7]; p = 0.406). There was no significant difference in EPIC domain scores between the PRN and placebo group at the end of DBT (Figures 1,2).

No significant group differences between tadalafil OaD and placebo were observed for the other EPIC domain scores (Figure 2).

A significant interaction (p ≤ 0.1) between age group and treatment was observed for EPIC sexual (p = 0.083) and urinary incontinence (p = 0.084) domain scores. In older patients (61-68 years), EPIC urinary incontinence domain scores improved significantly with tadalafil OaD versus placebo (Figure 3; overall treatment effect across all visits: 8.3 [0.4, 16.1]; p = 0.040). Unadjusted EPIC

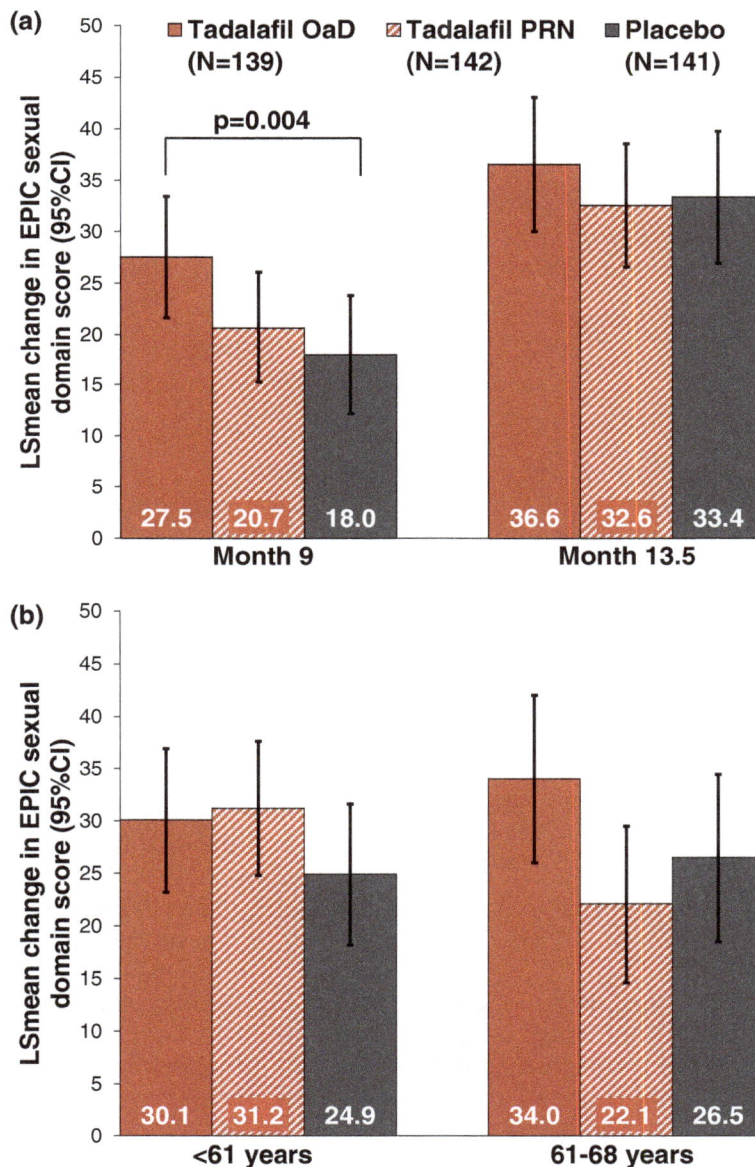

Figure 1 EPIC Sexual Domain Score Changes from Baseline: **(a)** at the end of DBT (Month 9) and OLT (Month 13.5), and **(b)** overall mean change in younger (<61 years) versus older (61–68 years) patients, as estimated from MMRM. MMRM model adjusted for baseline domain score, treatment, country, visit, visit-by-treatment interaction, age group, and age-group-by-treatment interaction. EPIC scores range from 0–100; higher scores indicate better values.

Score	LSmean treatment group difference [95% CI] of score changes versus placebo			
	Tadalafil OaD		Tadalafil PRN	
	End of DBT (Month 9)	End of OLT (Month 13.5)	End of DBT (Month 9)	End of OLT (Month 13.5)
IIEF-EF	+2.8 [0.8,4.8]**	+1.6 [-0.8, +4.0], n.s.	+1.6 [-0.4,+3.6], n.s.	+0.8 (-1.5,+3.2], n.s.
EPIC				
Sexual function	+9.6 [3.1,16.0]**	+3.2 [-4.3,10.7], n.s.	+2.7 [-3.6,+9.0], n.s.	-0.8 [-8.1,+6.5], n.s.
Urinary incontinence	+3.5 [-1.8,+8.8], n.s.	+2.0 [-3.5,+7.4], n.s.	+0.5 [-4.7,+5.8], n.s.	+0.1 [-5.2,+5.4], n.s.
Men ≤60 years	-2.8 [-9.0,+3.5], n.s.[a]		-1.2 [-7.3,+5.0], n.s.[a]	
Men 61-68 years	+8.3 [+0.4,+16.1]*[a]		+1.8 [-5.9,+9.5], n.s.[a]	
Urinary irritative/obstructive	+1.6 [-1.0,+4.2], n.s.	+1.6 [-1.1,+4.2], n.s.	+1.0 [-1.5,+3.6], n.s.	+1.5 [-1.1,+4.1], n.s.
Bowel	-0.5 [-3.0,+2.0], n.s.	+0.1 [-2.4,+2.6], n.s.	-0.2 [-2.6,+2.2], n.s.	-0.3 [-2.7,+2.1], n.s.
Hormonal	+1.9 [-1.0,+4.8], n.s.	-0.5 [-3.2,+2.1], n.s.	+2.9 [+0.1,+5.7]*	-0.1 [-2.7, +2.5], n.s.
EDITS total	+0.3 [+0.1,+0.6]**	+0.3 [+0.02,+0.5]*	+0.2 [+0.01,+0.5]*	+0.1 [-0.1,+0.4], n.s.
SEAR sexual relationship	+1.8 [-0.3,+3.8], n.s.	+0.2 [-2.2,+2.5], n.s.	+0.5 [-1.5,+2.5], n.s.	-0.04 [-2.3,+2.3], n.s.
SEAR confidence	+0.4 [-1.2,+1.9], n.s.	+0.1 [-1.6,+1.8], n.s.	+0.4 [-1.1,+1.9], n.s.	+0.2 [-1.5,+1.8], n.s.

LS mean treatment group difference versus placebo: **: p <0.01 ; *: p <0.05; n.s.: not significant (p>0.05)

Figure 2 Summary of treatment group differences between tadalafil OaD and tadalafil PRN versus placebo at the end of DBT and OLT. [a]For men ≤ 60 years and 61–68 years, the overall treatment effect presented includes all visits from baseline to end of OLT. Data are from MMRM models, including baseline value (except for EDITS), treatment, country, visit, visit-by-treatment interaction, and age group (men ≤60 years, men 61–68 years). The MMRM assessing the combined sexual/incontinence score (post-hoc) additionally adjusted for body mass index, smoking status, nerve-sparing score, and type of surgery (open, conventional, robot-assisted, other). Age-group-by-treatment interaction was included in the models only if significant at the 10% level.

domain score data (Additional file 1: Table S2) were consistent with these findings.

EPIC domain scores – patient-partner agreement

Approximately one-third (N = 153) of patients' partners attended the study visits and completed the EPIC partner questionnaire. Patient-partner agreement could only be assessed for approximately one-third of patients (e.g., partner and patient baseline EPIC sexual domain score available for 140 of 422 patients, 33.2%). Agreement between patients and partners' ratings was poor (0 to 0.2) to moderate (0.4 to 0.6) for the different time points and domains assessed; no definite pattern of agreement was observed.

Treatment satisfaction

Treatment satisfaction (EDITS total scores) increased significantly in both tadalafil groups when compared with placebo at the end of DBT (OaD versus placebo: 0.33 [0.10,0.56]; p = 0.005, and PRN versus placebo: 0.23 [0.01,0.45]; p = 0.041) (Figure 2,4). At the end of OLT, improvement was only significant for tadalafil OaD versus placebo (p = 0.035). Unadjusted data for EDITS total scores were consistent (Additional file 1: Table S3).

No significant treatment group differences were observed for SEAR (Additional file 1: Tables S4 and S5).

Discussion

Any major surgery is expected to reduce overall patient QoL during the initial stages of healing and rehabilitation, this is enhanced by the psychosocial impact of a cancer diagnosis. Patients after nsRP face additional challenges, namely impaired EF and urinary continence, which may continue to affect their QoL long after the initial healing phase is complete [17,18]. This can be particularly difficult for younger patients who may be more sexually active than the elderly population. Patients are faced with a long period of time during which sexual and urinary function is not entirely regained, substantially impacting QoL not only for the patients recovering from nsRP but also for their partners [19].

As reported previously, 9 months of DBT with tadalafil OaD, but not tadalafil PRN, significantly increased and accelerated EF recovery when compared with placebo [9,20]; improvements in IIEF-EF and SEP-3 exceeded the minimum clinically relevant difference (MCID) [9]. Treatment with tadalafil OaD treatment was well tolerated; no new safety signals were detected in the prostate cancer patient population [9]. This analysis evaluated if tadalafil treatment affected the patients' perceived QoL in terms of sexual function and urinary incontinence, as assessed by the respective EPIC domain scores. During DBT, IIEF-EF, EPIC sexual domain score, and EDITS score improved with tadalafil

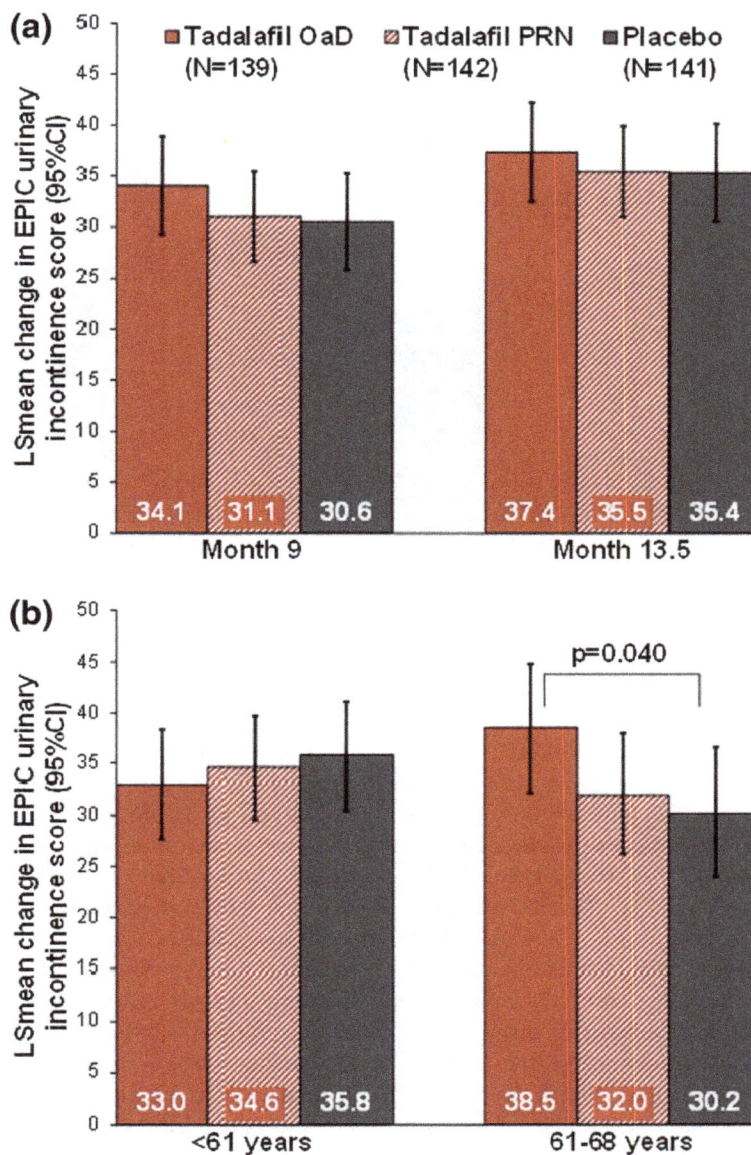

Figure 3 EPIC Urinary Incontinence Score Changes from Baseline: **(a)** at the end of DBT (Month 9) and OLT (Month 13.5), and **(b)** overall mean change in younger (<61 years) and older (61–68 years) patients, as estimated from MMRM. Data from MMRM model, adjusting for baseline domain score, treatment, country, visit, visit-by-treatment interaction, age group, and age-group-by-treatment interaction. EPIC scores range from 0–100; higher scores indicate better values.

OaD versus placebo but not with tadalafil PRN (Figure 2). This may be due to chronic (daily) tadalafil dosing that would lead to steady-state PDE5-inhibition [21] and may be associated with prolonged (continuous) periods of increased tissue oxygenation during the post-operative regenerative process.

During DBT, patient-rated EPIC sexual domain scores improved in all 3 treatment groups by 27.5% with tadalafil OaD, 20.7% with tadalafil PRN, and 18.0% with placebo. As for IIEF-EF and SEP-3 [9], the improvement

was statistically significant versus placebo (p = 0.004) in the tadalafil OaD group only.

The LS mean difference in EPIC sexual domain score changes between tadalafil OaD and placebo was 3.2 points; there is currently no general consensus on how to define the MCID for EPIC domain scores. During the 3 months of additional OLT with tadalafil OaD, EPIC sexual domain scores continued to improve, with overall improvements of more than 30% from baseline to the end of OLT in all 3 groups. The significant treatment

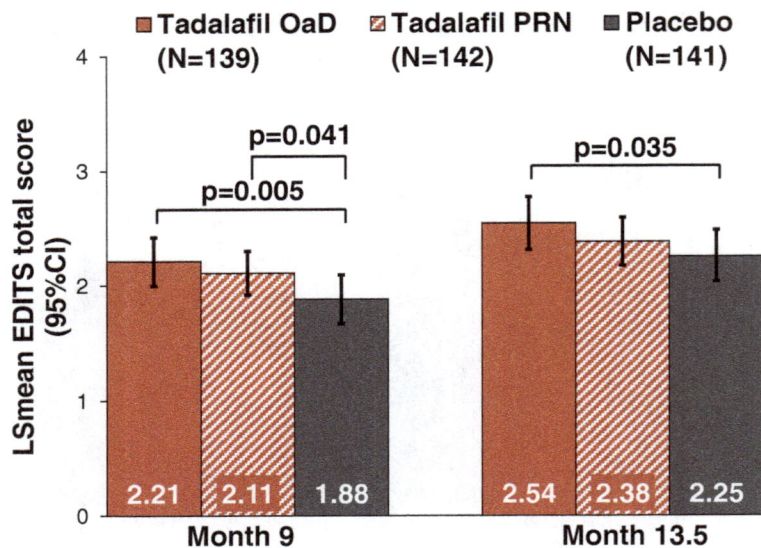

Figure 4 EDITS Total Scores at the End of DBT (Month 9) and OLT (Month 13.5). Data from MMRM model, adjusting for treatment, country, visit, visit-by-treatment interaction, age group, and age-group-by-treatment interaction. EDITS total score ranges from 0–4; higher score indicates better value.

group differences from DBT were not maintained as all groups received active tadalafil OaD during OLT.

A significant age group-by-treatment interaction (p = 0.084) indicated that in older patients only (61–68 years of age), EPIC urinary incontinence scores also significantly improved with tadalafil OaD compared with placebo (no significant effect with PRN). The effect was not observed in younger patients (<61 years of age), potentially because they were less affected by urinary incontinence symptoms. There are currently competing hypotheses for the etiology of post-prostatectomy incontinence [22]. Apart from the experience of the surgeon and the surgical technique employed, the most relevant pre-operative predictors of urinary incontinence following robot-assisted nsRP as identified by a meta-analysis included age, body mass index (BMI), comorbidity index, lower urinary tract symptoms, and prostate volume [23]. Urinary incontinence after nsRP is known to be a long-term complication. In the prostate cancer outcome study, 8.4% of all patients were incontinent at ≥18 months after nsRP, even more (14%) had urinary incontinence symptoms after 5 years [12,17]. In a recent study by Nam et al. approximately 5% of patients required incontinence surgery within 15 years post-nsRP [24]. In both studies, the risk for late urinary complications post-nsRP also increased with age [17,24]. In the elderly patients, a fair correlation between EPIC urinary and sexual domain scores (highest at baseline: r = 0.39) was observed in the current study.

Several clinical trials show that PDE5 inhibitors, including tadalafil OaD, can reduce lower urinary tract symptoms in patients with benign prostate hyperplasia [25-27].

A positive effect for PDE5 inhibitors on urinary continence following nsRP was initially observed in a retrospective study by Gandaglia et al. [28]. More recently, Gacci et al. reported significantly improved urinary continence in patients using vardenafil (nightly) compared with placebo in a prospective 12-month study (39 patients) [29].

It is not fully understood how PDE5 inhibitors might act to improve bladder function, although improvements in sphincteric and/or pelvic floor blood supply could be responsible for this effect [28,29]. Moreover, the human bladder expresses high levels of PDE5, inhibition of which can modulate bladder contractility through induction of cyclic guanosine monophosphate [29,30]. The correlation between EPIC urinary incontinence and sexual domain scores decreased over time, potentially due to a differential improvement of sexual and urinary scores.

The perception of the partner during couples' sexual recovery after nsRP has not been extensively studied, although partners' needs should be addressed as legitimate aspect of patient care [31]. In this study, only 33.2% of patients' partners completed the EPIC questionnaire, no clear pattern of patient-partner agreement could be derived. Findings in other studies have indicated that partner QoL can be negatively impacted for at least as long as a patient's QoL following prostate cancer treatment [19,32].

Although significant improvements in the EPIC sexual and urinary incontinence domains were only observed for tadalafil OaD treatment, treatment satisfaction at the end of DBT, as measured by the EDITS questionnaire, was significantly improved following both tadalafil OaD and PRN administration relative to placebo. However, at the end of OLT, improvement in treatment satisfaction was only significant for tadalafil OaD versus placebo.

There were several potential limitations of the current study. One important consideration is that the patient group selected may not have been ideal for observing an effect on EF or urinary incontinence with chronic tadalafil administration. Patients were on average relatively young (58 years of age), sexually active, and had few comorbidities, thus possibly representing a population of patients who might have shown improvement of EF and urinary continence rates after nsRP without treatment [33]. This could result in dilution of an effect of tadalafil on QoL, and might explain why tadalafil OaD administration significantly improved EPIC urinary incontinence domain scores versus placebo in the elderly population (61 to 68 years) only. Thus, future studies with different patient populations (older, less fit) could help clarify the effect of tadalafil OaD treatment on QoL in post-nsRP patients.

Additional limitations were imposed by the study design. First, the 9-month DBT period may have been too short for optimal assessment of EF recovery, sexual function, urinary incontinence, and associated QoL. After 9 months of DBT, low EF recovery rates of 25.2%, 19.7%, and 14.2% for tadalafil OaD, tadalafil PRN, and placebo, respectively, were observed [9]. In contrast, a retrospective study from Briganti et al. found 3-year EF recovery rates following nsRP of 72% in patients receiving PDE5 inhibitors versus 38% in patients receiving placebo [1], and a recent sildenafil study found recovery rates of around 40% following 12 months of treatment [34]. Second, EPIC scores were not assessed at the end of the drug-free washout period, but only at the end of DBT and OLT. Thus, sexual function and urinary incontinence after treatment cessation could not be assessed. Also, no valid conclusions are possible regarding the patient-partner agreement for EPIC domain scores since only one-third of the partners completed the questionnaire. Finally, the only source for the data on urinary incontinence was the respective EPIC domain score. EPIC data were collected to evaluate patients' disease-specific QoL; standard instruments for assessment of urinary function, such as the International Prostate Symptom Score might be better suited to evaluate the impact of PDE5 inhibitor treatment on urinary function.

Conclusion

Chronic dosing of tadalafil started early after nsRP increases and accelerates EF recovery [9,20] and also improves patients' QoL. The improvement of urinary incontinence facilitated by tadalafil OaD specifically in elderly patients may contribute to this effect on QoL.

Additional file

Additional file 1: Table S1. List of Ethical Review Boards. Table S2. Arithmetic mean EPIC domain score changes (patient). Table S3. Arithmetic mean EDITS total scores. Table S4. LSmean changes [95% CI] in SEAR domain scores from baseline. Table S5. Arithmetic mean SEAR scores. Figure S1. Trial design. Figure S2. Patient disposition.

Abbreviations
CI: Confidence interval; DBT: Double-blind treatment; ED: Erectile dysfunction; EDITS: Erectile Dysfunction Inventory of Treatment Satisfaction; EF: Erectile function; EPIC: Expanded Prostate Cancer Index Composite (EPIC-26); IIEF: International Index of Erectile Function; LS mean: Least squares mean; MMRM: Mixed model for repeated measures; N: Number of patients in the ITT population; nsRP: Nerve-sparing radical prostatectomy; OaD: Once daily; OLT: Open-label treatment; PRN: "Pro-re-nata"/on-demand; QoL: Quality of life; SEP: Sexual Encounter Profile; SEAR: Self-Esteem and Relationship.

Competing interests
HRP has received speaker honoraria, as well as honoraria and travel expenses for coloplast educational programs from Eli Lilly. HB, CH, JBA, KHM, JBR and DI are employees of Eli Lilly and Company; HB, KHM and DI also own Lilly stock. NS, BC, DC, and RA have no conflicts of interest to disclose.

Authors' contributions
HB and CH contributed to drafting the manuscript, HB was also involved in the design of the study. HP, NS, BC, DC, and RA were study investigators, JBR was responsible for clinical trial management. CH was responsible for the statistical analysis. HRP, NS, BC, DC, RA, JBA, KHM, and DI revised the draft manuscript critically. All authors read and approved the final manuscript.

Acknowledgements
The study was funded by Eli Lilly and Company. We thank all patients for participating and all trial investigators for their contribution to data acquisition and patient care. We thank Julia Branicka and Tom Clayton, both Eli Lilly and Company, for supporting the conduct of the trial. We thank Joaquin Casariego and Kraig Kinchen, Eli Lilly and Company, for medical advice. We thank Clare Barker, Bruce Basson, Ann Gibb, Pepa Polavieja, and Xiao Ni, all from Eli Lilly and Company, for statistical support. Statistical analyses were programmed by PSI CRO LTD, St. Petersburg, Russia. We thank Jasmine Smith and Karin Helsberg, Trilogy Writing and Consulting GmbH, Frankfurt, Germany, for providing medical writing services on behalf of Eli Lilly.

Author details
[1]Department of Urology, University Hospital North Norway, Sykehusvegen 38, 9038 Tromsø, Norway. [2]Lilly UK, Basingstoke, UK. [3]Addenbrooke's Hospital, Cambridge, UK. [4]Department of Urology, Edouard Herriot University Hospital, Lyon, France. [5]South Tees Hospitals NHS Foundation Trust, Stockton-on-Tees, UK. [6]Centre Hospitalier Universitaire de Liège, Service d'Urologie, Belgium. [7]Lilly Deutschland GmbH, Bad Homburg, Germany. [8]Eli Lilly Polska, Warsaw, Poland.

References
1. Briganti A, Di Trapani E, Abdollah F, Gallina A, Suardi N, Capitanio U, et al. Choosing the best candidates for penile rehabilitation after bilateral nerve-sparing radical prostatectomy. J Sex Med. 2012;9:608–17.
2. Ficarra V, Novara G, Ahlering TE, Costello A, Eastham JA, Graefen M, et al. Systematic review and meta-analysis of studies reporting potency rates after robot-assisted radical prostatectomy. Eur Urol. 2012;62:418–30.
3. Mulhall JP, Donatucci CF, Chiles KA, Büttner H. Management of erectile dysfunction after radical prostatectomy. In: Patel HRH, Mould T, Joseph J, Delaney C, editors. Pelvic cancer surgery: modern breakthroughs and future advances. Verlag London: Springer; 2015. in press.
4. Montorsi F, Nathan HP, McCullough A, Brock GB, Broderick G, Ahuja S, et al. Tadalafil in the treatment of erectile dysfunction following bilateral nerve

sparing radical retropubic prostatectomy: a randomized, double-blind, placebo controlled trial. J Urol. 2004;172:1036–41.

5. Montorsi F, Brock G, Lee J, Shapiro J, Van Poppel H, Graefen M, et al. Effect of nightly versus on-demand vardenafil on recovery of erectile function in men following bilateral nerve-sparing radical prostatectomy. Eur Urol. 2008;54:924–31.

6. Hatzimouratidis K, Burnett AL, Hatzichristou D, McCullough AR, Montorsi F, Mulhall JP. Phosphodiesterase type 5 inhibitors in postprostatectomy erectile dysfunction: a critical analysis of the basic science rationale and clinical application. Eur Urol. 2009;55:334–47.

7. Padma-Nathan H, McCullough AR, Levine LA, Lipshultz LI, Siegel R, Montorsi F, et al. Randomized, double-blind, placebo-controlled study of postoperative nightly sildenafil citrate for the prevention of erectile dysfunction after bilateral nerve-sparing radical prostatectomy. Int J Impot Res. 2008;20:479–86.

8. Mulhall JP, Burnett AL, Wang R, McVary KT, Moul JW, Bowden CH, et al. A phase 3, placebo controlled study of the safety and efficacy of avanafil for the treatment of erectile dysfunction after nerve sparing radical prostatectomy. J Urol. 2013;189:2229–36.

9. Montorsi F, Brock G, Stolzenburg JU, Mulhall J, Moncada I, Patel HRH, et al. Effects of tadalafil treatment on erectile function recovery following bilateral nerve-sparing radical prostatectomy: a randomised placebo-controlled study (REACTT). Eur Urol. 2014;65:587–96.

10. Wei JT, Dunn RL, Litwin MS, Sandler HM, Sanda MG. Development and validation of the expanded prostate cancer index composite (EPIC) for comprehensive assessment of health-related quality of life in men with prostate cancer. Urology. 2000;56:899–905.

11. Sanda MG, Wei JT, Litwin MS. Scoring Instructions for the Expanded Prostate cancer Index Composite Short Form (EPIC-26). [http://www.med.umich.edu/urology/research/EPIC/EPIC-26-Scoring-1.2007.pdf]

12. Penson DF, McLerran D, Feng Z, Li L, Albertsen PC, Gilliland FD, et al. 5-year urinary and sexual outcomes after radical prostatectomy: results from the prostate cancer outcomes study. J Urol. 2005;173:1701–5.

13. Potosky AL, Davis WW, Hoffman RM, Stanford JL, Stephenson RA, Penson DF, et al. Five-year outcomes after prostatectomy or radiotherapy for prostate cancer: the prostate cancer outcomes study. J Natl Cancer Inst. 2004;96:1358–67.

14. Althof SE, Corty EW, Levine SB, Levine F, Burnett AL, McVary K, et al. EDITS: development of questionnaires for evaluating satisfaction with treatments for erectile dysfunction. Urology. 1999;53:793–9.

15. Cappelleri JC, Althof SE, Siegel RL, Shpilsky A, Bell SS, Duttagupta S. Development and validation of the self-esteem and relationship (SEAR) questionnaire in erectile dysfunction. Int J Impot Res. 2004;16:30–8.

16. Cappelleri JC, Rosen RC, Smith MD, Mishra A, Osterloh IH. Diagnostic evaluation of the erectile function domain of the international index of erectile function. Urology. 1999;54:346–51.

17. Stanford JL, Feng Z, Hamilton AS, Gilliland FD, Stephenson RA, Eley JW, et al. Urinary and sexual function after radical prostatectomy for clinically localized prostate cancer: the prostate cancer outcomes study. JAMA. 2000;283:354–60.

18. Kilminster S, Müller S, Menon M, Joseph JV, Ralph DJ, Patel HRH. Predicting erectile function outcome in men after radical prostatectomy for prostate cancer. BJU Int. 2012;110:422–6.

19. Harden JK, Sanda MG, Wei JT, Yarandi H, Hembroff L, Hardy J, et al. Partners' long-term appraisal of their caregiving experience, marital satisfaction, sexual satisfaction, and quality of life 2 years after prostate cancer treatment. Cancer Nurs. 2013;36:104–13.

20. Moncada I, De Bethencourt FR, Lledó-Garcia E, Romero J, Turbi C, Büttner H, et al. Effects of tadalafil once daily or on-demand versus placebo on time to recovery of erectile function in patients after bilateral nerve-sparing radical prostatectomy. World J Urol. 2014, Aug 26. [Epub ahead of print]

21. Forgue ST, Patterson BE, Bedding AW, Payne CD, Phillips DL, Wrishko RE, et al. Tadalafil pharmacokinetics in healthy subjects. Br J Clin Pharmacol. 2006;61:280–8.

22. Cameron AP, Suskind AM, Neer C, Hussain H, Montgomery J, Latini JM, et al. Functional and anatomical differences between continent and incontinent men post radical prostatectomy on urodynamics and 3T MRI: a pilot study. Neurourol Urodyn. 2014, Apr 21. [Epub ahead of print].

23. Ficarra V, Novara G, Rosen RC, Artibani W, Carroll PR, Costello A, et al. Systematic review and meta-analysis of studies reporting urinary continence recovery after robot-assisted radical prostatectomy. Eur Urol. 2012;62:405–17.

24. Nam RK, Herschorn S, Loblaw DA, Liu Y, Klotz LH, Carr LK, et al. Population based study of long-term rates of surgery for urinary incontinence after radical prostatectomy for prostate cancer. J Urol. 2012;188:502–6.

25. McVary KT, Monnig W, Camps Jr JL, Young JM, Tseng LJ, van den Ende G. Sildenafil citrate improves erectile function and urinary symptoms in men with erectile dysfunction and lower urinary tract symptoms associated with benign prostatic hyperplasia: a randomized, double-blind trial. J Urol. 2007;177:1071–7.

26. McVary KT, Roehrborn CG, Kaminetsky JC, Auerbach SM, Wachs B, Young JM, et al. Tadalafil relieves lower urinary tract symptoms secondary to benign prostatic hyperplasia. J Urol. 2007;177:1401–7.

27. Stief CG, Porst H, Neuser D, Beneke M, Ulbrich E. A randomised, placebo-controlled study to assess the efficacy of twice-daily vardenafil in the treatment of lower urinary tract symptoms secondary to benign prostatic hyperplasia. Eur Urol. 2008;53:1236–44.

28. Gandaglia G, Albersen M, Suardi N, Gallina A, Abdollah F, Castiglione F, et al. Postoperative phosphodiesterase type 5 inhibitor administration increases the rate of urinary continence recovery after bilateral nerve-sparing radical prostatectomy. Int J Urol. 2013;20:413–9.

29. Gacci M, Ierardi A, Rose AD, Tazzioli S, Scapaticci E, Filippi S, et al. Vardenafil can improve continence recovery after bilateral nerve sparing prostatectomy: results of a randomized, double blind, placebo-controlled pilot study. J Sex Med. 2010;7(1 Pt 1):234–43.

30. Filippi S, Morelli A, Sandner P, Fibbi B, Mancina R, Marini M, et al. Characterization and functional role of androgen-dependent PDE5 activity in the bladder. Endocrinology. 2007;148:1019–29.

31. Wittmann D, Carolan M, Given B, Skolarus TA, An L, Palapattu G, et al. Exploring the role of the partner in couples' sexual recovery after surgery for prostate cancer. Support Care Cancer. 2014;22:2509–15.

32. Wittmann DA, West B, Skolarus T, Montie J. Couples' sexual recovery trajectory after surgery for prostate cancer: change in sexual function, sexual satisfaction and dyadic satisfaction [abstract]. Soc Social Work Res. 2014 Annual Conference, San Antonio, Tx, January 15-19, 2014.

33. Castiglione F, Nini A, Briganti A. Penile rehabilitation with phosphodiesterase type 5 inhibitors after nerve-sparing radical prostatectomy: are we targeting the right patients? Eur Urol. 2014;65:673–4.

34. Pavlovich CP, Levinson AW, Su LM, Mettee LZ, Feng Z, Bivalacqua TJ, et al. Nightly vs on-demand sildenafil for penile rehabilitation after minimally invasive nerve-sparing radical prostatectomy: results of a randomized double-blind trial with placebo. BJU Int. 2013;112:844–51.

MMP9 overexpression is associated with good surgical outcome in children with UPJO

Sabrina Thalita Reis[*], Kátia R. M. Leite, Nayara Izabel Viana, Roberto Iglesias Lopes, Caio Martins Moura, Renato F. Ivanovic, Marcos Machado, Francisco Tibor Denes, Amilcar Giron, William Carlos Nahas, Miguel Srougi and Carlo C. Passerotti

Abstract

Background: Ureteropelvic junction obstruction (UPJO) diagnosed prenatally occurs in 1:150 – 1:1200 pregnancies. Although many studies investigating the molecular changes of this obstructed segment have been performed, the underlying mechanisms are still unclear. The role of extracellular matrix (ECM) components remains controversial, and the investigations in the field of ECM changes, might help the better understanding of the pathogenesis of this common condition. The aim of the present study was to investigate for the first time in the literature whether MMP9 and its specific inhibitors, TIMP1 and RECK, are expressed in a reproducible, specific pattern in UPJ.

Methods: UPJO specimens were obtained from 16 children at the time of dismembered pyeloplasty due to intrinsic UPJ stenosis. Expression levels of the three genes (MMP9, TIMP1 and RECK) were analyzed by quantitative real-time polymerase chain reaction (qRT-PCR). Then correlated the expression levels of the genes according to grade study population that was divided in 2 categories according to Society of Fetal Urology classification, grade 3 (moderate) and 4 (severe). For DTPA we subdivided the childrens in 2 groups, obstructive (T 1/2 more than 20 min) and partial obstructive (T 1/2 between 10 and 20 min) and success in a surgery was defined as decrease in T 1/2 to less than 20 min, absence of symptoms, improving renal function and decreasing dilatation on successive exams.

Results: MMP9 was underexpressed and TIMP1 and RECK were overexpressed in children with obstructive DTPA but the differences were not statistically significant. Overexpression of MMP9 was higher among patients with severe grade of UPJ compared to those with moderate grade. Surprisingly expression levels of MMP-9 was three times higher in children who were successfully treated by surgery ($n = 10$) ($p = 0.072$), so those who were followed for at least 1 year after surgery and remained with improvement in renal function and decreasing dilation on intravenous urogram and TIMP-1 was underexpressed in 100 % of this cases ($p = 0.00$).

Conclusions: We showed an increase in expression of MMP9 and a decrease in expression of TIMP1 in children who improving renal function and decreasing dilation after surgery. We believe that the higher expression of MMP9 in these cases can reflect an increase in degradation and remodeling process that could be used as a marker for surgical outcome.

Keywords: UPJO, Metaloproteinases, Children

* Correspondence: sasareis@gmail.com
Urology Department, Laboratory of Medical Investigation (LIM55), University of Sao Paulo Medical School, Av. Dr. Arnaldo 455, 2° floor, room 2145, 01246-903 Sao Paulo, Brazil

Background

Ureteropelvic junction obstruction (UPJO) diagnosed prenatally occurs in 1:150–1:1200 pregnancies [1, 2]. Hydronephrosis can be a result of anatomical or functional obstruction. It is diagnosed almost twice as often in boys and can affect either one (most often the left) or both kidneys [3–7].

Although many studies investigating the molecular changes of this obstructed segment have been performed, the underlying mechanisms are still unclear. The studies revealed abnormal innervation patterns and abnormalities of smooth muscle or collagen composition as well as reduction in the number of interstitial cells of Cajal [8, 9]. The role of extracellular matrix (ECM) components and neural distribution remains controversial, and the investigations in the field of ECM changes, and innervation patterns might help the better understanding of the pathogenesis of this common condition.

ECM is a biologically active composition of structural and adhesive proteins embedded in a hydrated ground substance of glycosaminoglycans and proteoglycans. Matrix metalloproteinases (MMPs) are secreted from connective tissue cells of mesenchymal origin, part of a family of closely related proteolytic enzymes, able to degrade most component of the ECM [10]. The MMPs are proteolytic enzymes present in both normal and pathologic tissues in which matrix remodeling occurs. The gelatinase (MMP9) degrades the basal membrane. Studies have explored the role of ECM in primary obstructed and primary refluxing megaureters showing both a decrease in smooth muscle and an increase in the ECM [11], and higher ECM turnover in refluxing ureteral endings [12]. Early descriptions of the UPJ alterations were those of extensive fibrosis and muscular attenuation. Innervation abnormalities at the UPJ have been suggested as another cause for UPJ obstruction, based on findings of reduced nerve distribution at this location [13].

The aim of the present study was to investigate whether MMP9 and its specific inhibitors, Tissue inhibitors of metalloproteinases 1 (TIMP1) and Reversion-inducing cysteine-rich protein with Kazal motifs (RECK), are expressed in a reproducible, specific pattern in UPJO. Additionally, we evaluated the correlation between the expression of these genes and important clinical parameters (Grade and DTPA) and surgical outcome in childrens with UPJ submitted to pyeloplasty.

Methods

Patient selection

After obtaining institutional ethic board approval, UPJ specimens were obtained from 16 children (11 boys, 5 girls) at the time of dismembered pyeloplasty due to intrinsic UPJ stenosis (median age, 4.0 years, range, 1–16 years). All cases of UPJ obstruction were confirmed on the basis of radiological, scintigraphic, and operative findings.

We first analyzed MMP9, TIMP1 and RECK expression levels in fresh tissue specimens from the 16 children using quantitative real-time polymerase chain reaction (qRT-PCR). Tissue sample was taken at the time of the surgery and a small fragment of 1 by 1 cm from the transition between ureter and pelvis were analysed.

Then correlated the expression levels of the genes with important clinical parameters (Grade and DTPA) and surgical outcome in children with UPJO. According to grade study population was divided in 2 categories according to Society of Fetal Urology classification, grade 3 (moderate) and 4 (severe). For DTPA we subdivided the childrens in 2 groups, obstructive (T 1/2 more than 20 min) and partial obstructive (T 1/2 between 10 and 20 min) and success in a surgery is defined as decrease in T 1/2 to less than 20 min, absence of symptoms, improving renal function and decreasing dilatation on successive exams.

RNA isolation and cDNA synthesis

All tissue samples were obtained from surgical specimens and immediately frozen at −170 °C in liquid nitrogen. Total RNA was isolated with an RNA aqueous Kit (Applied Biosystems, CA, USA) according to the manufacturer's instructions. RNA concentration was determined by 260/280 nM absorbance using a Nanodrop ND-1000 spectrophotometer (Thermo Scientific). cDNA was generated using a High Capacity cDNA Reverse Transcription Kit (Applied Biosystems, CA, USA). The reactions were incubated at 25 °C for 10 min, followed by 37 °C for 120 min and 85 °C for 5 min. The cDNA was stored at −20 °C until further use.

Quantitative real-time PCR and gene expression

Expression levels of the three genes were analyzed by qRT-PCR using an ABI 7500 Fast Real-Time PCR System (Applied Biosystems). Target sequences were amplified in a 10-µl reaction containing 5 µl of TaqMan Universal PCR Master Mix, 0.5 µl of TaqMan Gene Expression Assays (primers and probes; see Table 1), 1 µl of cDNA and 3.5 µl of DNase-free water. The PCR cycling conditions were 2 min at 50 °C, 10 min at 95 °C, and then 40 cycles of 15 s at 95 °C and 1 min at 60 °C. A TaqMan B2M assay was utilized as the endogenous control (Table 1).

Table 1 Primers utilized

Gene symbol	Assays ID
MMP9	Hs00957562_m1
TIMP1	Hs00212624_m1
RECK	Hs01019179_m1
B2M	Hs99999907_m1

Statistical analysis

We used the $\Delta\Delta CT$ method to calculate the relative expression of the three target genes using the formula $\Delta\Delta CT$. The fold change in gene expression was calculated as $2^{-\Delta\Delta CT}$. To compare the clinical characteristics of children with UPJ, we used the Mann–Whitney test. Statistical analysis was performed using SPSS 19.0 for Windows using a significance of $p \leq 0.05$.

Results

The children were grouped according to DTPA, grade and success of treatment. 13 children with obstructive DTPA were compared to 3 children with a partial obstruction, and as demonstrated in Fig. 1a we showed that MMP9 was underexpressed and TIMP1 and RECK were overexpressed in children with obstructive DTPA but

the differences were not statistically significant (MMP9, $p = 0.170$; TIMP1, $p = 0.389$; RECK, $p = 0.389$).

Our analysis of MMP9, TIMP1 and RECK expression levels according to grade of obstruction is shown in Fig. 1b. Overexpression of MMP9 was higher among patients with severe grade of UPJ ($n = 12$) compared to those with moderate grade ($n = 4$). However, statistical analysis revealed that these differences were not significant ($p = 0.694$). TIMP1 and RECK did not significantly differ considering grade of UPJ (TIMP-1, $p = 0.684$, RECK, $p = 0.684$).

When MMP9, TIMP1 and RECK expression levels were analyzed according to surgical outcome, surprisingly we found that the median expression levels of MMP-9 was three times higher in children who were successfully treated by surgery ($n = 10$) compared to

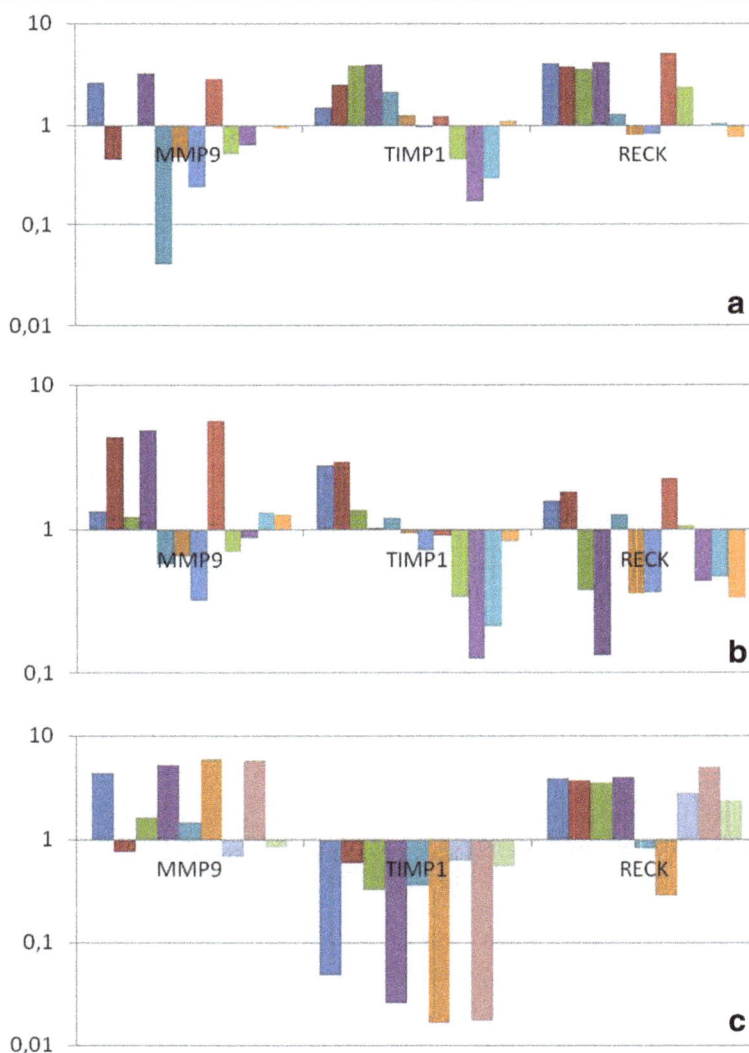

Fig. 1 Expression profile of MMP9, TIMP1 and RECK according to DTPA (**a**), grade (**b**) and success of treatment (**c**) in tissue of UPJ children

those did not have success ($n = 6$), with a marginal significance ($p = 0.072$), TIMP-1 was underexpressed in 100 % of this cases ($p = 0.00$) and RECK was overexpressed in 80 % of this same cases ($p = 0.082$). This results is shown in Fig. 1c.

Discussion

UPJ obstruction is mostly considered as a functional obstruction originating from abnormalities in the smooth muscle of the pelvis and ureter [14]. Although surgery in UPJ obstruction is efficient to protect the patient against renal function lost, results obtained in both experimental and human-studies suggest that UPJ obstruction induces permanent modifications of the renal parenchyma.

The nature of the abnormalities at the UPJ in children with congenital intrinsic UPJ obstruction remains controversial. Many studies revealed that UPJ obstruction is associated with a significant difference in the collagen and smooth muscle structural components [15]. The finding of the increased tissue matrix ratio was believed to decrease the ureteral distensibility resulting in damage to muscle cells influencing the contractility [16]. Furthermore, a variety of intrarenal factors lead to progressive interstitial and renal parenchyma fibrosis in patients with Congenital anomalies of the kidney and urinary tract, like UPJ, including growth factors, cytokines, chemokines and adhesion molecules, which are produced by the hydronephrotic kidney. An altered renal expression of growth factors and cytokines modulates cell death by apoptosis or phenotypic transition of glomerular, tubular, and vascular cells. Mediators of cellular injury include hypoxia, ischemia, and reactive oxygen species, while fibroblasts undergo myofibroblast transformation with increased deposition of extracellular matrix [17].

The present study is the first to investigate the expression of MMP9 and its negative controllers in obstructed UPJ tissue. The change in expression of ECM components could be an alternative mechanism leading to UPJ obstruction together with the reduction of interstitial cells of Cajal. The reduction in peristalsis, result of the reduced number of Cajal's cells associated to reduction in distensibility, result of alteration in ECM components could be the physiopathology of the disease [18]. MMPs have many important functions in wound healing processes and angiogenesis. In the case of deregulation of their production, matrix degradation and turnover are the consequences [19] and It has been shown that an increase in ECM turnover influences the neuronal network within the ureteral wall. Also, some MMPs have been proved to be neurotoxic degrading ECM proteins like collagen type 1, which are normally able to protect cultured neurons from cytotoxic cell death [20].

Defective collagen production from smooth muscle cells has been held responsible for this pathology and decreased neural cells have been thought to play an important role, especially in intrinsic type obstructions [21]. There are other studies showing that this disintegration in the configuration of smooth muscle and overdeposition of collagen may be an etiologic factor, and collagen to smooth muscle ratio may have a prognostic value [15].

There are some limitation that should be pointed out. Our small number of cases would interfere in our findings and may affect in our subgroups analysis (successful against failure and intrinsic against crossing vessel group). Since it refers to a low incidence disease with decreasing surgical indication it may be of difficult to increase sample size in a small period of time. Also the lack of control group because of the absence normal tissue also may impact in our findings. At last, there is an intentional bias in selection, including a higher number of failure cases does not reflects the overall success in the surgical approach.

Conclusion

Here, curiously we showed an increase in expression of MMP9 and a decrease in expression of TIMP1 in children who were successfully treated by surgery. UPJ obstruction is associated with a significant difference in the collagen, and MMPs are potent proteolytic enzymes that are known to play a key role in the degradation of this component, therefore, we believe that the higher expression of MMP9 in these cases can reflect an increase in degradation of collagen and remodeling process that could be used as a marker for surgical outcome.

Abbreviations
cDNA, complementary deoxyribonucleic *acid*; ECM, extracellular matrix; MMP, matrix metalloproteinase; qRT-PCR, quantitative real-time polymerase chain reaction; RECK, reversion-inducing cysteine-rich protein with Kazal motif; *RNA*, ribonucleic *acid*; TIMP-1, tissue inhibitor of metalloproteinases 1; UPJO, ureteropelvic junction obstruction

Acknowledgements
None.

Authors' contributions
Conception and design: STR, KRL, CCP ; acquisition of patients and data: RIL, MM, AG, FTD; Drafting of the manuscript: STR, KRL; molecular genetic studies: STR, NIV, CMM; Administration support: NIV, CMM; Statistical Analysis: STR; critical revision and important intellectual content: CCP, KRL; supervision: MS, WCN. We confirm that all authors read and aproved the final manuscript.

References

1. Elder JS. Antenatal hydronephrosis. Pediatr Clin North Am. 1997;44:1299–332.
2. Chevalier RL, Thornhill BA, Chang AY, et al. Recovery from release of ureteral obstruction in the rat: relationship to nephrogenesis. Kidney Int. 2002;61:2033–43.
3. Lee RS, Cendron M, Kinnamon DD, et al. Antenatal hydronephrosis as a predictor of postnatal outcome: a meta-analysis. Pediatrics. 2006;118:586–93.
4. Carr MC, El-Ghoneimi A. Anomalies and surgery of the ureteropelvic junction in children. In: Wein AJ, Kavoussi LR, Novick AC, editors. Campbell-Walsh urology. Philadelphia: Saunders; 2007. p. 3359.
5. Gawłowska A, Niedzielski J. Obstructive uropathy in children – chosen aspects. Przegl Pediatr. 2003;33:282–5.
6. Johnston J, Evans J, Glassberg K, et al. Pelvic hydronephrosis in children: a review of 219 personal cases. J Urol. 1977;117:97–101.
7. Choi YJ, Baranowska-Daca E, Nguyen V, et al. Mechanism of chronic obstructive uropathy: increased expression of apoptosis-promoting molecules. Kidney Int. 2000;58:1481–91.
8. Koleda P, Apoznanski W, Wozniak Z, et al. Changes in interstitial cell of Cajal-like cells density in congenital ureteropelvic junction obstruction. Int Urol Nephrol. 2012;44:7–12.
9. Lang RJ, Tonta MA, Zoltkowski BZ, et al. Pyeloureteric peristalsis: role of atypical smooth muscle cells and interstitial cells of Cajal-like cells as pacemakers. J Physiol. 2006;576(Pt3):695–705.
10. Toi M, Ishigaki S, Tominaga T. Metalloproteinases and tissue inhibitors of metalloproteinases. Breast Cancer Res Treat. 1998;52:113–24.
11. Lee BR, Partin AW, Epstein JI, et al. A quantitative histological analysis of the dilated ureter of childhood. J Urol. 1992;148:1482–6.
12. Oswald J, Schwentner C, Brenner E, et al. Extracellular matrix degradation and reduced nerve supply in refluxing ureteral endings. J Urol. 2004; 172:1099–102.
13. Zhang PL, Peters CA, Rosen S. Ureteropelvic junction obstruction: morphological and clinical studies. Pediatr Nephrol. 2000;14:820–6.
14. Mendelsohn C. Functional obstruction: the renal pelvis rules. J Clin Invest. 2004;113:957–9.
15. Murakumo M, Nonomura K, Yamashita T, et al. Structural changes of collagen components and diminution of nerves in congenital ureteropelvic junction obstruction. J Urol. 1997;157:1963–8.
16. Kim WJ, Yun SJ, Lee TS, et al. Collagen-to-smooth muscle ratio helps prediction of prognosis after pyeloplasty. J Urol. 2000;163:1271–5.
17. Silva AC S e, Pereira AB, Teixeira MM, Teixeira AL. Chemokines as potential markers in pediatric renal diseases. Dis Markers. 2014;2014:278715.
18. Solari V, Piotrowska AP, Puri P. Altered expression of interstitial cells of cajal in congenital ureteropelvic junction obstruction. J Urol. 2003;170:2420–2.
19. Matsui Y, Maeda M, Nakagami W, et al. The involvement of matrix metalloproteinases and inflammation in lumbar disc herniation. Spine. 1998;23:863–8.
20. Vos CM, Sjulson L, Nath A, et al. Cytotoxicity by matrix metalloproteinase-1 in organotypic spinal cord and dissociated neuronal cultures. Exp Neurol. 2000;163:324–30.
21. Kim WJ, Yun SJ, Lee TS, Kim CW, Lee HM, Choi H. Collagen-tosmooth muscle ratio helps prediction of prognosis after pyeloplasty. J Urol. 2000; 163:1271e5.

A pilot randomized trial of conventional versus advanced pelvic floor exercises to treat urinary incontinence after radical prostatectomy

Daniel Santa Mina[1,2,3*], Darren Au[1,4], Shabbir M. H. Alibhai[1,3], Leah Jamnicky[1], Nelly Faghani[5], William J. Hilton[1,4], Leslie E. Stefanyk[1,2], Paul Ritvo[6,7], Jennifer Jones[1,3], Dean Elterman[1,3], Neil E. Fleshner[1,3], Antonio Finelli[1,3], Rajiv K. Singal[3,8], John Trachtenberg[1,3] and Andrew G. Matthew[1,3]

Abstract

Background: Radical prostatectomy is the most common and effective treatment for localized prostate cancer. Unfortunately, radical prostatectomy is associated with urinary incontinence and has a significant negative impact on quality of life. Pelvic floor exercises are the most common non-invasive management strategy for urinary incontinence following radical prostatectomy; however, studies provide inconsistent findings regarding their efficacy. One potential reason for sub-optimal efficacy of these interventions is the under-utilization of regional muscles that normally co-activate with the pelvic floor, such as the transverse abdominis, rectus abdominis, and the diaphragm. Two novel approaches to improve urinary continence recovery are 'Pfilates' and 'Hypopressives' that combine traditional pelvic floor exercises with the activation of additional supportive muscles. Our study will compare an advanced pelvic floor exercise training program that includes Pfilates and Hypopressives, to a conventional pelvic floor exercises regimen for the treatment of post-radical prostatectomy urinary incontinence.

Methods/Design: This is a pilot, randomized controlled trial of advanced pelvic floor muscle training versus conventional pelvic floor exercises for men with localized prostate cancer undergoing radical prostatectomy. Eighty-eight men who will be undergoing radical prostatectomy at hospitals in Toronto, Canada will be recruited. Eligible participants must not have undergone androgen deprivation therapy and/or radiation therapy. Participants will be randomized 1:1 to receive 26 weeks of the advanced or conventional pelvic floor exercise programs. Each program will be progressive and have comparable exercise volume. The primary outcomes are related to feasibility for a large, adequately powered randomized controlled trial to determine efficacy for the treatment of urinary incontinence. Feasibility will be assessed via recruitment success, participant retention, outcome capture, intervention adherence, and prevalence of adverse events. Secondary outcomes of intervention efficacy include measures of pelvic floor strength, urinary incontinence, erectile function, and quality of life. Secondary outcome measures will be collected prior to surgery (baseline), and at 2, 6, 12, 26-weeks post-operatively.

Discussion: Pfilates and Hypopressives are novel approaches to optimizing urinary function after radical prostatectomy. This trial will provide the foundation of data for future, large-scale trials to definitively describe the effect of these advanced pelvic floor exercise modalities compared to conventional pelvic floor exercise regimes for men with prostate cancer undergoing radical prostatectomy

* Correspondence: Daniel.santamina@utoronto.ca
[1]University Health Network, Toronto, Ontario, 200 Elizabeth Street, Toronto, Ontario M5G 2C4, Canada
[2]University of Guelph-Humber, 207 Humber College Boulevard, Toronto, Ontario M9W 5L7, Canada
Full list of author information is available at the end of the article

Background

Radical prostatectomy (RP) is the most common treatment for localized prostate cancer (PCa) [1, 2] with a >90 % 15-year disease-specific survival for men with localized disease [3]. Unfortunately, RP is associated with post-operative urinary incontinence (UI) that can persist for two years or longer and is related to significant reductions in overall health-related quality of life (QoL) [4–7]. Moreover, UI can be an important economic burden to patients due to the cost of pads and lost work productivity [8]. Given the prevalence of RP in the management of PCa and the associated psychosocial, functional, and economic adversity caused by UI, expediting the recovery of urinary control is a major priority for patients and their clinicians.

Normally, the pelvic floor muscles (comprised of the internal sphincter, levator ani, coccygeus, striated urogenital sphincter, external anal sphincter, ischiocavernosus, and bulbospongiousus) work in a coordinated fashion to promote urinary control [9, 10]. While the exact etiology of post-RP UI is not well understood, it is hypothesized to result from injury to the internal sphincter and/or an onset of bladder detrusor hyperactivity that can cause urge incontinence through pressure on the bladder walls [10–16]. Consequently, continence becomes dependent on the pelvic floor musculature that supports the *external* urethral sphincter [12, 17, 18], and thus voluntary conditioning of these muscles is considered a primary, non-invasive UI management strategy post-RP [19, 20].

Conventional pelvic floor muscle exercises (PFMX) are intended to improve urinary control by increasing the strength, endurance, and coordination of the pelvic floor muscles and functional activation of the external urethral sphincter [21–23]. Moreover, chronic performance of PFMXs is suggested to cause hypertrophy of the periurethral striated muscles, a resultant stiffening and strengthening of the pelvic floor muscles and connective tissues,

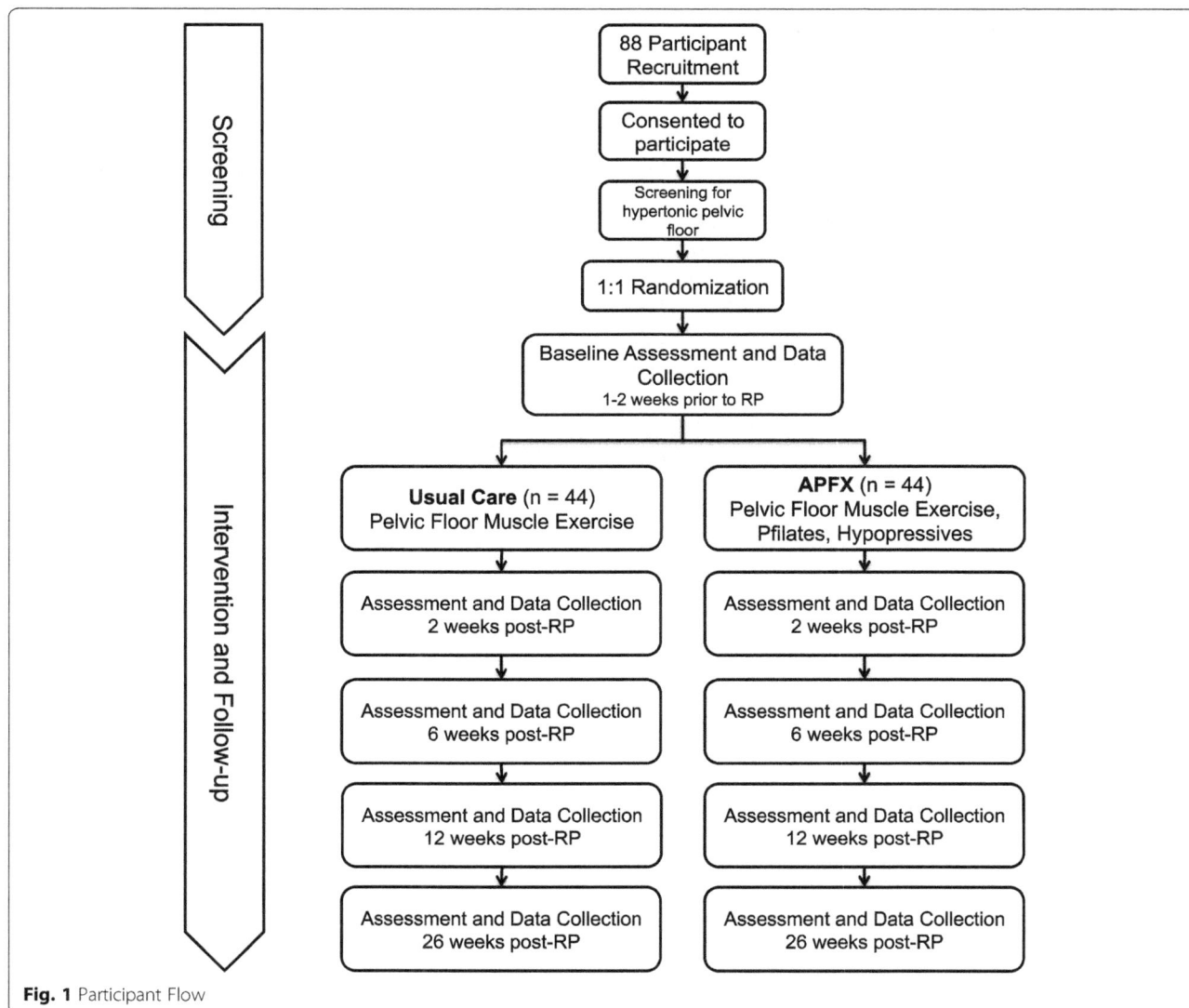

Fig. 1 Participant Flow

and an inhibition reflex of the detrusor muscles [24–26]. Collectively, the PFMXs facilitate improved capability for external urethral constriction [9] and relaxed detrusor activity to aid in the recovery of post-RP UI [27, 28]. PFMXs typically involve instructions to 'lift up' the pelvic floor to stop the flow of urine [17, 21, 29]. PFMX training starts with pelvic floor muscle identification through biofeedback, typically through active urinary flow control (i.e. voluntarily starting and stopping urination) and cueing (using imagery to identify and activate the correct muscles). Once appropriate control is observed, patients are instructed to practice the same contractions routinely with a target volume, intensity, frequency, and/or duration [23].

A recent Cochrane review on the management of UI after RP found a small to moderate benefit of conventional PFMXs; however, none of the included studies incorporated training of the surrounding muscles [21]. The paucity of evidence and modest benefits related to the management of UI with the engagement of surrounding muscle to the pelvic floor is salient because of the growing literature demonstrating that pelvic floor muscle contraction is optimized with co-activation of the abdominals and other regional muscles [30–34]. In particular, the transverse abdominis (TrA), rectus abdominis, and diaphragm muscles are often neglected in PMFX approaches despite their requirement for optimal pelvic floor activation [30, 33]. The relationship between the TrA and diaphragm with pelvic floor activation is described in several lines of research. First, Neumann et al. [33] observed that relaxation of the abdominal wall during pelvic floor muscle contraction only elicits 25 % of the maximal voluntary contraction of the pelvic floor. Second, research has indicated that the likelihood of poor pelvic floor tonic activity (autonomic contraction), and consequent risk of UI, is apparent when the ability of the TrA to maintain a contraction is impaired [30–32]. Third, improved tonic activity of the pelvic floor may improve the autonomic urethral constriction that could prevent leakage without conscious intervention [35, 36]. Similarly, 'deep belly' breathing exercises that emphasize diaphragmatic contraction and relaxation have been shown to improve pelvic floor muscle activation and reduce intra-abdominal pressure in women with incontinence [30, 37, 38].

More recent PFMX paradigms incorporate techniques aimed at optimizing pelvic floor muscle responsiveness and contraction quality through the utilization of other regional muscles. One such approach is "Pfilates" ('Pelvic Floor Pilates') that incorporates the fundamental elements of Pilates (a form of exercise that focuses on core strength, stability, flexibility, and muscle control, as well as posture and breathing) [39, 40] with targeted pelvic floor activation [41]. Pfilates includes several static poses that activate the TrA, hip adductors, gluteal, and pelvic floor muscles with instructions to pulse (small range of motion) with short, maximal effort contractions of the engaged muscles.

A recent study by Culligan et al. [40] demonstrated comparable improvements in pelvic floor strength measured by perineometry after 12 weeks of conventional PFMX versus Pilates in 62 women with little or no pelvic floor muscle dysfunction. Although UI was not measured, this study suggests that Pilates may produce similar benefits for UI as traditional PFMXs.

Another novel approach to PFMXs is known as 'Hypopressive' exercises. Hypopressive exercises emphasize engaging the TrA with conscious coordination of the diaphragm with breathing that is hypothesized to increase muscle tone of the pelvic floor muscles and subsequently cause urethral constriction [30, 42–45]. While executing the prescribed Hypopressive techniques, the use of deep breathing followed by a brief breath-hold causes relaxation of the diaphragm, decrease in intra-abdominal pressure, and a reflex contraction of the pelvic floor muscles, unconsciously maximizing a contraction and consequently improving reconditioning of these muscles [43, 45]. Caufriez [46] communicated this technique in 1997 and described the steps as follows: slow diaphragmatic inspiration, followed by total expiration and, after glottal closure, a gradual contraction of the abdominal wall muscles, with superior displacement of the diaphragm cupola (referred to as diaphragmatic aspiration). There is significant attention drawn to the distension of the ribs, breathing, and body positions, so that even though one is aware of their pelvic floor, it is an unconscious movement [30, 38, 43]. Early research on the effects of Hypopressive exercise programs have demonstrated increased tonic activity, strength, and size of the pelvic floor muscles via ultrasonography imaging [44].

To date, no study has assessed the effect of a comprehensive PFMX regimen that includes Pfilates and Hypopressives for UI. This represents a major gap in our understanding of non-invasive UI management strategies for PCa patients especially since the benefits of PFMX are modest and emerging literature suggests that the pelvic floor muscles are suboptimally activated during more focused pelvic floor training.

Methods

This study is a 2-arm, pilot randomized controlled trial (RCT) that compares the effect of a conventional PFMX program, considered usual care (UC), to an advanced pelvic floor exercise program (APFX) including Pfilates, and Hypopressive for the management of UI after RP for PCa. The primary objective of this study is to assess the feasibility of conducting a full-scale RCT of similar design. Feasibility will be determined via recruitment success, participant retention, outcome capture, intervention adherence, and prevalence of adverse events. Our secondary objectives are to compare the efficacy of APFX to UC in UI, pelvic floor strength, erectile function, and QoL after RP. This study will be conducted at the Wellness and

Exercise for Cancer Survivors (WE-Can) program at the Princess Margaret Cancer Centre. WE-Can is a multidisciplinary team of physicians, physiotherapists, kinesiologists, and other exercise professionals that provide exercise and physical activity programming for cancer survivors.

This study has been approved by the ethics boards of the participating institutions and all participants will be asked to provide voluntary and informed consent.

Study population/participants

Eighty-eight participants will be recruited for this trial. We anticipate an attrition rate of 20 % by the 26-week follow-up assessment to yield 70 participants (35 participants per group) for main efficacy estimate analyses that is aligned with recommended pilot and feasibility study sample sizes for treatment effect estimates [47–49]. *Inclusion Criteria*: Patients that: i) have localized PCa who have consented for RP (open retropubic, laparoscopic, or robot-assisted laparoscopic); ii) are between the ages of 40 and 80 years; and iii) are proficient in English. *Exclusion Criteria*: Patients that: i) are diagnosed with a known neurological disease, autoimmune connective tissue disorder; ii) have prior experience with pelvic floor training by a healthcare provider; iii) have uncontrolled hypertension; iv) have diagnosed chronic obstructive pulmonary disease (COPD) and/or chronic restrictive respiratory disease; v) have a history of inguinal herniation; or vi) have hypertonic pelvic floor muscles upon baseline evaluation. Pelvic floor tonicity will be assessed by a specially trained pelvic floor physiotherapist via digital rectal examination. Hypertonic pelvic floor is determined by the physical examination findings of extrapelvic musculoskeletal and connective tissue examination, as well as the elements of patient history [50]. These patients who exhibit levator ani hypertonicity (tension myalgia) will be excluded as they can experience pelvic, urogenital, and rectal pain; tightness and spasticity; and adverse effects on sexual, urinary, and bowel function that may be exacerbated with contraction-based pelvic floor training [51, 52].

Study recruitment and randomization

Recruitment will occur in the Greater Toronto Area (total population 4.5 million) in urological oncology clinics and through presentations and/or information stands [52] set-up at local PCa support group meetings. These peer-support meetings often include men who have been recently diagnosed and are considering various treatments for PCa, including RP. Men who self-identify as eligible will receive further verbal and written information about the study. Those deemed eligible and are interested will be asked to provide written consent.

Participants will be 1:1 randomized to the UC and APFX groups, stratified by age (±60 years). Blinded allocation of the participants to their treatment groups will be performed via a process consisting of placing the intervention assignments into opaque envelopes, sealing and shuffling the envelopes, and sequentially numbering them with each new participant receiving an envelope in sequence of recruitment. The envelopes will be opened by the research coordinator with the participant following the baseline assessment, prior to RP Fig. 1.

Study arms

The two groups will begin participation in their respective interventions immediately following post-operative catheter removal until 26-weeks post-operatively. The physiotherapist assessment of pelvic floor muscle activity and strength will be assessed during each visit in order to optimize the quality of the contractions. Instructions to correctly contract their pelvic floor will be provided verbally and with biofeedback via the Modified Oxford Scale (MOS). Grading of this scale is described below. The research coordinator, who is a Registered Kinesiologist with training and experience in pelvic floor strengthening, Pfilates, and Hypopressives, will be providing the intervention prescription for both study arms and will communicate weekly with the participants to support and quantify program compliance (# of completed contractions/# prescribed contractions), facilitate prescribed progression, and address any barriers to program participation. Furthermore, both groups will receive a manual that includes detailed information and instructions relevant to their training regimens (Tables 1 and 2).

Usual care

The UC group will receive generic PFMX exercise instructions and demonstrations from the research coordinator at the initial post-operative time point (post-operative day #10-14) comparable to standard practice for RP patients at the study site. Participants will be instructed on how to contract the pelvic floor using verbal cues and biofeedback (self-observation of urinary control at the toilet). After the pelvic floor muscles have

Table 1 UC, conventional pelvic floor muscle exercise prescription

Week	Positions	Reps each position	Sets	Contractions daily
1 & 2	Lying and sitting	15-20	2-3	30-60
3 & 4	Lying, sitting, and standing	30-40	2-3	60-120
5 & 6		40-50	3	120-150
7 – 26		50-60	3	150-180

Table 2 Advanced pelvic floor muscle exercise prescription

Week	Exercise	Position/pose	Reps	Sets	Hold (sec)	Pulses (Pfilates only)
1	Kegels	Lying and sitting	10-12	3	5-10	
	Pfilates	Butterfly	5	3	3-5	5
	Hypopressive	Diaphragmatic breathing (lying)	3	3	Fully inhale and exhale	
2	Kegels	Lying and sitting	10-12	3	5-10	
	Pfilates	Butterfly	5	2	5-8	5
		Bridge	5	2	3-5	5
	Hypopressive	Standing	3	3	5-10	
3	Kegels	Lying, sitting, and standing	10-12	2	8-10	
	Pfilates	Butterfly	5-10	2	8-10	5-10
		Bridge	5-10	2	5-8	5-10
		Lunge	5-10	2	3-5	5-10
	Hypopressive	Standing	3	2	10-15	
		Kneeling	3	2	5-10	
4	Kegels	Lying, sitting, standing	10-12	3	8-10	
	Pfilates	Butterfly	8-10	2	10	8-10
		Bridge	8-10	2	10	8-10
		Lunge	8-10	2	5-8	8-10
	Hypopressive	Standing	3	1	10-20	
		Kneeling	3	1	10-15	
		Downward kneel	3	1	10-15	
5	Kegels	Lying, sitting, standing	10-12	3	8-10	
	Pfilates	Butterfly	10-12	2	10	10-12
		Bridge	10-12	2	10	10-12
		Lunge	10-12	2	10	10-12
	Hypopressive	Standing	3	1	10-30	
		Kneeling	3	1	10-20	
		Downward Kneel	3	1	10-20	
		Sitting	3	1	10-15	
6-12	Kegels	Lying, sitting, standing	10-12	3	8-10	
	Pfilates	Butterfly	10-12	3	10	10-12
		Bridge	10-12	3	10	10-12
		Lunge	10-12	3	10	10-12
	Hypopressive	Standing	3	1	10-30	
		Kneeling	3	1	10-30	
		Downward Kneel	3	1	10-30	
		Sitting	3	1	10-30	
12-24	Kegels	Lying, sitting and standing	10-15	3	8-10	
	Pfilates	Butterfly	10-15	3	10	10-15
		Bridge	10-15	3	10	10-15
		Lunge	10-15	3	10	10-15
	Hypopressive	Standing	3	1	10-30	
		Kneeling	3	1	10-30	
		Downward Kneel	3	1	10-30	
		Sitting	3	1	10-30	

been identified, the UC prescription will consist of maximal voluntary contractions with escalating repetition volume every 2 weeks. Repetition volume will start at 30–60 repetitions per day during weeks 1–2; 60-120/day during weeks 3–4; and 120-150/day during weeks 5–6, and 150-180/day for weeks 7–26. Total daily contractions will be divided into multiple sets over the course of the day, aiming for 10–20 repetitions per set. The total number of repetitions will be divided equally between rhythmic (contract and relaxed over one second) and sustained contractions (contract and hold for up to 10s and relax). Table 1 provides a detailed description of the UC PFMX prescription and progression.

Advanced Pelvic Floor Exercise (APFX)

Participants will start with the introduction of basic PFMX (comparable to UC) with a gradual integration of Pfilates and Hypopressive exercises until week 12. The Pfilates exercises will progressively integrate postures that engage and activate supportive abdominal muscles including the TrA, hip adductors, and gluteals. During each pose, participants will be asked to perform a series of pulses within a small range of motion while maximally contracting their pelvic floor simultaneously. Similarly, the Hypopressive techniques are gradually integrated in the prescription and progressed over 12 weeks. These exercises focus on diaphragmatic breathing and TrA activation in various static postures. Participants are instructed to perform three successive slow diaphragmatic inspirations, followed by a total expiration and apnea (breath hold). Each apnea will be performed for approximately 10–30 seconds while activating their TrA and intercostal muscles and rising of their hemidiaphragm [45]. APFX participants will be gradually progressed in postures and repetition volume, varying between PFMX, Pfilates, and Hypopressives. Weeks 13–26 comprise the maintenance stage where patients will maintain their prescription until the end of the trial. A detailed week-by-week description of the program is provided in Table 2 and Appendix A. Total APFX contraction volume reflects the volume prescribed in the UC group following post-operative weeks.

Feasibility assessment

Prior pelvic floor training trials in PCa patients undergoing RP have observed recruitment rates of 21-70 % [21]. We will measure recruitment success through participant recruitment per week and record reasons for non-participation from those who inquire about the study and are eligible to participate but refuse. Adherence to the UC and APFX program will be measured through a logbook that is included in their respective manuals as well as a logbook completed by the research coordinator during the weekly telephone communication that will compare prescribed to completed volume of contractions. Retention

will be assessed by measuring attrition throughout the intervention period and at each assessment. We will monitor and record non-severe and severe adverse events that occur to participants during the course of this study using the National Cancer Institute Common Terminology Criteria for Adverse Events version 4.0 [53].

Outcome measures

Participants will complete five study assessments: baseline (approximately 1 week prior to RP), and at 2, 6, 12, 26-weeks post-operatively. Each assessment session will take place in Toronto, Ontario at the Princess Margaret Cancer Centre in the WE-Can Program. Participant demographics and self-reported disease and treatment-related variables will be collected at the baseline assessment.

Urinary incontinence

UI will be assessed using the 24-hour pad test, a 3-day, bladder diary, and a single-item on the Patient-Oriented Prostate Utility Scale (PORPUS). The 24-hour pad test will be used to measure UI by assessing the quantity of urine lost in one day. A urinary leakage pad is measured after a 24-hour period and compared to the unused pad weight and is used to assess the severity of UI [54–56]. Patients will receive their pre-weighed pads (TENA® Men's Protective Guards [57]) at baseline with accompanying plastic zipper storage bags which will be collected at their scheduled assessments. Additional pads per assessment will be provided in case of severe leakage. The pads will be individually weighed on an Ohaus® SP2001 (Ontario, Canada) scale, accurate to +/– 0.1 g. Continence is defined as a loss of ≤ 2 g of urine or the use of one or less pad per day [56, 58–60]. During the 24-hour period that the pad is worn, the participants will complete a frequency volume chart including urination frequency, times of UI, and if the pad was ever removed for a period of time. The 3-day bladder diary is a standard instrument for self-reporting voiding patterns. Items include fluid intake, frequency of toilet voids, episode of urine loss, nocturia, number of pads used, and activity during event for the three-day period. Bladder diaries are widely used in clinical trials assessing UI after prostatectomy [18, 29, 61–63]. Participants will be instructed to complete these 3 days prior to their scheduled assessment appointments. Finally, a single item regarding urinary leakage and bladder control is selected from the PORPUS as an additional self-reported measure of Post-RP UI that has been used in previous studies [64, 65].

Pelvic floor muscle strength

Digital rectal examination of the pelvic floor by a specially trained pelvic floor physiotherapist is currently the standard clinical method for assessing pelvic floor strength and function [9, 17, 66]. Pelvic floor strength will be performed in the crook lying position and participants are instructed to lift and squeeze the pelvic floor muscles as strongly as possible for a maximum of 5 seconds. The best of 3 maximum contractions is recorded. The quality of contractions are graded using the 6-point Modified Oxford Scale (MOS) [67-69]: 0 = no discernible PFM contraction; 1 = flicker, or pulsing under the examining finger, a very weak contraction; 2 = a weak contraction, an increase in tension in the muscle without any discernible lift or squeeze; 3 = a moderate contraction characterized by a degree of lifting of the posterior pelvic wall and squeezing on the base of the finger with in-drawing of the perineum; 4 = a good PFM contraction producing elevation of the posterior pelvic wall against resistance and in-drawing of the perineum; 5 = a strong contraction of the PFM; strong resistance can be given against elevation of the posterior pelvic wall. This will be measured at baseline (approximately 1 week prior to surgery), and post-operatively at 6, 12, 26-weeks. The MOS has been used in multiple studies assessing pelvic floor muscle strength following RP [56, 59, 70, 71].

Body composition

Research has shown that men who are overweight reported lower post-operative urinary function [72, 73]. Body mass index (kg/m^2) will be calculated using participant's height (m) and weight (kg). Body fat percentage will be assessed by bioelectrical impedance analysis (Tanita© 3000A, Tokyo, Japan). Waist to hip circumference ratio will be measured according to the World Health Organization protocol [74]. Waist circumference will be measured with the measuring tape positioned at the midpoint between lowest margin of the last palpable rib and the top of the iliac crest and hip circumference will be measured at the widest girth of the gluteal region.

Quality of life

PCa-specific QOL will be measured using two widely used and psychometrically valid and reliable measures: the Functional Assessment of Cancer Treatment-Prostate (FACT-P) [75] and the PORPUS [75-78]. Additional urological symptoms are assessed using the valid and reliable, 7-item International Prostate Symptom Score (IPSS) [79, 80]. Erectile function is assessed using the 5-item International Index of Erectile Function (IIEF) scale, a widely used, psychometrically validated multidimensional self-report instrument evaluating male sexual function [81, 82].

Physical activity

Recreational physical activity volume will be measured through the reliable and valid 3-item Godin Leisure-Time Exercise Questionnaire – Leisure Score Index (GLTEQ-LSI) [83, 84]. The GLTEQ-LSI assesses the frequency of mild, moderate, and strenuous bouts of leisure physical activity or exercise performed for at least 15 minutes over

the past week and has been previously used in trials with PCa survivors [65, 85].

Statistical analysis

Participant characteristics at baseline will be compared using independent sample t-tests or chi-square tests. We will report retention and compliance rates for the sample and their associated 95 % CI as well as reasons for non-participation of eligible patients. To calculate outcome capture, we will calculate the proportion of participants who have complete data on each outcome at each time point divided by the total number of study participants. Estimates of efficacy (Group and Time main effect, as well as Group x Time interactions) will be analyzed using a repeated-measure analysis of covariance (ANCOVA), controlling for the baseline value of the outcome of interest. We will examine the effect size (Cohen's d) of the intervention on the clinical outcomes by dividing the observed mean between-group difference in change in the outcome measure from baseline to follow-up (UC vs. APFX) by its standard deviation.

Discussion

PFMX continues to be the mainstay for conservative management of UI after RP; however, its efficacy is modest. One hypothesis for ineffective PFMX regimens is that the pelvic floor muscles are not adequately activated because ancillary pelvic and abdominal muscles are not concurrently engaged. Novel techniques to address UI secondary to pelvic floor muscle weakness and/or RP involve a more comprehensive strengthening of the pelvic floor and its surrounding structures. Studies have reported a higher maximal voluntary contraction of the pelvic floor when training the pelvic floor muscles and its surrounding muscles simultaneously (i.e. TrA, hip adductors, gluteal, diaphragm) [30–34]. These advanced pelvic floor training techniques include Pfilates and Hypopressives that also engage the TrA, rectus abdominis, gluteals, diaphragm, and hip abductors that enhance pelvic floor contraction. Synergistic training of abdominal and pelvic floor muscles presents a newer approach to the rehabilitation of pelvic floor dysfunction following RP.

The primary outcome of this pilot study is to determine the feasibility of conducting a full-scale RCT of a comprehensive pelvic floor conditioning program compared to conventional PFMX. Measures of outcome efficacy will also be measured in urinary function, pelvic floor muscle strength, and QoL. To our knowledge, this is the first study to examine the effect of a comprehensive PFMX regimen that includes Pfilates and Hypopressives for UI. The above-mentioned training techniques may prove to be an effective alternative in the conservative management of UI and the early recovery of continence after RP.

Appendix A. Sample cueing instructions for Pfilates and Hypopressives exercises

Pfilates exercises

Pfilates exercise incorporates a series of poses and plyometric exercises to compliment pelvic floor muscle training. This form of neuromuscular conditioning is a therapeutic alternative for basic pelvic floor muscle exercise that can be easily integrated into any regular exercise routine. In these exercises, the engagement of the external hip rotators, adductors of the thigh, transversus abdominis, and gluteal muscles will facilitate or induce pelvic floor activation.

For each Pfilates pose will follow a series of identical phases:

I. The positioning/movement: Here you will position yourself in the Pfilates pose and perform the movement a series of repetitions
II. The hold: during this phase you engage the active muscles and contract your pelvic floor muscles
III. The pulse (plyometric): In this last phase, you will perform a series of pulses, matching the number of repetitions in the first phase. (i.e. If you performed 10 repetitions in the movement phase, you will perform another 10 repetitions in the pulse phase).

Hypopressive exercises

Hypopressives are performed mainly via the transversus abdominis activation. The goal of these exercises is to relax the diaphragm, which in turn decreases the intra-abdominal pressure and may activate the abdominal and pelvic floor muscles simultaneously.

Each pose will follow a series of identical phases:

I. Positioning of the pose
II. Three diaphragmatic breaths (rest breaths), described below
III. Apnea (breath hold) of 5-30 seconds
IV. Repeat these steps a total of three times for each pose

Diaphragmatic breathing (rest breaths) – practice pose

1. Lie on your back on a flat surface with your knees bent and place your hands on the bottom of your ribs.
2. Breathe in slowly through your nose and open your upper chest as much as possible. You should feel your chest flare out ward with your hands.
3. Exhale fully through pursed lips.

Apnea

To perform a correct apnea (breath hold) you must close your nose and mouth (glottal stop). When you are performing the apnea phase of the exercise, you will have fully **exhaled** from your last rest breath. At this point, with a glottal stop, perform an inhalation without taking air in. You should feel your stomach and abdomen lift and squeeze up to your ribcage. Each apnea is held for 10 to 30 seconds.

Abbreviations
ANCOVA: Analysis of covariance; APFX: Advanced pelvic floor exercise; FACT-P: Functional assessment of cancer therapy-prostate; GLTEQ-LSI: Godin leisure time exercise questionnaire – leisure score index; IIEF: International index of erectile function; IPSS: International prostate symptom score; MOS: Modified Oxford scale; PCa: Prostate cancer; PFMX: Pelvic floor muscle exercise; PORPUS: Patient-oriented prostate utility scale; QOL: Quality of life; RP: Radical prostatectomy; TrA: Transverse adominis; UC: Usual care; UI: Urinary incontinence; WE-Can: Wellness and Exercise for Cancer Survivors Program.

Competing interests
The authors declare that they have no competing interests.

Authors' contributions
DSM, AGM, DA, WJH, and AGM collaboratively conceptualized the study objectives and methodology. SMHA, LJ, NF, LES assisted in further development of the protocol. JT, NEF, AF, DE, JJ, RKS and LJ support the project through protocol consultation and data collection. DSM, DA, AGM, LJ, and WJH will implement the protocol and oversee collection of the data. All authors have contributed to and approved this final manuscript.

Authors' information
DSM is the Program Lead for the Wellness and Exercise for Cancer Survivors Program (WE-Can) in ELLICSR at the Princess Margaret Cancer Centre and an Assistant Professor in the Faculty of Kinesiology and Physical Education at the University of Toronto. DA is an MSc candidate at the University of Guelph and Kinesiologist at WE-Can in ELLICSR at the Princess Margaret Cancer Centre. SMHA is a Staff Physician in the Department of Medicine at the University Health Network and a Senior Scientist with the Toronto General Research Institute. LJ is a Urologic Nurse at the Prostate Centre of the Princess Margaret Cancer Centre. NF is a Physiotherapist at Pelvic Health Solutions. WJH is an MSc candidate at the University of Guelph and Kinesiologist at WE-Can in ELLICSR at the Princess Margaret Cancer Centre. LES is the Assistant Program Head at the University of Guelph-Humber and a Kinesiologist at WE-Can in ELLICSR at the Princess Margaret Cancer Centre. PR is a Professor in the Faculty of Health at York University and a Senior Scientist with Cancer Care Ontario. JJ is an Associate Professor in the Department of Psychiatry, Faculty of Medicine at the University of Toronto and the Director of ELLICSR at the Princess Margaret Cancer Centre. DE is a Staff Urologist and the Medical Director of the Prostate Cancer Rehabilitation Clinic at the University Health Network. NEF is a Staff Surgeon, Clinician Scientist, and Head of the Division of Urology at the University Health Network and the Princess Margaret Cancer Centre, and a Professor in the Department of Surgery at the University of Toronto. AF is a Staff Surgeon and Clinician Scientist in the Division of Urology at the University Health Network, and an Assistant Professor in the Department of Surgical Oncology with the University of Toronto. RKS is a urologic surgeon at Toronto East General Hospital and Assistant Professor in the Department of Surgery at the University of Toronto. JT is a Professor of Surgery and Medical Imaging at the University of Toronto, a Staff Surgeon and Clinician Scientist in the Division of Urology and Director of the Prostate Centre at the Princess Margaret Cancer Centre. AGM is Senior Staff Psychologist and Clinician-Scientist in the Department of Surgery and the Department of Psychosocial Oncology and Palliative Care at the Princess Margaret Cancer Centre.

Funding
This study is made possible through funding from the Movember Discovery Grant Fund from Prostate Cancer Canada (Grant Number D2014-20).

Author details
[1]University Health Network, Toronto, Ontario, 200 Elizabeth Street, Toronto, Ontario M5G 2C4, Canada. [2]University of Guelph-Humber, 207 Humber College Boulevard, Toronto, Ontario M9W 5L7, Canada. [3]University of Toronto, 27 King's College Circle, Toronto, Ontario M5S 2W6, Canada. [4]University of Guelph, 50 Stone Rd E, Guelph, Ontario N1G 2W1, Canada.

[5]Pelvic Health Solutions, 372 Hollandview Trail, Aurora, Ontario L4G 0A5, Canada. [6]York University, 4700 Keele St, Toronto, Ontario M3J 1P3, Canada. [7]Cancer Care Ontario, Toronto, Ontario, Canada. [8]Toronto East General Hospital, Toronto, Ontario M4C 5T2, Canada.

References

1. Han M, Partin AW, Pound CR, Epstein JI, Walsh PC. Long-term Biochemical Disease-free and Cancer-specific Survival Following Anatomical Radical Retropubic Prostatectomy. The 15-year Johns Hopkins Exerience. Urol Clin North Am. 2001;28:555–65.

2. Bo K, Berghmans B, Morkved S, Kampen MV. Evidence-Based Physical Therapy for the Pelvic Floor: Bridging Science and Clinical Practice. Philadelphia: Elsevier Ltd.; 2007.

3. Shikanov S, Kocherginsky M, Shalhav AL, Eggener SE. Cause-Specific Mortality Following Radical Prostatectomy. Prostate Cancer Prostatic Dis. 2012;15:106–10.

4. Penson DF, McLerran D, Feng Z, Li L, Albertsen PC, Gilliland FD, et al. 5-Year Urinary and Sexual Outcomes After Radical Prostatectomy: Results from the Prostate Cancer Outcomes Study. J Urol. 2005;173:1701–5.

5. Weber BA, Roberts BL, Mills TL, Chumbler NR, Algood CB. Physical and Emotional Predictors of Depression After Radical Prostatectomy. Am J Mens Health. 2008;2:165–71.

6. Sanda MG, Dunn RL, Michalski J, Sandler HM, Northouse L, Hembroff L, et al. Quality of Life and Satisfaction with Outcome among Prostate-Cancer Survivors. N Engl J Med. 2008;358:1250–61.

7. Steineck G, Helgesen F, Adolfsson J, Dickman PW, Johansson J-E, Norlen BJ, et al. Quality of Life after Radical Prostatectomy or Watchful Waiting. N Engl J Med. 2002;347:790–6.

8. Newschaffer CJ, Otani K, McDonald MK, Penberthy LT. Causes of Death in Elderly Prostate Cancer Patients and in a Comparison Nonprostate Cancer Cohort. J Natl Cancer Inst. 2000;92:613–21.

9. Price N, Dawood R, Jackson SR. Pelvic Floor Exercise for Urinary Incontinence: A Systematic Literature Review. Maturitas. 2010;67:309–15.

10. Messelink B, Benson T, Berghmans B, Bo K, Corcos J, Fowler C, et al. Standardization of Terminology of Pelvic Floor Muscle Function and Dysfunction: Report From the Pelvic Floor Clinical Assessment Group of the International Continence Society. Neurourol Urodyn. 2005;24:374–80.

11. Centemero A, Rigatti L, Giraudo D, Lazzeri M, Lughezzani G, Zugna D, et al. Preoperative Pelvic Floor Muscle Exercise for Early Continence After Radical Prostatectomy: A Randomised Controlled Study. Eur Urol. 2010;57:1039–44.

12. Ficazzola MA, Nitti VW. The Etiology of Post-Radical Prostatectomy Incontinence and Correlation of Symptoms with Urodynamic Findings. J Urol. 1998;160:1317–20.

13. Mangera A, Patel AK, Chapple CR. Pathophysiology of Urinary Incontinence. Surgery. 2011;29:249–53.

14. Mariotti G, Sciarra A, Gentilucci A, Salciccia S, Alfarone A, Pierro GD, et al. Early Recovery of Urinary Continence After Radical Prostatectomy Using Early Pelvic Floor Electrical Stimulation and Biofeedback Associated Treatment. J Urol. 2009;181:1788–93.

15. Staskin D, Tubaro A, Norton PA, Ashton-Miller JA. Mechanisms of Continence and Surgical Cure in Female and Male SUI: Surgical Research Initiatives. Neurourol Urodyn. 2011;30:704–7.

16. Parekh AR, Feng MI, Kirages D, Bremner H, Kaswick J, Aboseif S. The Role of Pelvic Floor Exercises on Post-Prostatectomy Incontinence. J Urol. 2003;170:130–3.

17. Dorey G. Pelvic Floor Muscle Exercise for Men. Nurs Times. 2003;99:46–8.

18. Franke JJ, Gilbert WB, Grier J, Koch MO, Shyr Y, Smith Jr JA. Early Post-Prostatectomy Pelvic Floor Biofeedback. J Urol. 2000;163:191–3.

19. Burgio KL. Update on Behavioral and Physical Therapies for Incontinence and Overactive Bladder: The Role of Pelvic Floor Muscle Training. Curr Urol Rep. 2013;14:457–64.

20. Glazener C, Boachie C, Buckley B, Cochran C, Dorey G, Grant A, et al. Conservative treatment for urinary incontinence in Men After Prostate Surgery (MAPS): two parallel randomised controlled trials. Health Technol Assess. 2011;15:1–290.

21. Campbell SE, Glazener CMA, Hunter KF, Cody JD, Moore KN. Conservative Management for Postprostatectomy Urinary Incontinence (Review). Cochrane Database Syst Rev. 2012;1:CD001843.

22. Dorey G, Glazener C, Buckley B, Cochran C, Moore K. Developing a Pelvic Floor Muscle Training Regimen for Use in a Trial Intervention. Physiotherapy. 2009;95:199–208.

23. MacDonald R, Fink HA, Huckabay C, Monga M, Wilt TJ. Pelvic Floor Muscle Training to Improve Urinary Incontinence after Radical Prostatectomy: A Systematic Review of Effectiveness. BJU Int. 2007;100:76–81.

24. Dorey G. Pelvic Dysfunction in Men: Diagnosis and Treatment of Male Incontinence and Erectile Dysfunction. Chichester: John Wiley & Sons Ltd; 2006.

25. Mahony DT, Laferte RO, Blais DJ. Integral Storage and Voiding Reflexes: Neurophysiologic Concept of Continence and Micturition. Urology. 1977;9:95–106.

26. Berghmans LCM, Hendriks HJM, De Bie RA, Van Doorn VW, Bo K, Van Kerrebroeck P. Conservative Treatment of Urge Urinary Incontinence in Women: A Systematic Review of Randomized Clinical Trials. BJU Int. 2000;85:254–63.

27. Bø K, Berghmans LCM. Nonpharmacologic treatments for overactive bladder - pelvic floor exercises. Urology. 2000;55:7–11.

28. Ahmed S, Shafik IA. Overactive bladder inhibition in response to pelvic floor muscles exercises. World J Urol. 2003;20:374–7.

29. Chapman MM. Pelvic Muscle Exercise/Biofeedback for Urinary Incontinence after Prostatectomy: An Education Program. J Cancer Educ. 1997;12:218–23.

30. Sapsford R. Rehabilitation of Pelvic Floor Muscles Utilizing Trunk Stabilization. Man Ther. 2004;9:3–12.

31. Sapsford R, Hodges PW. Contraction of the Pelvic Floor Muscles during Abdominal Maneuvers. Arch Phys Med Rehabil. 2001;82:1081–8.

32. Sapsford R, Hodges PW, Richardson CA, Cooper DH, Markwell SJ, Jull GA. Co-activation of the Abdominal and Pelvic Floor Muscles During Voluntary Exercises. Neurourol Urodyn. 2001;20:31–42.

33. Neumann P, Gill V. Pelvic Floor and Abdominal Muscle Interaction: EMG Activity and Intra-Abdominal Pressure. Int Urogynecol J Pelvic Floor Dysfunct. 2002;13:125–32.

34. Madill S, McLean L. Quantification of Abdominal and Pelvic Floor Muscle Synergies in Response to Voluntary Pelvic Floor Muscle Contractions. J Electromyogr Kinesiol. 2008;18:955–64.

35. Vereeken RL, Derluyn J, Verduyn H. Electromyography of the Perineal Striated Muscles During Cystometry. Urology International. 1975;30:92–8.

36. Deindl FM, Vodusek DB, Hesse U, Schussler B. Activity Patterns of Pubococcygeal Muscles in Nulliparous Continent Women. Br J Urol. 1993;72:46–51.

37. Carrière B. Fitness for the Pelvic Floor. New York, NY, USA: Thieme; 2002.

38. Hung HC, Hsiao SM, Chih SY, Li HH, Tsauo JY. An Alternative Intervention for Urinary Incontinence: Retraining Diaphragmatic, Deep Abdominal and Pelvic Floor Muscle Coordinated Function. Man Ther. 2010;15:273–9.

39. Wells C, Kolt GS, Bialocerkowski A. Defining Pilates Exercise: A Systematic Review. Complement Ther Med. 2012;20:253–62.

40. Culligan PJ, Scherer J, Dyer K, Priestley JL, Guingon-White G, Delvecchio D, et al. A Randomized Clinical Trial Comparing Pelvic Floor Muscle Training to a Pilates Exercise Program for Improving Pelvic Muscle Strength. Int Urogynecol J Pelvic Floor Dysfunct. 2010;21:401–8.

41. Crawford, B. Pfilates: Pelvic Floor Pilates. 2015. http://www.pfilates.com. Accessed 27 Apr 2015.

42. Latorre GFS, Seleme MR, Resende APM, Stupp L, Berghmans B. Hipopressive Gymnastics: Evidences for an Alternative Training for Women with Local Proprioceptive Deficit of the Pelvic Floor Muscle. Fisioterapia Brasil. 2011;12:463–6.

43. Resende APM, Stupp L, Bernardes BT, Oliveira E, Castro RA, Girao MJBC, et al. Can Hypopressive Exercise Provide Additional Benefits to Pelvic Floor Muscle Training in Women With Pelvic Organ Prolapse? Neurourol Urodyn. 2012;31:121–5.

44. Bernardes BT, Resende APM, Stupp L, Oliveria E, Castro RA, Bella ZIKJ, et al. Efficacy of Pelvic Floor Muscle Training and Hypopressive Exercises for treating Pelvic Organ Prolapse in Women: Randomized Controlled Trial. Sao Paulo Med J. 2012;130:5–9.

45. Stüpp L, Resende APM, Petricelli CD, Uchiyama M, Alexandre SM, Zanetti MRD. Pelvic Floor Muscle and Transversus Abdominis Activation in Abdominal Hypopressive Technique Through Surface Electromyography. Neurourol Urodyn. 2011;30:1518–21.

46. Caufriez M. Gymnastique Abdominale Hypopressive. M. Caufriez: Bruxelles; 1997.

47. Hertzog MA. Considerations in determining sample size for pilot studies. Res Nurs Health. 2008;31:180–91.

48. Piantadosi S. Clinical Trials: A Methodologic Perspective. Second Editionth ed. Hoboken, NJ, USA: John Wiley & Sons, Inc; 2005.

49. Sim J, Lewis M. The size of a pilot study for a clinical trial should be calculated in relation to considerations of precision and efficiency. J Clin Epidemiol. 2012;65:301–8.

50. FitzGerald MP, Kotarinos R. Rehabilitation of the short pelvic floor. I: Background and patient evaluation. Int Urogynecol J. 2003;14:261–8.

51. Siegel AL. Pelvic Floor Muscle Training in Males: Practical Applications. Urology. 2014;84:1–7.

52. FitzGerald MP, Kotarinos R. Rehabilitation of the short pelvic floor. II: Treatment of the patient with the short pelvic floor. Int Urogynecol J. 2003;14:269–75.

53. U.S. Department of Health and Human Services: Common Terminology Criteria for Adverse Events (CTCAE) Version 4.0. National Cancer Institute 2009.

54. Bettez M, Tu LM, Carlson K, Corcos J, Gajewsi J, Jolivet M, et al. Update: Guidelines for Adult Urinary Incontinence Collaborative Consensus Document for the Canadian Urological Association. Canadian Urological Association. 2012;2012(6):354–63.

55. O'Sullivan R, Karantanis E, Stevermuer TL, Allen W, Moore KH. Definition of Mild, Moderate and Severe Incontinence on the 24-Hour Pad Test. BJOG. 2004;111:859–62.

56. Moore KN, Griffiths D, Hughton A. Urinary Incontinence After Radical Prostatectomy: A Randomized Controlled Trial Comparing Pelvic Muscle Exercises With or Without Electrical Stimulation. BJU Int. 1999;83:57–65.

57. Karantanis E, O'Sullivan R, Moore KH. The 24-Hour Pad Test in Continent Women and Men: Normal Values and Cyclical Alterations. BJOG. 2003;110:567–71.

58. Ribeiro LHS, Prota C, Gomes CM, Jose De Bessa J, Boldarine MP, Dall'Oglio MF, et al. Long-Term Effect of Early Postoperative Pelvic Floor Biofeedback on Continence in Men Udergoing Radical Prostatectomy: A Prospective, Randomized, Controlled Trial. J Urol. 2010;184:1034–9.

59. van Kampen M, Weerdt WD, Poppel HV, Ridder DD, Feys H, Baert L. Effect of Pelvic-Floor Re-Education on Duration and Degree of Incontinence After Radical Prostatectomy: A Randomised Controlled Trial. Lancet. 2000;355:98–102.

60. Lucas MG, Bedretdinova D, Bosch JLHR, Burkhard F, Cruz F, Nambiar AK, et al. Guidelines on Urinary Incontinence. Arnhem, Netherlands: European Association of Urology; 2013.

61. Burgio KL, Goode PS, Urban DA, Umlauf MG, Locher JL, Bueschen A, et al. Preoperative Biofeedback Assisted Behavioral Training to Decrease Post-Prostatectomy Incontinence: A Randomized, Controlled Trial. J Urol. 2006;175:196–201.

62. Goode PS, Burgio KL, Johnson TMI, Clay OJ, Roth DL, Markland AD, et al. Behavioral Therapy With or Without Biofeedback and Pelvic Floor Electrical Stimulation for Persistent Postprostatectomy Incontinence: A Randomized Controlled Trial. JAMA. 2011;305:151–9.

63. Meaglia JP, Joseph AC, Chang M, Schmidt JD. Post-Prostatectomy Urinary Incontinence: Response to Behavioral Training. J Urol. 1990;144:674–6.

64. Toren P, Alibhai SMH, Matthew AG, Nesbitt M, Kalnin R, Fleshner NE, et al. The effect of nerve-sparing surgery on patient-reported continence post-radical prostatectomy. Canadian Urological Association journal = Journal de l'Association des urologues du Canada. 2009;3:6.

65. Santa Mina D, Guglietti CL, Alibhai SMH, Matthew AG, Kalnin R, Ahmad N, et al. The Effect of Meeting Physical Activity Guidelines for Cancer Survivors on Quality of Life Following Radical Prostatectomy for Prostate Cancer. J Cancer Surviv. 2013;8:190–8.

66. Nahon I, Waddington G, Adams R, Dorey G. Assessing Muscle Function of the Male Pelvic Floor using Real Time Ultrasound. Neurourol Urodyn. 2011;30:1329–32.

67. Frawley HC, Galea MP, Phillips BA, Sherburn M, Bo K. Reliability of Pelvic Floor Muscle Strength Assessment using Different Test Positions and Tools. Neurourol Urodyn. 2006;25:236–42.

68. Dorey G. Pelvic Floor Exercises After Radical Prostatectomy. Br J Nurs. 2013;22:s4–9.

69. Haslam J, Laycock J. Therapeutic Management of Incontinence and Pelvic Pain. Springer-Verlag London Limited: London, England; 2008.

70. Jackson J, Emerson L, Johnston B, Wilson J, Morales A. Biofeedback: A Non-Evasive Treatment for Incontinence after Radical Prostatectomy. Urol Nurs. 1996;16:50–4.

71. Manassero F, Traversi C, Ales V, Pistolesi D, Panicucci E, Valent F, et al. Contribution of Early intensive Prolonged Pelvic Floor Exercises on Urinary Continence Recovery After Bladder Neck-Sparing Radical Prostatectomy: Results of a Prospective Controlled Randomized Trial. Neurourol Urodyn. 2007;26:985–9.

72. van Roermund JGH, van Basten JPA, Kiemeney LA, Karthaus HFM, Witjes JA. Impact of Obesity on Surgical Outcomes following Open Radical Prostatectomy. Urol Int. 2009;82:256–61.

73. Ahlering TE, Eichel L, Edwards R, Skarecky DW. Impact of obesity on clinical outcomes in robotic prostatectomy. Urology. 2005;65:740–4.

74. World Health Organization. Waist Circumference and Waist-Hip Ratio. Geneva: World Health Organization; 2008.

75. Esper P, Mo F, Chodak G, Sinner M, Cella D, Pienta KJ. Measuring Quality of Life in Men with Prostate Cancer using the Functional Assessment of Cancer Therapy-Prostate Instrument. Urology. 1997;50:920–8.

76. Krahn M, Ritvo P, Irvine J, Tomlinson G, Bezjak A, Trachtenberg J, et al. Contruction of the Patient-Oriented Prostate Utility Scale (PORPUS): A Multiattribute Health State Classification SYstem for Prostate Cancer. J Clin Epidemiol. 2000;53:920–30.

77. Cella D, Hernandez L, Pharm D, Bonomi AE, Corona M, Vaquero M, et al. Spanish Language Translation and Initial Validation of the Functional Assessment of Cancer Therapy Quality-of-Life Instrument. Med Care. 1998;36:1407–18.

78. Overcash JARNP, Extermann M, Parr J, Perry JMS, Balducci L. Validity and Reliability of the FACT-G Scale for Use in the Older Person With Cancer. Am J Clin Oncol. 2001;24:591–6.

79. Barry MJ, Fowler Jr FJ, O'Leary MP, Bruskewitz RC, Holtgrewe HL, Mebust WK, et al. The American Urological Association Symptom Index for Benign Prostatic Hyperplasia. The Measurement Committee of the American Urological Association. J Urol. 1992;148:1549–57.

80. Gray M. Psychometric Evaluation of the International Prostate Symptom Score. Urol Nurs. 1998;18:175–83.

81. Rosen RC, Cappelleri JC, Gendrano III N. The International Index of Erectile Function (IIEF): A State-of-the-Science Review. Int J Impot Res. 2002;14:226–44.

82. Rosen RC, Cappelleri JC, Smith MD, Lipsky J, Pena BM. Development and Evaluation of an Abridged, 5-item Version of the International Index of Erectile Function (IIEF-5) as a Diagnostic TOol for Erectile Dysfunction. Int J Impot Res. 1999;11:319–27.

83. Godin G, Shephard RJ. A Simple Method to Assess Exercise Behavior in the Community. Can J Appl Sport Sci. 1985;10:141–6.

84. Jacobs Jr DR, Ainsworth BE, Hartman TJ, Leon AS. A Simultaneous Evaluation of 10 Commonly Used Physical Activity Questionnaires. Med Sci Sports Exerc. 1993;25:81–91.

85. Culos-Reed SN, Robinson JL, Lau H, O'Connor K, Keats MR. Benefits of a physical activity intervention for men with prostate cancer. J Sport Exerc Psychol. 2007;29:118–27.

Physical activity before radical prostatectomy reduces sick leave after surgery

E. Angenete[1*], U. Angerås[1], M. Börjesson[3,4], J. Ekelund[1], M. Gellerstedt[2], T. Thorsteinsdottir[5], G. Steineck[6,7] and E. Haglind[1]

Abstract

Background: Studies have reported that early physical rehabilitation after surgical procedures is associated with improved outcome measured as shorter hospital stay and enhanced recovery. The aim of this study was to explore the relationship between the preoperative physical activity level and subsequent postoperative complications, sick-leave and hospital stay after radical prostatectomy for prostate cancer in the setting of the LAPPRO trial (LAParoscopic Prostatectomy Robot Open).

Methods: LAPPRO is a prospective controlled trial, comparing robot-assisted laparoscopic and open surgery for localized prostate cancer between 2008 and 2011. 1569 patients aged 64 or less with an occupation were included in this sub-study. The Gleason score was <7 in 52 % of the patients. Demographics and the level of self-assessed preoperative physical activity, length of hospital stay, complications, quality of life, recovery and sick-leave were extracted from clinical record forms and questionnaires. Multivariable logistic regression, with log-link and logit-link functions, was used to adjust for potential confounding variables.

Results: The patients were divided into four groups based on their level of activity. As the group with lowest engagement of physical activity was found to be significantly different in base line characteristics from the other groups they were excluded from further analysis. Among patients that were physically active preoperativelly (n = 1467) there was no significant difference between the physical activity-groups regarding hospital stay, recovery or complications. However, in the group with the highest self-assessed level of physical activity, 5-7 times per week, 13 % required no sick leave, compared to 6.3 % in the group with a physical activity level of 1-2 times per week only (p < 0.0001).

Conclusions: In our study of med operated with radical prostatectomy, a high level of physical activity preoperatively was associated with reduced need for sick leave after radical prostatectomy compared to men with lower physical activity.

Keywords: Prostatic neoplasm, Prostatectomy, Physical fitness

* Correspondence: eva.angenete@vgregion.se
[1]Department of Surgery, Institute of Clinical Sciences, Sahlgrenska Academy at University of Gothenburg, SSORG, Sahlgrenska University Hospital/Östra, SE-416 85 Gothenburg, Sweden
Full list of author information is available at the end of the article

Background

Physical activity has gained increasing focus, as a lifestyle factor of importance with a number of studies have confirming its positive effects on cardiovascular and overall health [1]. It has been shown that self-assessed physical activity concurs well with the actual physical fitness of the individual [2].

In regard to cancer, physical activity may reduce the risk of cancer development, as shown by a review summarizing nearly 170 studies stating that the scientific evidence for the association between lack of physical activity and the development of cancer is convincing for breast and colon cancer and probably also for prostate cancer [3]. A high level of physical activity has also recently been reported to reduce overall and prostate-specific mortality in patients diagnosed with prostate cancer [4].

For postoperative rehabilitation, the benefits from preoperative physical activity in addition to a postoperative early rehabilitation schedule have been reported for spinal surgery [5] and is suggested for several types of cancer surgery [6], including prostate cancer [7]. In colorectal surgery the benefits of enhanced recovery programs, including early postoperative mobilization [8], have been clearly demonstrated. The impact of preoperative prehabilitation has been evaluated showing an improved cardiopulmonary function [9, 10], however most studies have not used clinically important outcome measures such as complications, postoperative morbidity or length of hospital stay, although studies are underway and there are several indications that prehabilitation reduces hospital stay [11] [12].

Localized prostate cancer can be treated with radical prostatectomy [13], which can be performed either by open, laparoscopic or robot-assisted laparoscopic surgery [14, 15]. Radical prostatectomy is associated with a low overall operative morbidity and mortality and hospital stay is two days or less [15, 16], but there is still considerable long-term morbidity with urinary incontinence and decreased sexual health [17]. In recent years self-assessment evaluations on recovery have been developed in addition to measurements such as length of hospital stay [18, 19]. Another more precise measurement of recovery is time to return to work or total time of sick-leave. For patients operated with radical prostatectomy studies in the United States have indicated that 50 % were back to work after a two week period and to unrestricted activity within one month although these figures may vary between countries and between different types of surgery [20–22].

In the large prospective Swedish trial, LAPPRO (LAParoscopic Prostatectomy Robot Open), comparing robot-assisted laparoscopic radical prostatectomy to open radical prostatectomy as a definitive treatment for localized prostate cancer, patients answered detailed questionnaires on many aspects of quality of life including self-assessed physical activity and sick leave [23]. Short-term results have been published, indicating that robot-assisted laparoscopic prostatectomy is a safe procedure and that it has some advantages compared to open surgery, such as shorter hospital stay and less risk of reoperation during initial hospital stay [24] and long-term results show no statistical difference in urinary incontinence at one year, but somewhat less erectile dysfunction in the robot-assisted laparoscopically radical prostatectomy compared to open (70 % vs. 75 %) [25].

The aim of the present study was to determine the relationship between the patients' self-assessed preoperative physical activity level and the postoperative course, including hospital stay and sick leave, after radical prostatectomy for localized prostate cancer in the setting of the LAPPRO trial.

Methods

Study design

The study-population derives from LAPPRO (LAParoscopic Prostatectomy Robot Open), a prospective, non-randomized controlled clinical trial comparing outcomes after open retropubic and robot-assisted laparoscopic radical prostatectomy [23]. Fourteen Swedish urological departments well established in performing radical prostatectomy included patients in the trial. Patient-reported data were collected before surgery as well as 3, 12 and 24 months after surgery. In addition, clinical record forms gathered information preoperatively, surgical data, follow-up data 6-12 weeks, 12 and 24 months after surgery. The study protocol has been published [23] and is available at www.ssorg.net.

Patients

A total of 3715 patients operated with a radical prostatectomy for clinically localized prostate cancer between September 2008 and November 2011 gave informed consent, and were included in the study (Fig. 1). For the pupose of this analysis, we focused on patients who could be in need of sick-leave. Thus we selected employed or un-employed patients, but did not include retired patients or those with full, chronic disability. To identify our target population out of the entire trial population we used results in questions asked in the baseline questionnaire, with the ensuing definitions based on answering categories. ($n = 1576$). Patients in the target population who did not answer the questionnaire in general or specifically the question regarding physical activity were excluded ($n = 7$). Left to analyze were 1569 patients, 397 patients were operated with open retropubic prostatectomy and 1170 patients were operated with robot-assisted laparoscopy, and two with an unidentified procedure. All patients were treated according to the local

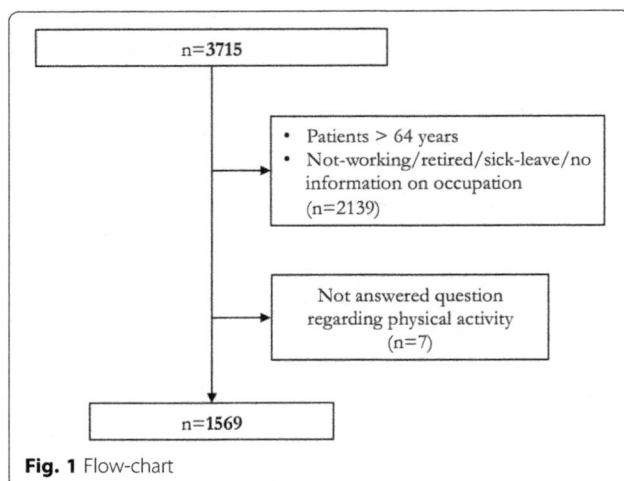

Fig. 1 Flow-chart

hospital routines, regarding preoperative and postoperative care. The patients were assigned a standardized period of short sick leave, with a possibility of additional sick leave by a simple phone call.

Data collection

Patients were given questionnaires prior surgery in the outpatient clinic and at 3, 12 and 24 months. In this substudy only questionnaires prior surgery and at three months were analyzed. The questionnaires with patient-reported data were modified from previous studies [26, 27]. Questions concerning primary and secondary endpoints, possible confounders and effect modifiers were included and most questions had been used previously in other studies [28]. Qualitative open interviews with prostate cancer patients before and after surgery revealed new topics that resulted in adjustments of the questions. The questionnaires were face-to-face validated with prostate cancer patients and content validated by experts in urology. A detailed description of the study design, the procedure and development of the clinical record forms and the validation of the questionnaires has been published previously [23]. Two research nurses monitored the recruiting sites and all means for collecting data were standardized. In the questionnaire there are questions regarding QoL in general prior surgery that have been included in this study to describe the study population. Physical and psychological well being as well as self-assessed global quality of life were assessed on seven-point Likert type scale from 1 to 7 anchored by for example, no physical well-being and the best possible physical well-being. The questions were dichotomized according to previous studies by Steineck et al [29] with the lowest five of seven possible categories collapsed.

Physical activity measurement

The questionnaires included a question regarding the patient's self-assessed level of physical activity: "How

often have you been physically active for 30 min or more with for example riding a bike, walking, gymnastics or similar the last month?" The available options were; "Never"; "Sometimes" (one to two times a week); "Often" (three to four times a week); and "Daily or almost daily" (five to seven times a week). The highest two levels of self-assessed activity (>three to four times/week) corresponds to fulfilling the national and international criteria for recommended levels of regular physical activity, established to be associated with health benefits [30].

Outcome measures

The primary outcome measure sick-leave was reported by the patients in the three-month postoperative questionnaire. The question read: "How long were you on sick-leave after the operation? The answering options were: "Not applicable, I was not on sick-leave", "0 weeks", "1-3 weeks", "4-6 weeks", "7-9 weeks", "10-12 weeks", "longer than 13 weeks (I am still on sick-leave)".

In Sweden the legislation does not require doctor's note, if sick-leave it is less than one week, thus "not applicable" and "0 weeks" were combined and used as a cut-off to define "no sick leave".

In the questionnaire patients were asked to assess their time until full recovery, given as number of weeks. The question was: "How long time do you estimate that it took until you were back in your normal acitivy level after surgery?" Answering options were "Not applicable", 0 weeks", "1-3 weeks", "4-6 weeks", "7-9 weeks", "10-12 weeks", "longer than 13 weeks (I am still not back to normal activity level)". This was then dichotomized into fully recovered prior to 4 weeks and not recovered at 13 weeks.

Regarding other outcome variables, the clinical record form at 6-12 weeks and the three-month postoperative questionnaire were used to assess hospital stay and adverse events. The adverse events were divided into five groups as follows; infection, cardiovascular, surgical, gastrointestinal and psychological events (Table 2). Sexual health and urinary incontinence were measured at one year, and were not the primary outcome of this study and are thus not reported in this study [25].

Statistical analysis

As this analysis is a sub-study of the LAPPRO trial no power calculation was performed. The primary end-point of the LAPPRO trial was urinary leakage at 12 months, and with a significance level $p = 0.05$, 80 % power, two-sided test it was calculated to require 1400 robot-assisted laparoscopic radical prostatectomies and 700 open prostatectomies. Quality-of-life measurements were dichotomized as previously described [29]. Postoperative stay was compared between groups using Kruskal-Wallis test. Categorical data were compared between groups using χ^2-tests, trends across groups were evaluated using Jonckheere-Terpstra's test. Two sided p-values ≤0.05 were considered statistically significant. We also calculated relative risk adjusted for possible confounders using multivariable logistic regression models both with logit-link and log-link functions. Possible confounders: age, level of education, smoking, body mass index (BMI), American Society of Anaesthesiologists (ASA) classification, and alcohol consumption were all evaluated in univariable analyses against the primary outcome sick leave. Factors being significant at the 5 % level in univariable analyses were all included in the base multivariable model; other factors were entered one at the time in order to evaluate their effect on the association between level of physical activity and sick leave.

Results

The demography is displayed in Table 1, with the patients being divided into the four groups, according to their self-assessed physical activity-level. The group answering "Never" was a minority, comprising of 102 patients (6.5 %). The patients in this group differed significantly from the others with a higher co-morbidity according to the American Society of Anaesthesiologists (ASA) classification and they reported smoking and drinking more often. To reduce the risk of including patients unable to exercise, these patients were excluded from the analyses regarding sick leave. Quality of life was higher in the patient group with a higher level of physical activity (Table 1) at base line. No other statistically significant differences were found at baseline between the three remainin groups of PA.

In Table 2 hospital stay, sick leave, and complications are displayed as well as current health status. A significantly larger proportion of patients (13 %) in the most active group reported a sick leave of shorter duration than one week. Most patients did not report full recovery within four weeks, but although statistically nonsignificant, it was slightly more common to be recovered within three months in the group with the highest level of self-assessed physical activity.

Higher age (mean 60.2 SD 3.5 vs. mean 57.9 SD 4.7, $p < 0.0001$) and higher educational level (521 patients with University degree reported 1 week or more compared to 760 patients with lower educational level, $p < 0.0001$) were both associated with shorter sick leave. However, when adjusting for these factors in a multivariate model (Table 3) the relationship between sick leave and level of physical activity remained, even when adding other potential confounders to the multivariate model one at a time.

Discussion

The main finding of the present study is that a higher level of self-assessed regular physical activity preoperatively was associated with a reduction in sick-leave after radical prostatectomy. Furthermore, we found that the self-assessed current health status was higher in the more physically active group, three months after surgery.

The finding that a higher level of physical activity preoperatively may reduce sick leave have important clinical implications. First of all, the quality of life for many patients still working, may be increased with an early return to work. Secondly, as many treatments and procedures aim to shorten hospital stay and reduce sick leave, increased levels of physical activity may reduce societal costs. While physical activity is known to have health benefits in patients with cancer [31], this study adds to the present knowledge by showing that also the postoperative recovery may be improved by having a higher level of physical activity before surgery.

The patients in our study in general had a shorter sick leave than what has previously been reported from in a similar setting [21], and this was especially true for the open prostatectomy group. This may be due to the standardized period of short sick leave, enabling patients to be on paid sick leave for a more exact time, as warranted, less influenced by any decision made by the doctor.

In this study no clear differences were found between the different groups of physical activity regarding postoperative complications or hospital stay, possibly due to the short hospital stay in itself.

In addition, the finding that the quality of life is associated with the level of preoperative physical activity is important as it is confirming earlier studies have shown that quality of life in general is improved in cancer patients with a higher level of physical activity [32, 33].

The strengths of this study include the prospective design and a large number of included patients. Furthermore, all patients we analysed answered a preoperative questionnaire, giving a baseline status. A limitation may be that we used a question to assess physical activity, that has not been validated in relation to long-term morbidity, such as the Saltin-Grimby scale has [34]. However, our questions uses a longer time frame (one month) than several other scales, which is good in this setting of patients with cancer waiting for surgery, as it may more clearly depict the patient's everyday habits, but this remains to be shown. One may speculate some occupations imply less need for a formal sick leave than other, and that in the same occupations the men are able to, or have the habit to, enrol in a high level of physical activity. We have no data to support this speculation. However, it is difficult to speculate upon to what extent this has affected our results. The two higher levels of physical activity on the scale correspond to national guidelines indicating their value in the clinical setting [35].

Another limitation may be that more than 70 % were operated with one technique (robot-assisted laparoscopic

Table 1 Demography. Men operated with open or robot-assisted laparoscopic prostatectomy between 2008-2011 age ≤ 65 years old at 14 centers in Sweden. Divided into the four different categories of physical activity[a]

	Never (n = 102)	Sometimes (1-2 times a week) (n = 598)	Often (3-4 times a week) (n = 466)	Daily or almost daily (5-7 times a week) (n = 403)	p-value	Missing
Type of surgery					p = 0.271	2 (0.1 %)
Open	27 (26.5 %)	151 (25.3 %)	107 (23.0 %)	112 (27.8 %)		
Robot-assisted	75 (73.5 %)	446 (74.6 %)	358 (76.8 %)	291 (72.2 %)		
Preoperative characteristics						
Age, median	58 (37-64)	59 (39-64)	59 (39-64)	59 (39-64)	p = 0.330	2 (0.1 %)
Level of Education					0 = 0.001	0 (0 %)
University	35 (34.3 %)	222 (37.1 %)	222 (47.6 %)	187 (46.4 %)		
Vocational school	13 (12.7 %)	73 (12.2 %)	48 (10.3 %)	32 (7.9 %)		
Secondary school	29 (28.4 %)	210 (35.1 %)	144 (30.9 %)	129 (32 %)		
Elementary school	24 (23.5 %)	91 (15.2 %)	47 (10.1 %)	52 (12.9 %)		
Other	1 (1 %)	2 (0.3 %)	5 (1.1 %)	3 (0.7 %)		
BMI, median	27.1 (19-38)	26.3 (19-40)	26.2 (19-41)	25.7 (19-54)	p = 0.041	0 (0 %)
Smoking					p = 0.0005	13 (0.8 %)
Non-smoker	38 (37.3)	237 (39.6 %)	230 (49.4 %)	171 (42.4 %)		
Former smoker	42 (41.2 %)	278 (46.5 %)	200 (42.9 %)	204 (50.6 %)		
Current smoker	15 (14.7 %)	56 (9 %)	30 (6.4 %)	19 (4.7 %)		
Current snuff user	16 (15.7 %)	93 (15.6 %)	71 (15.2 %)	63 (15.6 %)	p = 0.996	11 (0.7 %)
High alcohol consumption[b]	3 (2.9 %)	6 (1 %)	2 (0.4 %)	4 (1 %)	p = 0.121	17 (1.1 %)
American Society of Anaesthesiology (ASA) classification					p = 0.760	41 (2.6 %)
I	67 (65.7 %)	421 (70.4 %)	336 (72.1 %)	295 (73.2 %)		
II	32 (31.4 %)	154 (25.8 %)	109 (23.4 %)	99 (24.6 %)		
III	2 (2.0 %)	3 (0.5 %)	6 (1.3 %)	1 (0.2 %)		
Gleason score					p = 0.562	105 (6.7 %)
<7	54 (52.9 %)	314 (52.5 %)	245 (52.6 %)	198 (49.1 %)		
≥7	42 (41.2 %)	238 (39.8 %)	192 (41.2 %)	173 (42.9 %)		
Stroke	1 (1 %)	2 (0.3 %)	1 (0.2 %)	2 (0.5 %)	p = 0.774	10 (0.6 %)
Thromboembolic disease	1 (1 %)	8 (1.3 %)	6 (1.3 %)	5 (1.2 %)	p = 0.990	12 (0.8 %)
Neurologic disease	3 (2.9 %)	5 (0.8 %)	2 (0.4 %)	6 (1.5 %)	p = 0.245	11 (0.7 %)
Diabetes	4 (3.9 %)	28 (4.7 %)	20 (4.3 %)	17 (4.2 %)	p = 0.924	13 (0.8 %)
Hypertension	33 (32.4 %)	182 (30.4 %)	121 (26 %)	118 (29.3 %)	p = 0.269	11 (0.7 %)

Table 1 Demography. Men operated with open or robot-assisted laparoscopic prostatectomy between 2008-2011 age ≤ 65 years old at 14 centers in Sweden. Divided into the four different categories of physical activity[a] *(Continued)*

Diagnosed depression	3 (2.9 %)	15 (2.5 %)	11 (2.4 %)	5 (1.2 %)	16 (1.0 %)	$p = 0.363$
Angina pectoris	0 (0 %)	9 (1.5 %)	7 (1.5 %)	3 (0.7 %)	11 (0.7 %)	$p = 0.518$
Long-term pain, unspecified	12 (11.8 %)	48 (8.0 %)	33 (7.1 %)	24 (6 %)	15 (1 %)	$p = 0.472$
Low or moderate subjective quality of life[c]	62 (60.8 %)	314 (52.8 %)	217 (46.6 %)	174 (43.3 %)	4 (0.3 %)	$p = 0.004$
Low or moderate physical well-being[c]	59 (58.4 %)	281 (47.2 %)	168 (36.1 %)	126 (31.5 %)	7 (0.4 %)	$p < 0.0001$
Low or moderate psychological well-being[c]	60 (59.4 %)	333 (56.0 %)	227 (48.7)	177 (44.1 %)	6 (0.4 %)	$p = 0.003$
Decreased general physical capacity[c]	67 (65.7 %)	264 (44.4 %)	164 (35.2 %)	126 (31.3 %)	4 (0.3 %%)	$p < 0.0001$
Self assessment of current health status (median with range in parenthesis)[d]	80 (30-100)	83 (10-100)	85 (15-100)	90 (30-100)	27 (1.7 %)	$p < 0.0001$

[a]Unless otherwise stated data is given as number with percentages or range in parenthesis. [b] Risk consumption of alcohol is defined as more than 15 glasses/week. [c]The lowest five of seven possible categories. [d]On a scale from 0-100. Categorical data were compared between groups using chi-square-tests, trends across groups were evaluated using Jonckheere-Terpstra's test. Two sided p-values ≤0.05 were considered statistically significant

Table 2 Outcomes

	Sometimes (1-2 times a week) (n = 598)	Often (3-4 times a week) (n = 466)	Daily or almost daily (5-7 times a week) (n = 403)	p-value	Missing
Median length of post-op stay (days)	3 (1-18)	3 (2-15)	3 (1-8)	p = 0.561	130 (8.9 %)
Number of patients reporting no sick-leave or sick-leave less than one week	36 (6.3 %)	41 (9.2 %)	51 (13 %)	p < 0.001*	56 (3.8 %)
Feel fully recovered < 4 weeks postoperatively (%)	85 (14.9 %)	74 (16.9 %)	67 (17.5 %)	p = 0.214	56 (3.8 %)
Still not recovered at 3 months	76 (13.4 %)	53 (12.1 %)	42 (10.9 %)	p = 0.510	56 (3.8 %)
Any complication					
Infection[a]	118 (20.6 %)	93 (21.0 %)	73 (18.6 %)	p = 0.659	60 (4.1 %)
Cardiovascular[b]	28 (5.0 %)	22 (5.0 %)	21 (5.4 %)	p = 0.955	70 (4.8 %)
Surgical[c]	105 (18.5 %)	88 (20.0 %)	66 (16.8 %)	p = 0.493	64 (4.4.%)
Gastrointestinal[d]	72 (12.7 %)	56 (12.7 %)	47 (12.0 %)	p = 0.937	64 (4.4 %)
Psychological[e]	80 (14.2 %)	47 (10.8 %)	57 (14.7 %)	p = 0.182	78 (5.3 %)
Self assessment of current health status (median with range in parenthesis)	80 (5-100)	80 (19-100)	85 (19-100)	p = 0.02**	70 (4.7 %)

Postoperative stay, sick leave, evaluation of recovery and complications at 6-12 weeks postoperatively
Unless otherwise stated data are given as number with percentages or range in parenthesis. [a]On a scale from 0-100. n.s. denotes not statistically significant. Postoperative stay was compared between groups using Kruskal-Wallis test. Categorical data were compared between groups using χ^2-tests, trends across groups were evaluated using Jonckheere-Terpstra's test. Two sided p-values ≤0.05 were considered statistically significant. *Jonckheere-Terpstra's trend test. **Kruskall-Wallis test. [a]Infection in the operating wound, pneumonia or urinary tract infection. Number of patients in the analysis: 1407 [b] Pulmonary embolism, hypertension, acute myocardial infarction, arrhythmia or other heart diseases, deep venous thrombosis, stroke. Number of patients in the analysis: 1397. [c]Pain in the operating wound, pain in the lower abdomen, pain in the upper abdomen, bleeding from the operating wound, bleeding from the urinary tract, inguinal hernia. Number of patients in the analysis: 1403. [d]Nausea, impaired appetite, loose or frequent stools, constipation. Number of patients in the analysis: 1403. [e]Depressed mood, worry. Number of patients in the analysis: 1389

radical prostatectomy), however, surgical technique was included in the adjusted analysis and did not affect results. It is also possible that pre- and postoperative care differed between the different hospitals, however, due to the fact that center also was related to type of procedure this is difficult to fully cover in the adjusted statistical analysis. Another limitation is that the patients did not address whether their job was physically demanding or more office work prior to surgery, but to some extent this is made up for by the use of educational level as this often correlates well.

A future challenge is how to achieve a higher level of physical activity preoperatively for any patient group. Methods to increase the level of physical activity in patients have been introduced in recent years. The Swedish model of physical activity on prescription has been shown to increase the level of physical activity [36], and

to positively affect metabolic risk factors [37]. The National Board of Health and Welfare now recommend physical activity for all insufficiently physically active patients in Sweden (www.socialstyrelsen.se) [35]. The population of prostatectomy patients may be a target population for recommendations on similar physical activity interventions.

Conclusions

We found that a higher level of physical activity preoperatively was associated with a reduced sick leave for patients after radical prostatectomy in a Swedish setting. Further studies are required, but it is possible that a recommendation on individualised physical activity, prior to surgery, could be included in the preoperative programme aimed for patients being planned for prostatectomy.

Table 3 Unadjusted and adjusted analysis of the relationship between physical activity and sick leave

	Unadjusted OR (95 % CI)	p-value	Adjusted OR (95 % CI)[a]	p-value
Sometimes (1-2 times a week) versus Often (3-4 times a week)	0.66 (0.41-1.05)	p = 0.079	0.73 (0.45-1.20)	p = 0.215
Sometimes (1-2 times a week) versus Daily or almost daily (5-7 times a week)	0.45 (0.29-0.70)	p = 0.0004	0.49 (0.30-0.78)	p = 0.003
Often (3-4 times a week) versus Daily or almost daily (5-7 times a week)	0.68 (0.44-1.06)	p = 0.083	0.66 (0.42-1.05)	p = 0.080

[a]Adjusted for possible confounders using multivariable logistic regression models both with logit-link and log-link functions. Factors being significant at the five percent level in univariable analyses were all included in the base multivariable model; other factors were entered one at the time in order to evaluate their effect on the association between level of physical activity and sick leave. Adjusted for educational level, age, ASA-classification, alcohol consumption, smoking, BMI and surgical technique

Abbreviations
ASA-classification, American Society of Anaesthesiologists classification; BMI, body mass index; LAPPRO, LAParoscopic prostatectomy robot open.

Acknowledgements
Eva Haglind is the principal investigator and Gunnar Steineck the deputy principal investigator for LAPPRO.

Funding
The Swedish Society of Medicine, The Gothenburg Medical Society, Sahlgrenska University Hospital, Agreement concerning research and education of doctors, ALF 138751 and 146201, The Health & Medical Care Committee of the Regional Executive Board, Region Västra Götaland, The Tornspiran Foundation, Mrs Mary von Sydow Foundation, The Swedish Research Council (2012-1770), the Swedish Cancer Foundation (2013/497), HTA – VGR 6011 and Anna and Edvin Berger foundation.

Authors' contributions
EH, TT and GS participated in the conception and initial design as well as acquisition of data in the LAPPRO trial. EA, UA, MB, JE, MG, TT and EA participated in the design of this sub-study and analysis of data. EA, UA, MB, JE, MG, TT, GS and EH participated in interpretation of data. EA drafted the manuscript and UA, MB, JE, MG, TT, GS and EH participated in critical revision and final approval of the manuscript.

Competing interests
The authors declare that they have no competing interests.

Author details
[1]Department of Surgery, Institute of Clinical Sciences, Sahlgrenska Academy at University of Gothenburg, SSORG, Sahlgrenska University Hospital/Östra, SE-416 85 Gothenburg, Sweden. [2]University West, Trollhättan, Sweden. [3]Swedish School of Sport and Health Sciences, Stockholm, Sweden. [4]Department of Cardiology, Karolinska University Hospital, Stockholm, Sweden. [5]Faculty of Nursing, School of Health Sciences, University of Iceland, Reykjavik, Iceland. [6]Division of Clinical Cancer Epidemiology, Department of Oncology, Institute of Clinical Sciences, Sahlgrenska Academy at the University of Gothenburg, Gothenburg, Sweden. [7]Department of Oncology and Pathology, Division of Clinical Cancer Epidemiology, Karolinska Institutet, Solna, Sweden.

References
1. Woodcock J, Franco OH, Orsini N, Roberts I. Non-vigorous physical activity and all-cause mortality: systematic review and meta-analysis of cohort studies. Int J Epidemiol. 2011;40(1):121–38.
2. Wanderley FA, Silva G, Marques E, Oliveira J, Mota J, Carvalho J. Associations between objectively assessed physical activity levels and fitness and self-reported health-related quality of life in community-dwelling older adults. Qual Life Res. 2011;20(9):1371–8.
3. Friedenreich CM, Neilson HK, Lynch BM. State of the epidemiological evidence on physical activity and cancer prevention. Eur J Cancer. 2010;46(14):2593–604.
4. Bonn SE, Sjolander A, Lagerros YT, Wiklund F, Stattin P, Holmberg E, Gronberg H, Balter K. Physical activity and survival among men diagnosed with prostate cancer. Cancer Epidemiol Biomarkers Prev. 2015; 24(1):57–64.
5. Nielsen PR, Jorgensen LD, Dahl B, Pedersen T, Tonnesen H. Prehabilitation and early rehabilitation after spinal surgery: randomized clinical trial. Clin Rehabil. 2010;24(2):137–48.
6. Carli F, Scheede-Bergdahl C. Prehabilitation to enhance perioperative care. Anesthesiol Clin. 2015;33(1):17–33.
7. Santa Mina D, Guglietti CL, Alibhai SM, Matthew AG, Kalnin R, Ahmad N, Lindner U, Trachtenberg J. The effect of meeting physical activity guidelines for cancer survivors on quality of life following radical prostatectomy for prostate cancer. J Cancer Surviv. 2014;8(2):190–8.
8. Adamina M, Kehlet H, Tomlinson GA, Senagore AJ, Delaney CP. Enhanced recovery pathways optimize health outcomes and resource utilization: a meta-analysis of randomized controlled trials in colorectal surgery. Surgery. 2011;149(6):830–40.
9. Carli F, Charlebois P, Stein B, Feldman L, Zavorsky G, Kim DJ, Scott S, Mayo NE. Randomized clinical trial of prehabilitation in colorectal surgery. Br J Surg. 2010;97(8):1187–97.
10. Jack S, West M, Grocott MP. Perioperative exercise training in elderly subjects. Best Pract Res Clin Anaesthesiol. 2011;25(3):461–72.
11. Santa Mina D, Scheede-Bergdahl C, Gillis C, Carli F. Optimization of surgical outcomes with prehabilitation. Appl Physiol Nutr Metab. 2015;40(9):966–9.
12. Santa Mina D, Matthew AG, Hilton WJ, Au D, Awasthi R, Alibhai SM, Clarke H, Ritvo P, Trachtenberg J, Fleshner NE, et al. Prehabilitation for men undergoing radical prostatectomy: a multi-centre, pilot randomized controlled trial. BMC Surg. 2014;14:89.
13. Heidenreich A, Bellmunt J, Bolla M, Joniau S, Mason M, Matveev V, Mottet N, Schmid HP, van der Kwast T, Wiegel T, et al. EAU guidelines on prostate cancer. Part 1: screening, diagnosis, and treatment of clinically localised disease. Eur Urol. 2011;59(1):61–71.
14. Bill-Axelson A, Holmberg L, Ruutu M, Haggman M, Andersson SO, Bratell S, Spangberg A, Busch C, Nordling S, Garmo H, et al. Radical prostatectomy versus watchful waiting in early prostate cancer. N Engl J Med. 2005;352(19):1977–84.
15. Hugosson J, Stranne J, Carlsson SV. Radical retropubic prostatectomy: a review of outcomes and side-effects. Acta Oncol. 2011;50 Suppl 1:92–7.
16. Trinh QD, Sammon J, Sun M, Ravi P, Ghani KR, Bianchi M, Jeong W, Shariat SF, Hansen J, Schmitges J, et al. Perioperative outcomes of robot-assisted radical prostatectomy compared with open radical prostatectomy: results from the nationwide inpatient sample. Eur Urol. 2012;61(4):679–85.
17. Barry MJ, Gallagher PM, Skinner JS, Fowler Jr FJ. Adverse effects of robotic-assisted laparoscopic versus open retropubic radical prostatectomy among a nationwide random sample of medicare-age men. J Clin Oncol. 2012;30(5):513–8.
18. Kluivers KB, Riphagen I, Vierhout ME, Brolmann HA, de Vet HC. Systematic review on recovery specific quality-of-life instruments. Surgery. 2008;143(2):206–15.
19. Allvin R, Svensson E, Rawal N, Ehnfors M, Kling AM, Idvall E. The Postoperative Recovery Profile (PRP) - a multidimensional questionnaire for evaluation of recovery profiles. J Eval Clin Pract. 2011;17(2):236–43.
20. Sultan R, Slova D, Thiel B, Lepor H. Time to return to work and physical activity following open radical retropubic prostatectomy. J Urol. 2006;176(4 Pt 1):1420–3.
21. Hohwu L, Akre O, Pedersen KV, Jonsson M, Nielsen CV, Gustafsson O. Open retropubic prostatectomy versus robot-assisted laparoscopic prostatectomy: a comparison of length of sick leave. Scand J Urol Nephrol. 2009;43(4):259–64.
22. Bhayani SB, Pavlovich CP, Hsu TS, Sullivan W, Su LM. Prospective comparison of short-term convalescence: laparoscopic radical prostatectomy versus open radical retropubic prostatectomy. Urology. 2003;61(3):612–6.
23. Thorsteinsdottir T, Stranne J, Carlsson S, Anderberg B, Bjorholt I, Damber JE, Hugosson J, Wilderang U, Wiklund P, Steineck G, et al. LAPPRO: A prospective multicentre comparative study of robot-assisted laparoscopic and retropubic radical prostatectomy for prostate cancer. Scand J Urol Nephrol. 2011;45(2):102–12.
24. Wallerstedt A, Tyritzis SI, Thorsteinsdottir T, Carlsson S, Stranne J, Gustafsson O, Hugosson J, Bjartell A, Wilderang U, Wiklund NP, et al. Short-term results after robot-assisted laparoscopic radical prostatectomy compared to open radical prostatectomy. Eur Urol. 2015;67(4):660–70.
25. Haglind E, Carlsson S, Stranne J, Wallerstedt A, Wilderang U, Thorsteinsdottir T, Lagerkvist M, Damber JE, Bjartell A, Hugosson J, et al. Urinary incontinence and erectile dysfunction after robotic versus open radical prostatectomy: a prospective, controlled, nonrandomised trial. Eur Urol. 2015;68(2):216–25.
26. Steineck G, Bergmark K, Henningsohn L, al-Abany M, Dickman PW, Helgason A. Symptom documentation in cancer survivors as a basis for therapy modifications. Acta Oncol. 2002;41(3):244–52.
27. Steineck G, Hunt H, Adolfsson J. A hierarchical step-model for causation of bias-evaluating cancer treatment with epidemiological methods. Acta Oncol. 2006;45(4):421–9.

28. Johansson E, Steineck G, Holmberg L, Johansson JE, Nyberg T, Ruutu M, Bill-Axelson A, Investigators S. Long-term quality-of-life outcomes after radical prostatectomy or watchful waiting: the Scandinavian Prostate Cancer Group-4 randomised trial. Lancet Oncol. 2011;12(9):891–9.
29. Steineck G, Helgesen F, Adolfsson J, Dickman PW, Johansson JE, Norlen BJ, Holmberg L. Quality of life after radical prostatectomy or watchful waiting. N Engl J Med. 2002;347(11):790–6.
30. Haskell WL, Blair SN, Hill JO. Physical activity: health outcomes and importance for public health policy. Prev Med. 2009;49(4):280–2.
31. Barbaric M, Brooks E, Moore L, Cheifetz O. Effects of physical activity on cancer survival: a systematic review. Physiother Can. 2010;62(1):25–34.
32. Mishra SI, Scherer RW, Snyder C, Geigle PM, Berlanstein DR, Topaloglu O. Exercise interventions on health-related quality of life for people with cancer during active treatment. Cochrane Database Syst Rev. 2012;8:Cd008465.
33. Mishra SI, Scherer RW, Geigle PM, Berlanstein DR, Topaloglu O, Gotay CC, Snyder C. Exercise interventions on health-related quality of life for cancer survivors. Cochrane Database Syst Rev. 2012;8:Cd007566.
34. Saltin B, Grimby G. Physiological analysis of middle-aged and old former athletes. Comparison with still active athletes of the same ages. Circulation. 1968;38(6):1104–15.
35. Socialstyrelsen. The National Board of Health and Welfare: Nationella riktlinjer för sjukdomsförebyggande metoder 2011. Tobaksbruk, riskbruk av alkohol, otillräcklig fysisk aktivitet och ohälsosamma matvanor. Stöd för styrning och ledning. 2011. http://www.socialstyrelsen.se/Lists/Artikelkatalog/Attachments/18484/2011-11-11.pdf.
36. Kallings LV, Leijon M, Hellenius ML, Stahle A. Physical activity on prescription in primary health care: a follow-up of physical activity level and quality of life. Scand J Med Sci Sports. 2008;18(2):154–61.
37. Kallings LV, Sierra Johnson J, Fisher RM, Faire U, Stahle A, Hemmingsson E, Hellenius ML. Beneficial effects of individualized physical activity on prescription on body composition and cardiometabolic risk factors: results from a randomized controlled trial. Eur J Cardiovasc Prev Rehabil. 2009;16(1):80–4.

Comparison of patient-reported quality of life outcome questionnaire response rates between patients treated surgically for renal cell carcinoma and prostate carcinoma

David D. Thiel[1*], Andrew J. Davidiuk[1], Gregory A. Broderick[1], Michelle Arnold[2], Nancy Diehl[2], Andrea Tavlarides[2], Kaitlynn Custer[2] and Alexander S. Parker[2]

Abstract

Background: We sought to examine differences in response rates to quality of life (QoL) surveys in patients treated surgically for renal cell carcinoma (RCC) and prostate cancer (PCa) and to analyze factors associated with non-response of the surveys.

Methods: Patients who underwent surgery for RCC or PCa between 2006 and 2012 were offered enrollment in respective prospective cancer registries that included baseline and annual QoL assessments. We identified 201 RCC patients and 616 PCa patients who completed a baseline QoL survey and were mailed annual QoL surveys [RCC: SF-36, FACT–G (73 questions), PCa: EPIC, IIEF, Max-PC (80 questions)]. We compared patient characteristics between responders and non-responders using a Wilcoxon rank-sum test for continuous variables and a Fisher's Exact test for categorical variables.

Results: The overall response rates for the PCa and RCC groups were 63 and 48 % (p < 0.001), respectively. This difference in response rates remained when we limited analysis to only those with early stage disease (pT2 for PCa and pT1 RCC, 62 % vs. 52 %; $p = 0.03$). PCa characteristics associated with response included older age (64.1 vs 62.6 years, $p = 0.032$) and robotic versus open surgery (56 % vs 44 %; $p = 0.009$). There were no characteristics that were associated with response in RCC patients.

Conclusions: Surgically treated PCa patients have higher QoL mail-based survey response rates compared to patients treated surgically for RCC. This difference holds true for clinically localized cancers as well.

Keywords: Quality of life, Prostate cancer, Renal cell cancer, Oncology outcomes, Partial nephrectomy, Prostatectomy

Background

Five-year survival for surgically treated pT1 RCC is over 90 % [1, 2], and 10 year cancer specific survival for surgically treated intermediate risk PCa is over 95 % [3]. A downstream effect of these longer survival times has been a parallel increase in the desire to evaluate factors that affect post-surgical quality of life (QoL). Survey-based instruments to measure specific metrics related to patient QoL (eg, depression, cancer-specific anxiety, etc.) have been developed and validated. These same instruments have been shown to improve physician-patient communication and provide increased individualization of treatment and self-assessment of physician surgical outcomes [4, 5]. Despite the benefit to both research and clinical practice, only about 20 % of urologists report utilizing QoL assessments as part of their management of PCa patients, and patient response rates to these QoL assessments have been shown to vary considerably [6]. This underscores the need to improve our overall understanding of the response rates to QoL assessments in these

* Correspondence: thiel.david@mayo.edu
[1]Departments of Urology Mayo Clinic, 4500 San Pablo Road, Jacksonville, FL 32224, USA
Full list of author information is available at the end of the article

patient populations and to explore the factors that can predict patient response and non-response.

We harnessed resources at our institution to evaluate response to postoperative QoL surveys in PCa and RCC. We hypothesized that there is a difference in response rates to postoperative QoL surveys between PCa and RCC patients. To test our hypotheses, we utilized data collected as part of two cancer registry efforts at our institution (one for PCa and one for RCC), which include baseline QoL assessment followed by annual evaluations of QoL. We report herein our analysis of the response rates between the two patient populations as well as our assessment of factors associated with response rates for each group, respectively.

Methods

RCC Patients: Patients who underwent surgery for RCC at our institution between 2006 and 2012 were offered Mayo Clinic Institutional Review Board-approved enrollment in a prospective registry that included baseline and annual QoL assessment. Patients either underwent nephrectomy or partial nephrectomy that was completed laparoscopically or with an open incision. Patients gave written consent and completed QoL surveys at baseline and were mailed follow-up QoL surveys at postoperative year one and two. The QoL surveys mailed were the SF-36 and the FACT-G (Functional Assessment of Cancer Therapy-General). There were a total of 73 questions in the two surveys.

The SF-36 uses 36 questions to assess eight domains of functional health and well-being. It is non-specific to age, disease, and treatment, which is useful in both general and specific populations. All 36 questions on the SF-36 are scored on a scale from 0 to 100, with 100 as the highest level of functioning. Collective scores are calculated as a percentage of the total points possible. The scores from those questions that address each specific domain of functional health status are averaged together for a final score with each of the eight domains assessed [7].

The FACT-G is a 33-item questionnaire that measures four QoL domains; physical, social, emotional, and functional well-being, with nine additional questions dedicated to establishing QoL associated with RCC [8]. The FACT-G is scored by adding the individual scores (range 0 to 108), with higher scores indicating better QoL.

PCa patients: Patients who opted to enroll in the Institutional Review Board-approved PCa registry completed baseline QoL surveys prior to surgical therapy and were mailed follow-up questionnaires 6 months following surgery and then annually thereafter. PCa was treated surgically at our institution with radical retropubic prostatectomy (RRP) or robotic prostatectomy (RARP). The PCa surveys used were the EPIC, IIEF, and Max-PC surveys totalling 80 questions.

The EPIC (expanded prostate cancer index composite) is a prostate-specific instrument utilized to assess health related QoL with regard to function and bother. The instrument assesses urinary, bowel, sexual, and hormonal domains. Three scores are provided for each of the domains to provide a function score, a bother score, and a total score [9]. Higher scores reflect better function.

The IIEF (International Index for Erectile Function) is a brief, reliable, self-administered survey of erectile function that is cross-culturally valid and psychometrically sound. The IIEF addresses the relevant domains of male sexual function (erectile function, orgasmic function, sexual desire, intercourse satisfaction, and overall satisfaction) and has been linguistically validated in 10 languages. The IIEF demonstrates the sensitivity and specificity for detecting treatment-related changes in patients with erectile dysfunction [10].

The Max-PC survey (Memorial Anxiety Scale for Prostate Cancer) was developed to facilitate the identification and assessment of men with prostate cancer-related anxiety. This scale consists of three subscales that measure general prostate cancer anxiety, anxiety related to prostate specific antigen (PSA) levels in particular, and fear of recurrence [11]. It should be noted that patients who did not respond to the questionnaires were not contacted again until the following year. Patients were not contacted by phone or e-mail or sent another questionnaire if there was no response that year.

Study Analysis: We compared patient characteristics between responders (those who returned at least a one- or two-year follow-up survey) and non-responders (those who did not return any follow-up surveys). For the RCC registry, only RCC patients were included. Those with alternative pathology (such as oncocytoma, papillary adenoma, etc.) were excluded. All patients who underwent surgery for PCa were included. The PCa patients do receive a 6 month postoperative survey which was not included in the analysis. The analysis included patients treated surgically between 2006 and 2012 to allow for analysis of 1 year response rates.

Statistical analysis: Continuous variables were presented as median, minimum, and maximum values. Categorical data were presented as counts and percentages. Comparisons of patient characteristics between responders (who completed at least a one- or two-year annual follow-up) and non-responders were performed using a Wilcoxon rank-sum test for continuous variables and a Fisher's Exact test for categorical variables. The cumulative mortality rates were estimated using the Kaplan-Meier method and comparison between mortality of responders versus non-responders was evaluated using Cox Proportional Hazards models. All statistical tests were two-sided, with threshold of significance set at $a = 0.05$ and performed using SAS Version 9.2 (SAS Institute Inc., Cary, NC).

Results

We identified 201 patients in the RCC registry and 616 patients in the PCa registry who were surgically treated between 2006 and 2012 and were asked to fill out a baseline QoL survey and a follow-up QoL survey at 1 year following surgery and annually thereafter. The overall response rates for the PCa and RCC groups were 63 and 48 % (p < 0.001), respectively.

Table 1 outlines the patient and surgical characteristics in the 201 RCC patients stratified by non-response versus response rates. Surgery type (partial nephrectomy or radical nephrectomy), surgical approach (laparoscopic versus open surgery), T stage, or nuclear grade were not significantly associated with increased response rates.

Table 2 summarizes the 616 PCa patients in the PCa registry organized by response status and their association with the type of surgery performed, T stage, and Gleason score. Unlike RCC patients, there was an association with response rates with regard to age at surgery and surgery type (RRP versus RARP). Much like the RCC group, there was no association with response rates and prognostic variables, such as T stage or Gleason score.

Table 3 is a summary of the response rates of stage pT1 RCC patients compared to stage pT2 PCa patients.

Table 1 Association of patient and surgical characteristics in n = 201 RCC patients non-response versus response to QoL collected at one- or two-year follow-up

Variable[a]	Non-responder (n = 105)	Responder (n = 96)	P-value[b]
Age at surgery	65.2 (24.0, 87.5)	67.3 (35.3, 92.1)	0.48
Sex, male	75 (71 %)	62 (65 %)	0.36
Surgery type			
Partial	37 (35 %)	44 (46 %)	0.15
Radical	68 (65 %)	52 (54 %)	
Surgery type			0.88
Open	33 (31 %)	29 (30 %)	
LAP	72 (69 %)	67 (70 %)	
T stage			0.14
pT1	69 (68 %)	74 (79 %)	
pT2	9 (9 %)	8 (9 %)	
pT3, pT4	24 (24 %)	12 (13 %)	
Nuclear grade			0.098
1	4 (4 %)	9 (10 %)	
2	62 (60 %)	59 (63 %)	
3-4	37 (36 %)	26 (28 %)	

[a]Median [Minimum, Maximum] is given for continuous measures, and N (%) for categorical measures
[b]P-values for age at surgery and nuclear grade are based on Wilcoxon Rank Sum test. P-values given for Sex, Radical/partial surgical type, Open/LAP surgical type, and T-stage are based on Fisher's Exact test
RCC = renal cell carcinoma   QoL = quality of life
LAP = Laparoscopic

Table 2 Association of patient and surgical characteristics in n = 616 PCa patients versus response to QoL collected at one- or two-year follow-up

Variable[a]	Non-responder (n = 230)	Responder (n = 386)	P-value[b]
Age at surgery	62.6 (29.9, 76.8)	64.1 (42.9, 78.4)	0.032
Surgery type			
RRP	83 (36 %)	171 (44 %)	0.009
RARP	147 (64 %)	215 (56 %)	
T stage			0.51
pT1	0 (0 %)	3 (1 %)	
pT2	200 (87 %)	328 (85 %)	
pT3, pT4	30 (13 %)	54 (14 %)	
Pathological Gleason score			0.71
4-6	86 (37 %)	139 (36 %)	
7	123 (53 %)	211 (55 %)	
8-10	21 (9 %)	36 (9 %)	

[a]Median [Minimum, Maximum] is given for continuous measures, and N (%) for categorical measures
[b]P-values for age at surgery and Gleason score are based on Wilcoxon Rank Sum test. P-values given for T-stage are based on Fisher's Exact test
PCa = prostate cancer
QoL = quality of life
RRP = Radical Retropubic Prostatectomy
RARP = Robot-Assisted Radical Prostatectomy

Despite similar prognoses, the pT2 stage PCa patients are more likely to respond than pT1 RCC patients (62 % vs. 52 % p = 0.027).

Figure 1a and b demonstrate the survey response rates in relation to cancer specific mortality. It is obvious from both graphs that RCC patients were more likely to die (26 out of 201 RCC deaths) than PCa patients (7 out of 616 PCa deaths). Figure 1a demonstrates that RCC mortality was correlated with non-responder status, and this difference remains even when non-responders who died within the first year after surgery are excluded. Figure 1b illustrates that PCa mortality did not affect questionnaire response rates.

Discussion

QoL instruments have been shown to improve physician-patient communication, individualization of treatment, and physician self-assessment of surgical outcomes [4, 5]. Despite the advantages of QoL instruments, their use by urologists in addition to overall response rates by patients

Table 3 Questionnaire return rates of pT1 RCC patients and pT2 PCa patients

Variable	Non-responder (n = 269)	Responder (n = 402)	P-value
RCC pT1 only	69 (48 %)	74 (52 %)	0.027
PCa pT2 only	200 (38 %)	328 (62 %)	

RCC = renal cell carcinoma
PCa = prostate cancer

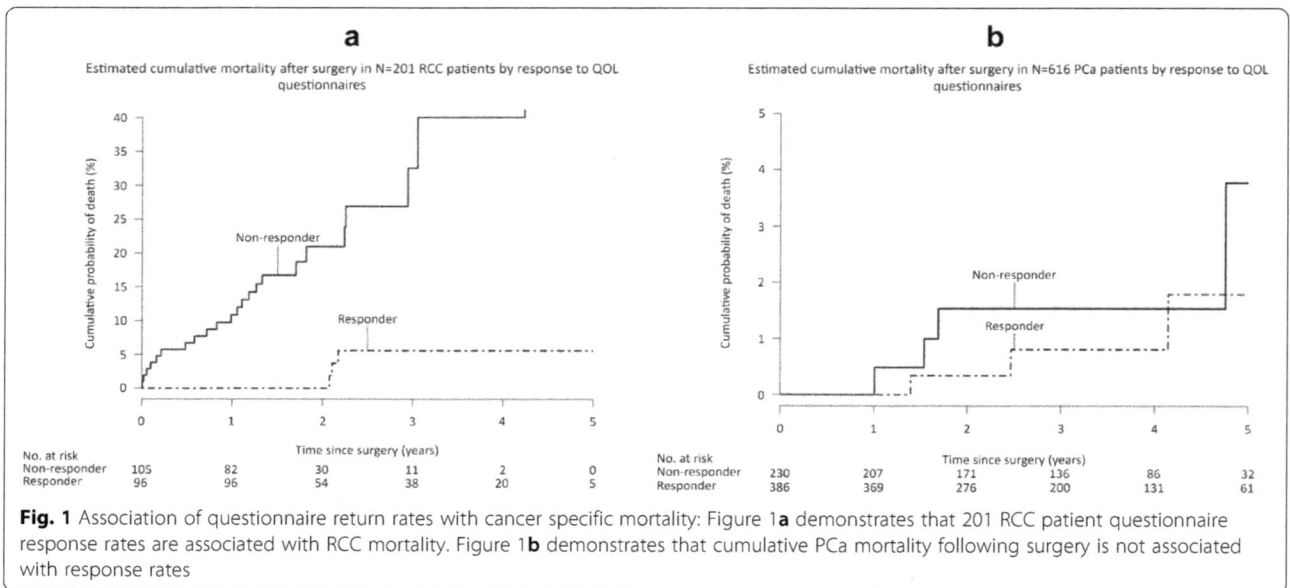

Fig. 1 Association of questionnaire return rates with cancer specific mortality: Figure 1**a** demonstrates that 201 RCC patient questionnaire response rates are associated with RCC mortality. Figure 1**b** demonstrates that cumulative PCa mortality following surgery is not associated with response rates

remains variable [6]. A common complaint regarding QoL instruments utilized for PCa is that these surveys are difficult to seamlessly integrate into practice and often take too much time to score and analyze [6]. Some have argued that these surveys may be too complex for the common patient; however, a recent analysis of the readability of QoL instruments utilized in urology practice for the most burdensome diseases notes that the reading level for these surveys is appropriate for the reading ability of most American adults [4].

A previous analysis of RCC patients at our institution revealed that RCC patients do not necessarily express high levels of concern following surgical treatment secondarily to feeling "cured" [8]. The study noted patients to have mood and anxiety changes early on following surgery, but those changes dissipated with longer-term follow-up. Our QoL instruments are mailed 1 year following surgery, and this time interval certainly allows patients time to recover from surgery and undergo follow-up imaging, possibly re-enforcing the feeling of being "cured." This may have contributed to the lower mail return rate for the QoL instruments in RCC patients. However, a man who has had a prostatectomy for clinically localized PCa has only a chance of approximately 2-3 % of dying from that disease within a decade, and this would certainly reinforce the feeling of being "cured" [3]. Figure 1 demonstrates that RCC patients are much more likely to die over this short follow-up period than their PCa counterparts. However, when patients with pT1 RCC (who have over 90 % 5 year survival) were compared to pT2 PCa patients in this study, a disparate number of questionnaire responses in favor of the PCa group remained.

One possible reason for the disparity in survey response rates seen in our study between PCa and RCC

patients may relate to the treatment decision-making process. RCC patients have few options other than surgery or ablation for their renal mass, which is especially true in clinically localized pT1 tumors. In contrast, patients with clinically localized PCa must decide between a multitude of treatment options such as active surveillance, cryoablation, ultrasound ablation, various radiotherapies, and surgery. The many choices make information gathering paramount and likely underlines the QoL return as a strong focus of PCa follow-up.

A Google search for "Prostate Cancer Treatment Options" currently results in 37 million hits compared to approximately 27 million hits for "Kidney Cancer Treatment Options." Media exposure and the high prevalence of PCa in aging males may make PCa more socially acceptable and easier to discuss in open forums compared to other cancers. The media exposure and the associated competitive marketing may also be setting men with PCa up for unreal expectations regarding post-therapy outcomes. One analysis demonstrated that men who had a RARP for PCa were more likely to experience treatment regret and dissatisfaction [12]. It is unknown what effect this may have on questionnaire return rates, but patients who had RARP were more likely to respond to QoL surveys than RRP patients.

Another possible reason for the disparity in return rates between RCC patients and PCa patients are the overall operative experiences of the two diseases. There may be a difference in postoperative expectations and QoL perception among patients with RCC and PCa. A diagnosis of RCC or PCa may each carry with it the fear of death. However, patients treated for PCa often carry the additional fear of recovering urinary continence and sexual potency [13]. This fact alone may explain why PCa patients are very in tune with their QoL recovery and with how long it may take to return to baseline QoL parameters. It also must be considered that full recovery of continence and potency following PCa surgery may take up to 24 months [14]. One concern with QoL questionnaire response rates is the length of the surveys. Patients may be unwilling to take the time to fill out lengthy surveys. The PCa and RCC question totals were similar in our registries (80 versus 73 questions) so we do not anticipate that survey length played a role in response rates between RCC and PCa.

One-year QoL response rates in patients surgically treated for PCa are reported as high as 93 % [15]. Two European studies analyzing the QoL of patients following surgery for RCC noted response rates of 71 and 72 % over a 6 month period, with one of the studies utilizing the same SF-36 survey used in this study [15, 16]. As evidenced by the studies above, the QoL response rates in both registries in our study are suboptimal. Our institution is looking into methods that may improve our overall QoL response rates. A 2012 examination of QoL outcomes following renal surgery gave patients the option of internet or paper-based follow-up [17]. Patients who did not respond were contacted by phone or e-mail up to three times. This led to a QoL response rate of 85 % over a 24 week period. Contacting patients via e-mail or phone calls may improve response rates, but it may also lead to inequality of data collection or recall bias, which may influence the results achieved. With regard to PCa, it has been noted that there is a wide gap between patient reported QoL outcomes and those assessed by physicians [18]. Therefore, we believe it is important to continue our current practice of mailing the surveys to the patients. One strategy to explore is direct emphasis to the patient by the surgeon on the importance of QoL survey return. Another option being explored is to deliver QoL survey material during follow-up visits. However, much of our patient population travels a great distance for surgery and receives their cancer follow-up locally, which may make this second option implausible.

Our RCC and PCa registries utilize mail surveys to collect QoL data and one strength of our study is that both surveys are collected in the same manner, which allows us to directly compare QoL return rates. However, this is a single-institution, retrospective study that has a few limitations as a result. One limitation of the study is the small sample size in both registries. This small sample size decreases our power to detect potentially meaningful differences between the PCa and RCC groups. Another limitation is that it involves a sample drawn from a tertiary care center, and the information may not be generalizable to the population as a whole. The respondents in the study were predominantly men, and it is unclear what effect this has on questionnaire response rates. In addition, patient-specific factors such as race and socioeconomic status were not included for analysis and may affect patient response rates. Another factor that may affect response rates that is not recorded is whether or not patients with recurrent cancer are undergoing adjuvant or salvage therapy. Also, it should be noted that the surveys for each population were different, with differing numbers of questions, which may have been another factor possibly impacting survey response rates.

Conclusions

At our institution, patients who are surgically treated for PCa are more likely to participate in QoL mail surveys than surgically treated RCC patients. QoL response rates for both groups of patients remains suboptimal, and other strategies may be necessary to achieve maximum assessment of postoperative QoL for RCC and PCa patients.

Abbreviations
EPIC: Expanded prostate cancer index composite; PCa: Prostate cancer; QoL: Quality of life; RARP: Robotic prostatectomy; RCC: Renal cell carcinoma; RRP: Radical retropublic prostatectomy.

Competing interests
DT: Invited speaker for Cooper Surgical, Inc. AD: None. GB: Participated in randomized clinical trial of botox vs. Vesicare for Allergan. MA: None. ND: None. AT: None. KC: None. AP: None.

Authors' contributions
DT: Conception and design, manuscript drafting. AD: Drafting of the manuscript. GB: Study design and manuscript design. MA: Data collection and manuscript revision. ND: Statistical analysis. AT: Data collection and manuscript revision. KC: Data collection and analysis. AP: Study design and manuscript revision. All authors read and approved the final manuscript.

Author details
[1]Departments of Urology Mayo Clinic, 4500 San Pablo Road, Jacksonville, FL 32224, USA. [2]Health Sciences Research at Mayo Clinic, 4500 San Pablo Road, Jacksonville, FL 32224, USA.

References
1. Permpongkosol S, Bagga HS, Romero FR, Sroka M, Jarrett TW, Kavoussi LR. Laparoscopic versus open partial nephrectomy for the treatment of pathological T1N0M0 renal cell carcinoma: a 5 year survival rate. J Urol. 2006;176:1984–8.
2. Rampersaud EN, Klatte T, Bass G, Patard JJ, Bensaleh K, Böhm M, Allhoff EP, Cindolo L, De La Taille A, Mejean A, Soulie M, Bellec L, Bernhard JC, Pfister C, Colombel M, Belldegrun AS, Pantuck AJ, George D. The effect of gender and age on kidney cancer survival: younger age is an independent prognostic factor in women with renal cell carcinoma. Urol Oncol. 2014;32:30.e9–30.e13.
3. Kibel AS, Ciezki JP, Klein EA, Reddy CA, Lubahn JD, Haslag-Minoff J, Deasy JO, Michalski JM, Kallogjeri D, Piccirillo JF, Rabah DM, Yu C, Kattan MW, Stephenson AJ. Survival among men with clinically localized prostate cancer treated with radical prostatectomy or radiation therapy in the prostate specific antigen era. J Urol. 2012;187:1259–65.
4. Bergman J, Gore JL, Singer JS, Anger JT, Litwin MS. Readability of health related quality of life instruments in urology. J Urol. 2010;183:1977–81.
5. Gazmararian JA, Baker DW, Williams MV, Parker RM, Scott TL, Green DC, Fehrenbach N, Ren J, Koplan JP. Health literacy among Medicare enrollees in a managed care organization. JAMA. 1999;281:545–51.

6. Kim SP, Karnes RJ, Nguyen PL, Ziegenfuss JY, Han LC, Thompson RH, Trinh QD, Sun M, Boorjian SA, Beebe TJ, Tilburt JC. Clinical implementation of quality of life instruments and prediction tools for localized prostate cancer: results from a national survey of radiation oncologists and urologists. J Urol. 2013;189:2092–8.

7. Ware JE, Snow KK, Kosinsnki M, et al. SF-36 health survey manual and interpretation guide. Boston, MA: The Health Institute, New England Medical Center Hospitals; 1993.

8. Ames SC, Parker AS, Crook JE, Diehl NN, Tan WW, Williams CR, Ames GE. Quality of life of patients undergoing surgical treatment for newly-diagnosed, clinically localized renal cell carcinoma. J Psychosoc Oncol. 2011;29:593–605.

9. Wei JT, Dunn RL, Litwin MS, Sandler HM, Sanda MG. Development and validation of the expanded prostate cancer index composite (EPIC) for comprehensive assessment of health-related quality of life in men with prostate cancer. Urology. 2000;56:899–905.

10. Rosen RC, Riley A, Wagner G, Osterloh IH, Kirkpatrick J, Mishra A. The international index of erectile function (IIEF): a multidimensional scale for assessment of erectile dysfunction. Urology. 1997;49:822–30.

11. Roth AJ, Rosenfeld B, Kornblith AB, Gibson C, Scher HI, Curley-Smart T, Holland JC, Breitbart W. The memorial anxiety scale for prostate cancer validation of a new scale to measure anxiety in men with with prostate cancer. Cancer. 2003;1;97:2910–8.

12. Huang KH, Carter SC, Hu JC. Does robotic prostatectomy meet its promise in the management of prostate cancer? Curr Urol Rep. 2013;14:184–91.

13. Klotz L. Active surveillance, quality of life, and cancer-related anxiety. Eur Urol. 2013;64:37–9.

14. Ludovico GM, Dachille G, Pagliarulo G, D'Elia C, Mondaini N, Gacci M, Detti B, Malossini G, Bartoletti R, Cai T. Bilateral nerve sparing robotic-assisted radical prostatectomy is associated with faster continence recovery but not with erectile function recovery compared with retropubic open prostatectomy: the need for accurate selection of patients. Oncol Rep. 2013;29:2445–50.

15. Beisland C, Beisland E, Hjelle KM, Bostad L, Hjermstad MJ, Aarstad AK, Aarstad HJ. Health-related quality of life in long-term survivors after renal cancer treatments. Scand J Urol. 2014;48:52–64.

16. Gratzke C, Seitz M, Bayrle F, Schlenker B, Bastian PJ, Haseke N, Bader M, Tilki D, Roosen A, Karl A, Reich O, Khoder WY, Wyler S, Steif CG, Staehler M, Bachmann A. Quality of life and perioperative outcomes after retroperitoneoscopic radical nephrectomy, open RN, and nephron-sparing surgery in patients with renal cell carcinoma. BJU Int. 2009;104:470–5.

17. Kim SB, Williams SB, Cheng SC, Sanda MG, Wagner AA. Evaluation of patient-reported quality-of-life outcomes after renal surgery. Urology. 2012;79:1268–73.

18. Sonn GA, Sadetsky N, Presti JC, Litwin MS. Differing perceptions of quality of life in patients with prostate cancer and their doctors. J Urol. 2013;189:S59–65.

3D vs 2D laparoscopic radical prostatectomy in organ-confined prostate cancer: comparison of operative data and pentafecta rates

Pierluigi Bove[*], Valerio Iacovelli, Francesco Celestino, Francesco De Carlo, Giuseppe Vespasiani and Enrico Finazzi Agrò

Abstract

Background: Currently, men are younger at the time of diagnosis of prostate cancer and more interested in less invasive surgical approaches (traditional laparoscopy, 3D-laparoscopy, robotics). Outcomes of continence, erectile function, cancer cure, positive surgical margins and complication are well collected in the pentafecta rate. However, no comparative studies between 4th generation 3D-HD vision system laparoscopy and standard bi-dimensional laparoscopy have been reported. This study aimed to compare the operative, perioperative data and pentafecta rates between 2D and 3D laparoscopic radical prostatectomy (LRP) and to identify the actual role of 3D LRP in urology.

Methods: From October 2012 to July 2013, 86 patients with clinically localized prostate cancer [PCa: age ≤ 70 years, prostate-specific antigen (PSA) ≤ 10 ng/ml, biopsy Gleason score ≤ 7] underwent laparoscopic extraperitoneal radical prostatectomy (LERP) and were followed for approximately 14 months (range 12–25). Patients were selected for inclusion via hospital record data, and divided into two groups. Their patient records were then analyzed. Patients were randomized into two groups: the former 2D-LERP (43 pts) operated with the use of 2D-HD camera; the latter 3D-LERP (43 pts) operated with the use of a 3D-HD 4th generation view system. The operative and perioperative data and the pentafecta rates between 2D-LERP and 3D-LERP were compared.

Results: The overall pentafecta rates at 3 months were 47.4% and 49.6% in the 2D- and 3D-LERP group respectively. The pentafecta rate at 12 months was 62.7% and 67% for each group respectively. 4th generation 3D-HD vision system provides advantages over standard bi-dimensional view with regard to intraoperative steps. Our data suggest a trend of improvement in intraoperative blood loss and postoperative recovery of continence with the respect of the oncological safety.

Conclusions: Use of the 3D technology by a single surgeon significantly enhances the possibility of achieving better intraoperative results and pentafecta in all patients undergoing LERP. Potency was the most difficult outcome to reach after surgery, and it was the main factor leading to pentafecta failure. Nevertheless, further studies are necessary to better comprehend the role of 3D-LERP in modern urology.

Keywords: Laparoscopic radical prostatectomy, Pentafecta, 3D laparoscopy, Prostatectomy

* Correspondence: pierluigi.bove@uniroma2.it
Department of Urology, Tor Vergata University of Rome, V.le Oxford 81,
00133 Rome, Italy

Background

Prostate cancer is the most common tumor in people aged over 50 and is the second leading cause of cancer death in Europe and in the United States. Worldwide, nearly 900,000 men were estimated to have been diagnosed with prostate cancer during 2008 and 258,000 men died for this reason [1]. Incidence in Western countries is higher than in less developed ones where it is slowly increasing. Furthermore, there were recent significant decreases in prostate cancer mortality in Europe and in the United States. In contrast, mortality rates have increased in other countries [2,3]. Decreasing mortality rates is mainly due to earlier diagnosis and improved treatment.

Laparoscopic radical prostatectomy (LRP) has become an established treatment for organ confined prostate cancer and is increasingly performed at selected centers worldwide even though open radical retropubic prostatectomy (RRP) is widely considered the treatment of choice. For the first time in 1992 Schuessler carried out a LRP in order to transfer the well-known advantages of the laparoscopic technique to the most common open surgical treatment for prostate cancer [4]. Only after years, Guillonneau and Valencien improved the techniques obtaining results similar to those of open surgery but, because of the steep learning curve, laparoscopic radical prostatectomy has slowly risen in popularity [5]. The advent of robotic surgery has further helped to confine laparoscopic surgery to a special niche. Shorter learning curve, three-dimensional view as well as the ease of movement offered by the Da Vinci® operating arms have made robot-assisted laparoscopic prostatectomy (RALP) more reproducible despite the higher costs. So RALP is easier to learn and is now the surgical treatment of choice in most centers of excellence in the United States [6].

Nowadays, laparoscopic surgery could be regenerated by the introduction of a high-resolution three-dimensional view (3D). 3D techniques have been improved in comparison to the first generation of 3D vision system introduced in the 90s and can even replace the classic bi-dimensional view [7]. 3rd-generation three-dimensional view was introduced about 10 years ago but few experiences were reported in literature probably due to some limit of this technique. The use of a quite heavy helmet with a head mounted display caused surgeon fatigue [8,9]. 4th-generation three-dimensional system uses more ergonomic glasses and an innovated technology.

Better knowledge of pelvic anatomy, improvements in surgical technique have led to improved oncological results and reduced adverse functional outcomes. Historically, outcomes of continence, erectile function, and oncologic control were the major surgical achievement and were called 'trifecta' outcomes. Nowadays, patients with a diagnosis of prostate cancer are younger, healthier and have higher expectations from the advanced minimally invasive surgical technologies. Hence, the 'pentafecta' was proposed as a new method of outcomes analysis by adding early complications and positive surgical margins (PSMs) to trifecta [10]. According to these theories, pentafecta has become a new cornerstone in the analysis of urological surgery results.

In this pilot randomized study, we aim to highlight the differences between the standard two-dimensional (2D) with the 4th-generation three-dimensional view (3D) applied to laparoscopic extraperitoneal radical prostatectomy (LERP) in order to assess if the 3D visualization of the operative field could really improve intraoperative and perioperative steps and the pentafecta outcomes.

Methods

Patients and technologies

From October 2012 to July 2013, all patients with clinical T1c prostate tumor, belonging to low/intermediate D'Amico risk group, were included in the study. 86 consecutive patients, who met these criteria, underwent LERP. Patients were selected for inclusion via hospital record data. The data were collected in a database and retrospectively analyzed. Fondazione PTV – Policlinico Tor Vergata Ethic Committee approved our clinical study and data collection. In accordance with our institution's Ethic Committee, informed and signed consent was obtained from each patient prior treatment. A statement of ethical approval covered permission to access patient records and use them for study purposes. All patients constituting the cohort had at least 1 yr follow-up.

Patients were randomized into two groups: the former 2D-LERP (43 pts) operated with the use of 2D-HD Storz® camera with a 10 mm 0° laparoscope; the latter 3D-LERP (43 pts) operated with the use of a 3D-HD Viking® camera with a 10 mm and 0° lens double-channel stereolaparoscope. The 3D view is achieved with the help of a 3DHD Viking® screen and with the use of polarized glasses. The glasses are filtered; each lens only lets one direction of light pass through the eye, thus maintaining two perspectives of the image and giving a tridimensional vision.

Procedures: surgery and rehabilitation

All 86 patients were operated by the same surgeon (P.B.) following the same surgical technique of LERP. A 1,5 cm cutaneous incision is made at 1 cm below the inferior margin of the umbilicus and a dilator device is inserted into the preperitoneal space and about 300 ml of air is inflated to develop the space of Retzius (pneumo-Retzius). 4 secondary trocars are then placed under laparoscopic view (2 for each iliac fossa, right and left) in the inverted fan configuration. The endopelvic fascia is incised on each side and bladder neck is dissected and isolated through the "bladder neck sparing" technique. Once the bladder neck is opened close to the prostate, the posterior lip of the bladder neck is lowered to provide access to the interprostatorectal plane. Vasa deferentes and seminal vesicles are isolated and dissected. Then, prostatic pedicles are incised in an anterograde mode with preservation of the neurovascular bundle when it is indicated. Finally, a meticulous preparation of the urethral stump introduces to the vesicourethral anastomosis which is collected in interrupted sutures [11].

The drainage is left in place until leakage is observed, and normally it is removed on second post-operative day. Urinary fistula is defined as prolonged drainage over postoperative day 10. The catheter is normally removed between 7 and 10 days after surgery; in case of urinary fistula a cystography is carried out on 14th and 21st postoperative day and both drainage and catheter are removed at the complete closure of the anastomosis.

Baseline sexual and urinary functions were assessed before LERP with self-administered, validated questionnaires: the International Index of Erectile Function 6 (IIEF-6) and the Incontinence Quality of Life (I-QoL) [12,13].

Pelvic floor muscles exercises were recommended for all patients immediately after catheter removal in order to facilitate continence recovery. After catheter removal, all patients received phosphodiesterase type 5 (PDE5) inhibitors at least three times a week and began penile rehabilitation no later than three weeks after radical surgery by using intracavernous pharmacotherapy (ICP) with Prostaglandin E1 (alprostadil).

Data collection
Operative and perioperative data. Operative time (OT – from skin to skin closure), anastomosis time (AT – time to complete the anastomosis till the catheter insertion), number of stitches used (NuS), estimated blood loss (EBL) and any intraoperative complication were recorded. Perioperative data include: days of drainage (DD), days of catheterization (DC), hospital stay (HS), pathological staging and complications. Histopathologic staging was performed according to the 2002 TNM system [14].

Pentafecta. The five outcomes included in the analysis of the pentafecta are complications, positive surgical margins (PSMs) and the trifecta outcomes (urinary continence, sexual potency, biochemical recurrence BCR-free survival rates). Pentafecta is achieved if there were no complications, negative surgical margins and if the patient was continent, potent and BCR-free.

Statistical analysis
Fisher test was used to analyze non-parametric data as appropriate. Student t-test was used to analyze parametric data such as patients' characteristics, intra and remaining perioperative data. Results were considered significant if the p value was ≤ 0.05.

Results
There were not significant differences between the two groups in terms of age, body mass index (BMI), preoperative PSA level and biopsy Gleason score. Patients' characteristics are summarized in Table 1.

Operative and perioperative data
Operative and perioperative data are presented in Table 2. Median OT for 3D-LERP was significantly shorter than that in 2D-LERP (162 versus 241 minutes, p 0.01). Moreover, in the 3D LERP group, median OT for the first 3 cases was significantly longer than the remaining cases due to the initial operator learning curve. Statistically significant differences were also recorded in median AT (24 versus 32 minutes, p 0.03) and median NuS (5.65 versus 6.45, p 0.018). Median EBL did not reach a statistical significance in the two groups with two patients requiring transfusion in the 2D group and 1 patient in the 3D group. No conversion to open surgery was necessary and no complications occurred requiring early re-intervention. Median HS was 7.6 and 5.5 days for the 2D-LERP and 3D-LERP respectively (p = 0.180). Median DD was 5 in the 2D-LERP and 4,5 in the 3D-LERP (p = 0.925). The median CT was of 10.55 days and 10.75 days for the 2D to 3D respectively (p = 0.880).

Complications
Complications can be considered as a perioperative outcome. We discussed complications apart from the other perioperative data in order to underline their role in the pentafecta.

Modified Clavien grading system was used to classify complications occurring during the surgical procedure or within 90 days after surgery (early complications) [15].

Twenty-three of 86 patients experienced complications. More specifically, perioperative complications were reported in 15 (34.8%) cases in the 2D-LRP and in 8 (18.6%) cases in the 3D-LRP. 2D-LRP and 3D-LRP complications

Table 1 Preoperative data

Variable	2D	3D
Age, yr, mean	60.1	63.9
BMI, mean	25.2	24.6
Preoperative PSA value (ng/mL)	6.7	6.2
Biopsy Gleason score	6.15	6.15

Table 2 Intraoperative and perioperative data

Intraoperative data

Variables	2D	3D	P value
Mean operative time (min)	241 (150–350)	162 (90–160)	0,01*
Mean anastomosis time (min)	32 (20–45)	24 (15–50)	0,03*
Number anastomosis stitches	6,45	5,65	0,018*
Mean blood loss (ml)	532 (200–2000)	383 (200–600)	0,11
Perioperative data			
Days of drainage	4.5	4.85	0.92
Days of catheterization	10.55	10.75	0.88
Hospital stay	7.6	5.5	0.18

*Statistically significant differences.

are summarized in Table 3. Minor complications (Clavien grade 1 and 2) represent respectively 80% and 63% for the two groups of all those reported. Major complications (Clavien grade ≥ 3) constituted respectively 20% and 37%. There were no cases of complications graded 4a, 4b and 5 according to the modified Clavien grading system. Data are depicted in Table 3.

Oncologic outcomes: biochemical recurrence and positive surgical margins

Oncological results are presented in Tables 4 and 5. The distribution of pathological stage and Gleason score was similar in the 2 groups.

Table 3 Complications

Modified Clavien grading system	2-D	3-D
	(n = 43)	(n = 43)
Grade 1	Penis and scrotum edema	Penis and scrotum edema
	(n = 7)	(n = 5)
	Hematuria (n = 1)	0
	bladder catheter exchange (n = 1)	0
Grade 2	transfusions (n = 2)	0
	Epididymitis (n = 1)	
Grade 3a	AUR (n = 1)	AUR (n = 1)
	Anastomotic stenosis (n = 2)	Anastomotic stenosis (n = 1)
Grade 3b	0	Urinary fistula (n = 1)
Grade 4a-b/5	0	0
Total (%)	34.8% (15)	18.6% (8)
	Minor 80%	Minor 63%
	Major 20%	Major 37%

Table 4 Histopathologic data

	2-D	3-D
	(n = 43)	(n = 43)
Pathologic stage		
pT2a	5 (12%)	6 (14%)
pT2b	3 (7%)	3 (7%)
pT2c	25 (58%)	23 (54%)
pT3a	7 (16%)	8 (18%)
pT3b	3 (7%)	3 (7%)
Specimen Gleason score		
6 (3 + 3)	23 (53%)	23 (53%)
7 (3 + 4)	8 (18%)	9 (21%)
7 (4 + 3)	11 (26%)	9 (21%)
8 (4 + 4)	1 (2%)	2 (5%)

The overall PSM rate was 9% in the 2D-LERP and 4% in the 3D-LERP. When stratified by pathological stage, PSM rate was significantly different in pT2c/pT3 disease between groups (halved in the 3D-LERP compared with the 2D-LRP group).

BCR was defined as two consecutive prostate-specific antigen (PSA) levels of >0.2 ng/ml [16]. The overall BCR-free rate at 3 months was 93% (2D-LERP, 40 patients) and 95% (3D-LERP, 41 patients). Reassessed at 12 months, the overall BCR-free rate was 88% (2D-LERP, 38 patients) and 91% (3D-LERP, 39 patients). Patients with recurrences underwent further salvage therapy with either radiation and/or hormonal treatment. Aligned with the literature data, 25% of the patients with BCR had PSMs.

Urinary continence

According to the European Association of Urology Guidelines (EAU Guidelines, 2013), urinary incontinence represents a postoperative complication that persists after 1 year in 7.7% of patients who underwent radical prostatectomy [17]. The American Urological Association Guidelines (AUA Guidelines, 2007 updated in 2011)

Table 5 Oncological results

	2-D	3-D
	(n = 43)	(n = 43)
Positive surgical margin	9% (4)	4% (2)
pT2c	2/25	1/23
pT3	2/10	1/11
BCR-free rate (%)		
3 months follow-up	93% (40)	95% (41)
12 months follow-up	88% (38)	91% (39)

report a rate of postoperative urinary incontinence that ranges between 3% and 74% [18].

Urinary continence was assessed with the self-administered, validated questionnaire Incontinence Quality of Life (I-QoL). The definition of continence was based on a specific question appropriate to reflect the range of incontinence severity: "How many pads per day did you usually use to control urine leakage during the last 4 weeks?". We considered "dry" patients without any loss of urine (no pads/day) or those who used a safety pad/day.

The overall continence rates did not reach a statistically significant difference although the trend is clearly favorable to the 3D-LERP group (89% and 92% vs 83% and 88% of patients were continent at 3 and 12 month follow-up in the 3D and 2D-LERP group respectively).

I-QoL questionnaire showed a significant quality of life improvement at the first month in the 3D (mean score 90,45) compared to the 2D-LERP group (mean score 81,8) (p = 0.01). These positive results are also confirmed at third (93.3 vs 83.6 - p = 0.01) and twelfth (95.4 vs 88.1 p = 0.03) month follow-up in the 3D compared to the 2D-LERP group respectively. Pre- and postoperative urinary continence data are depicted in Table 6.

Erectile function

It is widely recognized that the preoperative Erectile Function (EF) is an important prognostic factor for erectile dysfunction recovery after radical prostatectomy [19]. Several other factors are predictive for EF recovery after surgery: age, type of surgery, pre- and post-RP libido, adjuvant treatments, comorbidities, urinary continence, availability of a partner and sane mental health. Therefore, it is essential to determine the EF baseline. The International Consultation on Sexual Medicine (ICSM) Committee recommends the use of validated psychometric instruments such as IIEF. In our experience, potency rate has been assessed using the IIEF-6. After surgery, erectile function rehabilitation was recommended for all patients (scheme reported above) in order to preserve the functional smooth muscle tissue of

the corpora cavernosa and to avoid the effects of the surgical-related neuroapraxia [20].

Preoperative Potency was defined as the ability to achieve and maintain satisfactory erection for sexual activity or as a score IIEF-6 score ≥ 17 (without pharmacological or mechanical support). Post-operative potency was defined as the ability to achieve and maintain erections firm enough for sexual intercourse in more than 50% of attempts, with or without the use of iPDE5 and with eventual ICP (IIEF-6 score ≥ 17).

Patients were subjected to bilateral or unilateral nerve-sparing surgery (NSS). The overall potency rates were 60% and 67% at 3 months and 67% and 72% at 12 months in the 2D- and 3D-LERP group respectively. Type of surgery, pre-surgical evaluation of erectile function and potency outcomes are summarized in Tables 7 and 8.

Pentafecta outcomes

The overall pentafecta rate at 3 months was 47.4% and 49.6% in the 2D- and 3D-LERP group respectively. The pentafecta rate at 12 months was 62.7% and 67% for each group respectively.

The most common reasons for not achieving the pentafecta were erectile dysfunction (33% and 28% respectively in 2D-LERP and 3D-LERP; trifecta not achieved) and complication rate (34.8% and 18.6%, 2D vs 3D). Furthermore, urinary incontinence (12% and 8%, 2D vs 3D), BCR (12% and 9%, 2D vs 3D) and positive surgical margins (9% and 4%, 2D vs 3D). Results are shown in Table 9.

Discussion

In the past decade, a dramatic shift towards lower-stage tumors has become evident. Currently, men are younger at the time of diagnosis and more interested in less invasive surgical approaches (eg. Laparoscopy, robotics) than they are for the traditional approach [21]. At the same time and more importantly, normal continence and preserving sexual function are fundamental but not the only primary goals of radical prostatectomy. Patients want to know if the treatment option will render them cancer free with a minimum of complications and the shortest possible convalescence time while preserving continence and potency [10].

These observations highlight two main topics: on one hand, the possibility of considering a minimally invasive surgical approach with its innovative technical characteristics

Table 6 Continence data

Pad system	2-D	3-D
	n = 43	n = 43
Pre-operative	100% (43)	100% (43)
3 months follow-up	83% (36)	89% (38)
12 months follow-up	88% (38)	92% (40)
IQoL	2-D	3-D
	n = 43	n = 43
3 months follow-up	83,6	93,3
12 months follow-up	88,1	95,4

Table 7 Potency surgical approach

Nerve sparing surgery	2-D	3-D
Monolateral	42% (18)	37% (16)
Bilateral	58% (25)	63% (27)

Table 8 Potency data

Erectile Function IIEF 6 ≥ 17	2-D	3-D
	n = 43	n = 43
Pre-operatory	86% (37)	88% (38)
3 months follow-up	60% (26)	67% (29)
12 months follow-up	67% (29)	72% (31)

every time that it is possible and, on the other hand, the necessity of adopting a more comprehensive method of reporting peri- and post-operative outcomes.

By adopting the laparoscopic technique with adherence to established oncological principles, the aim is to duplicate the open surgical method in its entirety. LRP has slowly risen in popularity and has become, in some centers, the surgical approach of choice for the treatment of localized prostate cancer for its advantages. Lower blood loss and transfusion rate associated with the laparoscopic approach together with shorter hospital stay, reduced catheterization time, better pain control and faster return to everyday activities seem to be the most encouraging improvements obtained [22].

Unfortunately, classic laparoscopic surgery is limited by a two-dimensional vision that does not allow perception of the operative field as in open surgery. The lack of depth perception has repercussions both on the learning curve, which still constitutes a major obstacle to the development of laparoscopy [23], and in the possibility for the surgeon to maneuver the instruments with an accuracy comparable to that which would occur in the same "open" operation. Even if the experienced surgeon is able over time to regain some vision of depth, this will never be optimal [24].

For this reason and through the increasing popularity of laparoscopy, a three-dimensional display system was introduced in the early 90s, with the expectation that this technique could make laparoscopic interventions safer and faster[23]. Up to now, just a few studies on three-dimensional laparoscopy have been written without any definite conclusion about its utility. Some articles describe better results with 3D laparoscopic technique than with the 2D system

Table 9 Variables comprising the pentafecta success rates at 12 mo

Variable	2D LERP		3D LERP	
	Patients	%	Patients	%
Complication	28/43	65	35/43	81
PSM	39/43	91	41/43	96
BCR-free rate	38/43	88	39/43	91
Continence	38/43	88	40/43	92
Potency	29/43	67	31/43	72
Pentafecta	27/43	62,7	29/43	67

both in surgical training exercises and in different surgical procedures. Exercises like linear cutting and suturing, curved cutting and suturing, tubular suturing and dorsal vein complex suturing simulation have been performed and it has been suggested that the new-generation 3D system could be helpful in laparoscopy [25-27].

In the 90s, comparative studies were organized to evaluate the improvement and superiority of vision between traditional 2D and 3D system (3rd generation) in terms of dissection of the kidney, securing of the renal vessels and laparoscopic suturing, but the Authors found no differences between the two vision systems, either with respect to the accuracy and speed of surgical execution, nor as regards to the learning curve [28-32]. Gynecologists and general surgeons have described similar studies in the field of 3D laparoscopic surgery with discordant conclusions [33-35].

Robotic surgery had a great benefit from the three-dimensional view. The advent of Da Vinci® has further helped to confine laparoscopic prostatectomy to a special niche. Shorter learning curve, three-dimensional view as well as the ease of movement offered by the operating arms, makes robot-assisted laparoscopic prostatectomy (RALP) more reproducible despite the higher costs. This way, Robertson et al. recently underlined that RALP is easier to learn and is now the surgical treatment of choice in most centers of excellence in the United States [22].

This is the first study reported in urologic literature that aims to establish, after twenty years since the first 3D model was introduced, the utility of the 4th generation 3D vision system during LERP in terms of feasibility and potential advantages over the 2D vision system regarding operative and perioperative data and the pentafecta outcomes. Only one work reported by Good et al. in 2013 analyzed the pentafecta learning curve for laparoscopic radical prostatectomy [36].

Transition from the 2D to 3D vision system, requires an initial period of adaptation. This is demonstrated by longer operative time and the incidence of postoperative urinary fistula that occurred at the very beginning of our experience using the 3D vision system. This short learning curve is related to a new perception of the depth of the operative field that requires a different spatial assessment of instrument positioning rather than an initial difficulty in recognizing anatomical landmarks avoiding possible complications. Once adaptation to 3D view is reached, a more realistic visualization of the surgical field allows greater speed and precision in the movement of the surgical instrument. This translates in a better preparation of the bladder neck and the urethral stamp reducing anastomosis time. Although not resulting in a statistically significant difference, the easy identification of small vessels using the 3D vision may reduce blood loss.

Despite the necessary adaptation from 2D to 3D vision by an expert laparoscopist, on the other hand, the 3D vision may offer significant advantages in teaching laparoscopic skills to inexperienced individuals [37].

Meticulous handling and tissue dissection obtained with the auxilium of the 3D view have allowed earlier continence recovery. This could be mainly related to less trauma and greater sphincter- structures saving [38] as demonstrated by a better I-QoL and a decreased number of pads per day in the 3D LERP Group. One of the operating steps that gets more advantages from the 3D view is the dissection of seminal vesicles, vas deferens and prostatic pedicles. Dissection of these delicate structures makes 3D vision very effective. Basically, these operating stages and their higher accuracy might affect a possible earlier and better recovery of erectile function.

These encouraging results obtained with the 3D vision system were associated with a number of positive surgical margins and post-operative complications comparable in both groups demonstrating a good oncological and functional efficacy. From our point of view, some problems related to the prolonged use of 3D vision such as headaches, fatigue and nausea, already reported in previous studies, have still remained unresolved, but it is not an important limitation to its use [39,40].

Statistically significant differences were recorded for all intraoperative steps and data suggest a trend of improvement in intraoperative blood loss, postoperative recovery of continence and potency with the respect of the oncological safety for the 4th generation 3D-HD vision system of the 3D-LERP over standard bi-dimensional view in 2D-LERP.

One of the advantages of this study is that the comparison between the 2D and 3D surgical procedures was performed by a single surgeon making it more reliable and avoiding possible bias. Despite this fact, the extensive experience of the surgeon may have influenced the results and complication rates of our study and, as a result, the outcomes cannot be generalized.

However, this study has several limitations. First of all, being a pilot study, with a small number of procedures and a relatively short follow-up, it does not allow the definition of the definitive role of this technique. Data analysis was a retrospective. Some data may not reach a statistical significance between groups because the study was not powered to identify these differences; nevertheless, a trend of improvement in surgical and functional outcomes has been shown. Furthermore, we included both bilateral and monolateral NSS procedures. Another limitation is that we did not use the Expanded Prostate Cancer Index Composite (EPIC) questionnaire to better assess urinary symptoms. Finally, the study is limited by the short follow-up, which can affect BCR-free and functional outcomes.

Nowadays, all the laparoscopic prostatectomies in our Department are performed with the auxilium of 3D video system. If these preliminary data will be confirmed by larger follow-up of a greater number of patients, the 4th generation 3D laparoscopy may play an important role in the treatment of prostate cancer.

Conclusions

This preliminary study has shown that 4th generation 3D-HD vision system provides advantages over standard bi-dimensional view with regard to intraoperative steps. Our data suggest a trend of improvement in intraoperative blood loss and early postoperative recovery of continence along with the respect of the oncological safety. Pentafecta has been reached with a higher score for the 3D-HD LERP.

Given the large number of men diagnosed with prostate cancer and the exponential growth of the medical costs on a global level, it would be better that treatment options are not only effective but also less expensive. In this context, the 3D laparoscopy may be an intermediate step between the standard 2D laparoscopy and robot-assisted laparoscopy, allowing the combination of the low cost of the first with the 3D technology of the second. Further studies are necessary to better comprehend the role of 3D-LERP in modern urology.

Abbreviations

LRP: Laparoscopic radical prostatectomy; LERP: Laparoscopic extraperitoneal radical prostatectomy; RRP: Radical retropubic prostatectomy; RALP: Robot-assisted laparoscopic prostatectomy; 3D HD: High-definition three dimensional view; PSMs: Positive surgical margins; IIEF 6: International index of erectile function 6; IQoL: Incontinence quality of life; PDE5: Phosphodiesterase type 5; ICP: Intracavernous pharmacotherapy; OT: Operative time; AT: Anastomosis time; NuS: Number of stitches; EBL: Estimated blood loss; DD: Days of drainage; DC: Days of catheterization; HS: Hospital stay; BCR: Biochemical recurrence; BMI: Body mass index; EAU: European association of urology; AUA: American urological association; ICSM: International consultation on sexual medicine; NSS: Nerve-sparing surgery; EPIC: Expanded prostate cancer index composite.

Competing interests

The authors declared that they have no competing interests.

Authors' contributions

PB carried out the surgical procedures and drafted the manuscript. VI carried out the surgical procedures as assistant and drafted the manuscript. FC carried out the surgical procedures as assistant and participated in the design of the study. FDC collected all the data and performed the statistical analysis. GV carried out the surgical procedures. EFA conceived the study, participated in its design and coordination and helped to draft the manuscript. All authors read and approved the final manuscript.

References

1. International Agency for Research on Cancer (IARC) Ferlay J, Shin HR, Bray F, Forman D, Mathers C, Parkin DM. GLOBOCAN 2008 ver. 2.0. Cancer incidence and mortality worldwide: IARC CancerBase No. 10 Lyon: IARC; c2010. Cited 2012 Jul 12. http://globocan.iarc.fr.
2. Center M, Jemal A, Bray F, et al. International variation in prostate cancer incidence and mortality rates. Eur Urol. 2012;61:1079–92.

3. Baade PD, Youlden DR, Krnjacki LJ. International epidemiology of prostate cancer: geographical distribution and secular trends. Mol Nutr Food Res. 2009;53:171–84.

4. Schuessler W, Sculam P, Clayman R, Kavoussi L. Laparoscopic radical prostatectomy: initial short-term experience. Urology. 1997;50:854–7.

5. Guillonneau B, Vallancien G. Laparoscopic radical prostatectomy: the Montsouris technique. J Urol. 2000;163:1643–9.

6. Hakimi AA, Feder M, Ghavamian R. Minimally invasive approaches to prostate cancer a review of the current literature. Urol J. 2007;4:130–7.

7. Zobel J. Basics of three-dimensional endoscopic vision. Endosc Surg Allied Technol. 1993;1:36–9.

8. Bhayani SB, Andriole GL. Three-dimensional (3D) vision: does It improve laparoscopic skills? an assessment of a 3D head-mounted visualization system. Rev Urol. 2005;7(4):211–4.

9. Mueller MD, Camartin C, Dreher E. Ha¨nggi W.: three-dimensional laparoscopy gadget or progress? a randomized trial on the efficacy of three-dimensional laparoscopy. Surg Endosc. 1999;13:469–72.

10. Patel VR, Sivaraman A, Coelho RF, Chauhan S, Palmer KJ, Orvieto MA, et al. Pentafecta: a new concept for reporting outcomes of robot-assisted laparoscopic radical prostatectomy. Eur Urol. 2011;59(5):702–7.

11. Bove P, Iacovelli V. Laparoscopic radical prostatectomy. In: Laparoscopy – an interdisciplinary approach. Meinhold-Heerlein I, editor, InTech; ISBN: 978-953-307-299-9, Available from: http://www.intechopen.com/books/laparoscopy-an-interdisciplinary-approach/laparoscopic-radical-prostatectomy 2011.

12. Rosen RC, Cappelleri JC, Gendrano 3rd N. The international index of erectile function (IIEF): a state-of-the-science review. Int J Impot Res. 2002;14(4):226–44.

13. Wagner TH, Patrick DL, Bavendam TG, Martin ML, Buesching DP. Quality of life of persons with urinary incontinence: development of a new measure. Urology. 1996;47(1):67–71. discussion 71–2.

14. Greene FL, Page DL, Fleming ID, et al. American joint committee on cancer staging manual, ed 6. New York, NY: Springer; 2002. p. 77–87.

15. Dindo D, Demartines N, Clavien P. Classification of surgical complications. Ann Surg. 2004;240:205–13.

16. Heidenreich A, Aus G, Bolla M, et al. EAU guidelines on prostate cancer [in Spanish]. Actas Urol Esp. 2009;33:113–26.

17. Heidenreich A, Bellmunt J, Bolla M, et al. EAU guidelines on prostate cancer. Part 1: screening, diagnosis, and treatment of clinically localised disease. Eur Urol. 2011;59:61–71.

18. Thompson I, Thrasher JB, Aus G, Burnett AL, Canby-Hagino ED, Cookson MS, et al. American Urological Association. Guideline for the management of clinically localized prostate cancer: 2007 update. J Urol. 2007;177(6):2106–31.

19. Salonia A, Burnett AL, Grefen M, Montorsi F, et al. Prevention and management of Postprostatectomy sexual dysfunctions. Eur Urol. 2012;62:261–72.

20. Mulhall JP et al. Phosphodiesterase type 5 inhibitors in Postprostatectomy erectile dysfunction: a critical analysis of the basic science rationale and clinical application. Eur Urol. 2009;55:334–47.

21. Schroeck FR, Krupski TL, Sun L, et al. Satisfaction and regret after open retropubic or robot-assisted laparoscopic radical prostatectomy. Eur Urol. 2008;54:785–93.

22. Robertson C, Close A, Fraser C, Gurung T, Jia X, Sharma P, et al. Relative effectiveness of robot-assisted and standard laparoscopic prostatectomy as alternatives to open radical prostatectomy for treatment of localised prostate cancer: a systematic review and mixed treatment comparison meta-analysis. BJU Int. 2013;112(6):798–812.

23. Abdelshehid CS, Eichel L, Lee D, et al. Current trends in urologic laparoscopic surgery. J Endourol. 2005;19:15–20.

24. Hofmeister J, Frank TG, Cuschieri A, Wade NJ. Perceptual aspects of two dimensional and stereoscopic display techniques in endoscopic surgery: review and current problems. Semin Laparosc Surg. 2001;8:12–24.

25. Patel HRH, Ribal MJ, Arya M, et al. Is It worth revisiting laparoscopic three-dimensional visualization? a validated assessment. Urology. 2007;70:47–9.

26. Badani KK, Bhandari A, Tewari A, et al. Comparison of Two-dimensional and three-dimensional suturing: is there a difference in a robotic surgery setting? J Endourol. 2005;19:1212–5.

27. Peitgen K, Walz MV, Holtmann G, Eigler FW. A prospective randomized experimental evaluation of three-dimensional imaging in laparoscopy. Gastrointest Endosc. 1996;44:262–7.

28. Chiu AW, Babayan RK. Retroperitoneal laparoscopic nephrectomy utilizing three-dimensional camera case report. J Endourol. 1994;8:139–41.

29. Babayan RK, Chiu AW, Este-McDonald J, Birkett DH. The comparison between 2-dimensional and 3-dimensional laparoscopic video systems in a pelvic trainer. J Endourol. 1993;7:S195.

30. McDougall EM, Soble JJ, Wolf JS, Nakada SY, Elashry OM, Clayman RV. Comparison of three-dimensional and two-dimensional laparoscopic video systems. J Endourol. 1996;10:371–4.

31. Jones DB, Brewer JD, Soper NJ. The influence of three-dimensional video systems on laparoscopic task performance. Surg Laparosc Endosc. 1996;6:191–7.

32. Chan ACW, Chung SCS, Yim APC, et al. Comparison of two-dimensional vs three-dimensional camera systems in laparoscopic surgery. Surg Endosc. 1997;11:438–40.

33. Wenzl R, Lehner R, Vry U, Pateisky N, Sevelda P, Husslein P. Three-dimensional video endoscopy: clinical use in gynaecological laparoscopy. Lancet. 1994;344:1621–2.

34. Hanna GB, Shimi SM, Cuschieri A. Randomized study of the influence of two dimensional –versus three dimensional imaging on performance of laparoscopic cholecystectomy. Lancet. 1998;351:248–51.

35. Hanna GB, Cuschieri A. Influence of two-dimensional and three-dimensional imaging on endoscopic bowel suturing. World J Surg. 2000;24(4):444–8.

36. Good DW, Stewart GD, Stolzenburg JU, McNeill SA. Analysis of the pentafecta learning curve for laparoscopic radical prostatectomy. World J Urol. 2014;32(5):1225–33.

37. Votanopoulos K, Brunicardi FC, Thornby J, et al. Impact of three-dimensional vision in laparoscopic training. World J Surg. 2008;32:110–8.

38. Schlomm T, Huland H, et al. Full functional-length urethral sphincter preservation during radical prostatectomy. Eur Urol. 2011;60:320–9.

39. Pietrabissa A, Cancello E, Carobbi A, et al. Three-dimensional versus two-dimensional video system for the trained endoscopic surgeon and the beginner. Endosc Surg Allied Technol. 1994;2:315–7.

40. Taffinder N, Smith SGT, Huber J, et al. The effect of a second-generation 3D endoscope on the laparoscopic precision of novices and experienced surgeons. Surg Endosc. 1999;13:1087–92.

Comparison of continence outcomes of early catheter removal on postoperative day 2 and 4 after laparoscopic radical prostatectomy

Masashi Matsushima, Akira Miyajima*, Seiya Hattori, Toshikazu Takeda, Ryuichi Mizuno, Eiji Kikuchi and Mototsugu Oya

Abstract

Background: The optimal timing of catheter removal following laparoscopic radical prostatectomy (LRP) has not yet been determined. This prospective study was designed to compare the efficacy and safety of catheter removal on postoperative day (POD) 2 versus POD 4 after LRP and its impact on urinary continence outcomes.

Methods: One hundred and thirteen patients underwent LRP and were prospectively randomized into two groups: group 1 ($n = 57$) had the urinary catheter removed on POD 2 while group 2 ($n = 56$) had the catheter removed on POD 4. The urine loss ratio (ULR) was defined as the weight of urine loss in the pad divided by the daily micturition volume. Continence was defined as a pad-free status.

Results: No significant differences were observed in clinical features between groups 1 and 2. Acute urinary retention (AUR) after catheter removal occurred in 21 patients (18.6 %) (13 (22.8 %) in group 1 and 8 (14.3 %) in group 2 ($p = 0.244$). The first-day mean ULR values were 1.16 ± 4.95 in group 1 and 1.02 ± 3.27 in group 2 ($p = 0.870$). The last-day mean ULR values were 0.57 ± 1.60 in group 1 and 2.78 ± 15.49 in group 2 ($p = 0.353$). Continence rates at 3, 6, 9, and 12 months were 21.8, 41.1, 58.0, and 71.4 % in group 1 and 34.5, 66.0, 79.2, and 83.7 % in group 2 ($p = 0.138, 0.009, 0.024$, and 0.146, respectively). In AUR cases, continence rates at 3, 6, 9, and 12 months were 0, 23.1, 38.5, and 54.5 % in group 1 and 37.5, 75.0, 87.5, and 87.5 % in group 2 ($p = 0.017, 0.020, 0.027$, and 0.127, respectively). A multivariate analysis identified AUR after catheter removal on POD 2 as the only predictive factor for incontinence 6 and 9 months after LRP ($p = 0.030$ and 0.018, respectively).

Conclusions: Our results demonstrated that early catheter removal on POD 2 after LRP may increase the risk of incontinence.

Keywords: Laparoscopic radical prostatectomy, Early catheter removal, Urinary incontinence, Prostate cancer

* Correspondence: akiram@a8.keio.jp
Department of Urology, Keio University School of Medicine, 35
Shinanomachi, Shinjuku-ku, Tokyo 160-8582, Japan

Background

The management of patients after radical prostatectomy (RP) has historically been associated with a long period of catheterization to allow anastomotic healing. Traditionally, the duration of catheterization has averaged from 10 to 21 days at most urologic centers [1–3]. However, there is currently no objective evidence to support the use of indwelling urinary catheters for such long periods after RP [4]. Furthermore, previous studies on the feasibility of early catheter removal after RP have reported a low complication rate with a high rate of successful catheter removal [5–7].

Several studies reported that protracted catheterization was a major source of discomfort and irritation in patients after RP [4, 5]. Therefore, the indwelling urinary catheter needs to be removed as early as possible without jeopardizing the outcome. A recent study demonstrated that it was safe to remove catheters in most patients 3 to 4 days after RP if cystography showed no urinary extravasation [7].

The technique of laparoscopic radical prostatectomy (LRP) has gained worldwide acceptance as a treatment for localized prostate cancer since the first feasibility report by Schuessler et al. in 1997 and standardization of the technique by Guillonneau et al. in 1999 [8, 9]. The advantages of LRP have been supported by multiple studies and include a shorter inpatient stay, better pain control, faster return to everyday activities, and decreased short-term complications [10]. A definite advantage may be reduced catheterization time after LRP because vesicourethral anastomosis (VUA) is performed under direct vision, and there is better luminosity and magnification with no blind knotting [11]. Nadu et al. revealed the absence of contrast medium leakage in 84.9 % of patients 2-4 days after LRP, and also that urethral catheter removal could then be safely performed [11].

Urinary incontinence is one of the most feared complications of RP, LRP, and robot-assisted LRP (RALP). In a recent meta-analysis, continence rates 12 months after LRP ranged from 66 % to 95 % [12]. The time to continence after removal of a urinary catheter is a common clinical question. Therefore, the urine loss ratio (ULR) after catheter removal has been suggested as a reliable measure to predict the severity and duration of urinary incontinence [13–15].

To the best of our knowledge, the effects of the differential timing of early catheter removal have not yet been elucidated in detail. Therefore, the aim of the present study was to compare the efficacy and safety of urinary catheter removal on postoperative day (POD) 2 versus POD 4 after LRP and its impact on urinary continence outcomes.

Methods

Between March 2012 and September 2014, 125 patients with clinically localized prostate cancer underwent LRP performed by the same experienced surgeon ($\geq$300 LRP cases at study initiation) at Keio University Hospital. Inclusion criteria were as follows: localized prostate cancer without lymph node and distant metastasis and age <75 years. Exclusion criteria were as follows: previous radiotherapy; previous prostatic, bladder neck, urethral, or pelvic surgery; and the presence of an indwelling urinary catheter ($N = 6$). The remaining 119 patients were randomly divided into two groups (1:1) before surgery on the basis of the timing of their catheter removal after LRP. Randomization was carried out after consent using a computer generated random table by an independent researcher who was not directly involved with the study. Random blocks of different lengths were used. Group 1 had the urinary catheter removed on POD 2, while group 2 had the catheter removed on POD 4. Blinding was not possible in this trial because the timing of catheter removal was different. Cystography revealed leakage in three patients in group 1 (5.3 %) on POD 2 and in three patients in group 2 (5.4 %) on POD 4. These six patients with extravasation were excluded from the data analysis. We identified 113 patients who were followed-up for at least 3 months after LRP as our prospective study population. The primary end-point of this study was the continence rate, and secondary end-points were other complications. A study consort diagram of the randomization procedure is given in Fig. 1.

Ethical approval for the design of this study was granted by the Keio University Hospital Ethical Committee. Prior to undergoing surgery, all patients were informed of the objectives of the present study as well as the timing of catheter removal after LRP (POD 2 or POD 4). Written informed consent was obtained from all patients prior to participation in this study. This study was registered with the University Hospital Medical Information Network Clinical Trials Registry in Japan (UMIN000014944) on 12 March 2012.

Surgical technique

LRP was performed under general anesthesia using an extraperitoneal 5-port approach. Insufflation pressure was typically maintained at 10 mmHg during surgery. Bilateral dissection was limited to the lymph nodes along the external iliac vein and in the obturator fossa. Posterior reconstruction of the rhabdosphincter was performed before VUA, as described by Rocco et al. [16]. V-Loc 180 (barbed polyglyconate suture; Covidien, Mansfield, USA) was used for VUA, and a 20-Fr Foley catheter was inserted after VUA. The integrity of the anastomosis was tested intraoperatively by instilling 120 mL of saline into the bladder. At the end of surgery, an 8-mm drainage tube was placed in the prevesical space. The tube was removed when drainage was less than 100 mL per day, which in many cases was on POD 1.

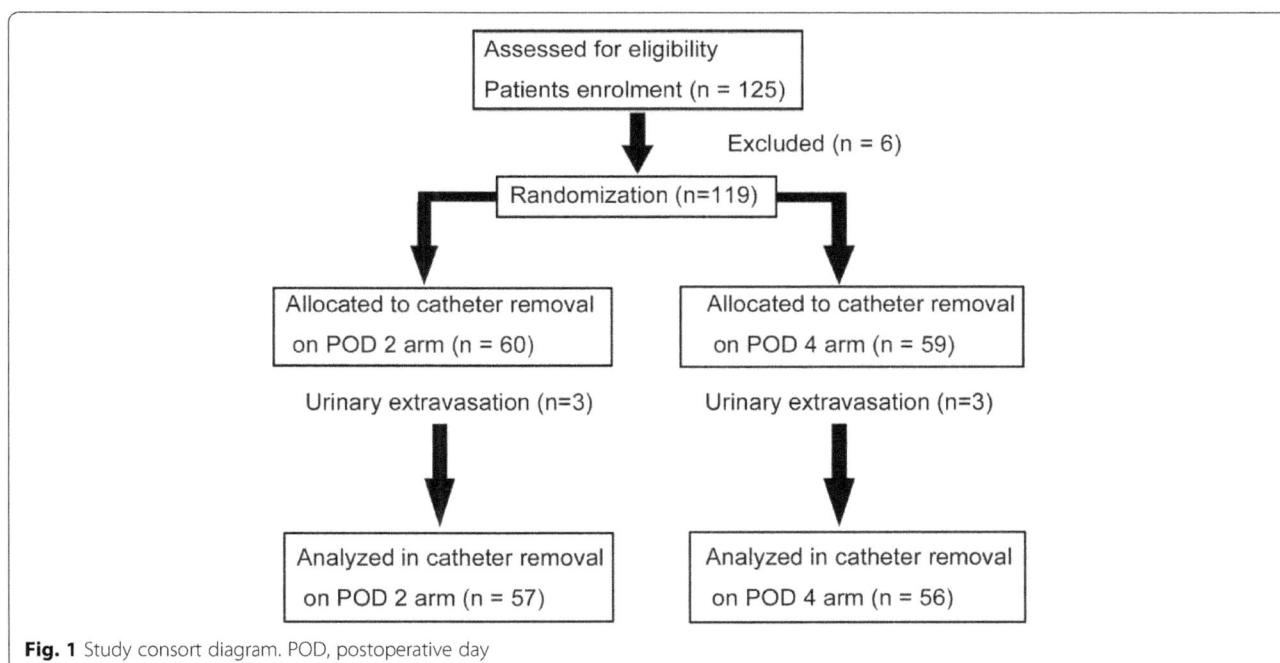

Fig. 1 Study consort diagram. POD, postoperative day

Gravitational cystography was performed on POD 2 or 4 after LRP to check VUA. During cystography, the catheter was advanced slightly to prevent it from compressing the bladder neck, and the bladder was filled with 140 mL of contrast media. Removal of the urinary catheter was performed when the cystogram was normal without any urinary extravasation. If any extravasation of contrast media was observed, the catheter was left in place, and cystography was repeated after a few days. If urinary retention was noted, the catheter was reinserted.

After catheter removal, the 24-h pad test was performed each day during the remaining hospital stay. The 24 hourly total micturition volume was also measured every day until discharge. ULR was defined as the weight of urine loss in the pad divided by the daily micturition volume, distinguishing between ULR on the first day after catheter removal and on the last day of the hospital stay. Previous studies reported that ULR predicted the time to continence [13–15]. The first-day ULR was defined as ULR on the day of catheter removal, and the last-day ULR was described as ULR on the last day of the hospital stay. The maximum ULR was defined as the maximum ULR during the hospital stay, while the minimum ULR was defined as the minimum ULR during the hospital stay. Patients did not take any therapeutic agents for urinary incontinence during the measurement of ULR.

During the follow-up, patients were asked how many pads they required daily. ULR during hospitalization and the number of pads 1, 3, 6, 9, and 12 months

postoperatively were analyzed. Urinary continence was defined as a pad-free status. Complications and continence during the immediate and late postoperative periods were assessed during a follow-up period that ranged from 3 to 30 months (mean 19.9 ± 7.0 months). The continence outcomes of men whose catheters were removed on POD 2 were compared with the outcomes of those whose catheters were removed on POD 4.

Statistical analysis

The power calculation for this study was based on the primary end-point of urinary continence. The minimum clinically important difference was estimated to be 25 %, based on our clinical judgment because no previous similar study has provided continence rates following early catheter removal on different days after LRP. A sample size of 43 patients per arm was required to provide a power of 80 % in order to detect a difference of 25 % with a 2-sided alpha error of 0.05, and adjusting by 20 % for potential dropouts gave a final sample size of 113.

All values are presented as the mean ± standard deviation (S.D.). The Student's t-test and Mann–Whitney U test were used to assess quantitative parametric and nonparametric variables, respectively. The chi-square test was used to assess differences in distributions between categorical parameters. A logistic regression analysis was used to identify a significant set of independent predictors of incontinence 6 and 9 months after LRP. Significance was determined as $p < 0.05$. All analyses were performed using IBM® SPSS® Statistics Version 21

(International Business Machines Corporation, New York, USA).

Results

All LRP procedures were performed safely with no serious complications and no open conversion. There was no intraoperative urinary leakage. The mean age of patients was 65.9 ± 5.5 years, the mean preoperative PSA level was 9.0 ± 6.7 ng/mL, and the median follow-up interval was 21 (3–30) months. The mean prostate volume was 30.2 ± 11.3 mL. The clinical stage was T1c in 38 patients, T2a in 53, T2b in 4, and T2c in 18. The biopsy Gleason score was ≤6 in 22 patients, 7 in 73, and ≥8 in 18. The mean operative time was 177.2 ± 37.4 min, including lymph node dissection. Average blood loss, including urine volume, was 208.2 ± 246.9 mL. Table 1 summarizes the characteristics of the patient population, including age, PSA, prostate volume, biopsy Gleason score, clinical T stage, presence of nerve sparing, operative time, and blood loss.

No significant differences were observed in clinical characteristics between groups 1 and 2 (Table 2). Acute urinary retention (AUR) after catheter removal occurred in 21 patients (18.6 %) (13 (22.8 %) in group 1 and 8 (14.3 %) in group 2 ($p = 0.244$)). These patients were treated with simple catheter replacement for a few days. In every case, the catheter was replaced easily without

Table 2 Comparison of clinical characteristics between group 1 (catheter removal on POD 2) and group 2 (catheter removal on POD 4)

		Group 1 (n = 57)	Group 2 (n = 56)	p value
Age	<65	16	21	0.286
	≥65	41	35	
PSA before LRP	<10	46	37	0.078
	≥10	11	19	
Prostate volume	<30	33	33	0.911
	≥30	24	23	
Gleason score	≤6	10	12	0.602
	≥7	47	44	
Clinical T stage	T1c	16	22	0.207
	T2a,b,c	41	34	
Nerve sparing	+	13	13	0.959
	–	44	43	
Operative time	<150	19	13	0.233
	≥150	38	43	
Blood loss	<100	24	18	0.273
	≥100	33	38	
AUR	+	13	8	0.244
	–	44	48	

POD postoperative day, *LRP* laparoscopic radical prostatectomy, *AUR* acute urinary retention

cystoscopy or fluoroscopy. None of the AUR patients developed hematuria or clots. Bladder neck contracture was not observed.

The first-day mean ULR values were 1.16 ± 4.95 in group 1 and 1.02 ± 3.27 in group 2 ($p = 0.870$). The last-day mean ULR values were 0.57 ± 1.60 in group 1 and 2.78 ± 15.49 in group 2 ($p = 0.353$). The maximum mean ULR values were 1.48 ± 5.13 in group 1 and 2.93 ± 15.47 in group 2 ($p = 0.558$). The minimum mean ULR values were 0.22 ± 0.35 in group 1 and 0.85 ± 3.24 in group 2 ($p = 0.206$). No significant differences were observed between the two groups (Table 3).

Continence rates 3, 6, 9, and 12 months after removal of the urinary catheter were 21.8, 41.1, 58.0, and 71.4 % in group 1 and 34.5, 66.0, 79.2, and 83.7 % in group 2 ($p = 0.138, 0.009, 0.024,$ and 0.146, respectively) (Table 3). Continence rates 6 and 9 months after LRP were significantly lower in group 1 than in group 2. However, if patients with AUR were excluded from this analysis, these differences became insignificant.

In AUR cases, continence rates 3, 6, 9, and 12 months after removal of the urinary catheter were 0, 23.1, 38.5, and 54.5 % in group 1 and 37.5, 75.0, 87.5, and 87.5 % in group 2 ($p = 0.017, 0.020, 0.027,$ and $0.127,$ respectively) (Table 4). In patients with AUR, continence rates

Table 1 Clinical characteristics of patients who underwent LRP

		No of Pts	%
Age	<65	37	32.7
	≥65	76	67.3
PSA before LRP	<10	83	73.5
	≥10	30	26.5
Prostate volume (mL)	<30	66	58.4
	≥30	47	41.6
Biopsy Gleason score	≤6	22	19.5
	7	73	64.6
	≥8	18	15.9
Clinical T stage	T1c	38	33.6
	T2a	53	46.9
	T2b	4	3.5
	T2c	18	15.9
Nerve sparing	+	26	23.0
	–	87	77.0
Operative time (min)	<150	32	28.3
	≥150	81	71.7
Blood loss (mL)	<100	42	37.2
	≥100	71	62.8
Total cases		113	

LRP laparoscopic radical prostatectomy, *Pts* patients

Table 3 Comparison of ULR and continence rates between group 1 (catheter removal on POD 2) and group 2 (catheter removal on POD 4)

		Group 1 ($n = 57$)	Group 2 ($n = 56$)	p value
ULR	First-day mean ULR	1.16 ± 4.95	1.02 ± 3.27	0.870
	Last-day mean ULR	0.57 ± 1.60	2.78 ± 15.49	0.353
	Maximum mean ULR	1.48 ± 5.13	2.93 ± 15.47	0.558
	Minimum mean ULR	0.22 ± 0.35	0.85 ± 3.24	0.206
Continence				
1 month after LRP	+	2 (3.6 %)	3 (5.4 %)	0.647
	-	54 (96.4 %)	53 (94.6 %)	
3 months after LRP	+	12 (21.8 %)	19 (34.5 %)	0.138
	-	43 (78.2 %)	36 (65.5 %)	
6 months after LRP	+	23 (41.1 %)	35 (66.0 %)	0.009
	-	33 (58.9 %)	18 (34.0 %)	
9 months after LRP	+	29 (58.0 %)	38 (79.2 %)	0.024
	-	21 (42.0 %)	10 (20.8 %)	
12 months after LRP	+	35 (71.4 %)	41 (83.7 %)	0.146
	-	14 (28.6 %)	8 (16.3 %)	

POD postoperative day, *ULR* urine loss ratio, *LRP* laparoscopic radical prostatectomy

3, 6, and 9 months after LRP were significantly lower in group 1 than in group 2.

A multivariate analysis (Table 5) identified AUR after catheter removal on POD 2 as the only independent predictor of incontinence 6 months after LRP (odds ratio, 4.472; $p = 0.030$). Age, PSA, prostate volume, the Gleason score, clinical stage, nerve sparing, operative time, blood loss, or AUR after catheter removal on POD 4 had no effect on the continence rate 6 months after LRP. Similar results were observed in the multivariate analysis of factors affecting incontinence 9 months after LRP (odds ratio, 4.313; $p = 0.018$).

Discussion

This prospective study was designed to compare the efficacy and safety of catheter removal on POD 2 versus POD 4 after LRP and its impact on urinary continence outcomes. In this study, 94.7 % of men undergoing cystography on POD 2 or 4 exhibited no evidence of urinary extravasation. The main complication associated with early catheter removal in this study was AUR. A total of 18.6 % of men who had catheters removed on POD 2 or 4 developed AUR. Although no significant differences were observed between the two groups in terms of clinical characteristics, AUR rate, or average ULR

Table 4 Comparison of continence rates in AUR cases between group 1 (catheter removal on POD 2) and group 2 (catheter removal on POD 4)

	Continence	AUR cases in group 1 ($n = 13$)	AUR cases in group 2 ($n = 8$)	p value
1 month after LRP	+	0 (0 %)	0 (0 %)	-
	-	13 (100 %)	8 (100 %)	
3 months after LRP	+	0 (0 %)	3 (37.5 %)	0.017
	-	13 (100 %)	5 (62.5 %)	
6 months after LRP	+	3 (23.1 %)	6 (75 %)	0.020
	-	10 (76.9 %)	2 (25 %)	
9 months after LRP	+	5 (38.5 %)	7 (87.5 %)	0.027
	-	8 (61.5 %)	1 (12.5 %)	
12 months after LRP	+	6 (54.5 %)	7 (87.5 %)	0.127
	-	5 (45.5 %)	1 (12.5 %)	

AUR acute urinary retention, *POD* postoperative day, *LRP* laparoscopic radical prostatectomy

Table 5 Analysis of factors affecting incontinence 6 months after LRP

	Univariate analysis (*p* value)	Multivariate analysis (*p* value)	Standard error	Odds ratio
Age <65 vs. ≥65	0.949			
PSA before LRP <10 vs. ≥10	0.851			
Prostate volume <30 vs. ≥30	0.566			
Gleason score ≤6 vs. ≥7	0.688			
Clinical T stage T1c vs. T2a,b,c	0.623			
Nerve sparing yes vs. no	0.293			
Operative time <150 vs. ≥150	0.203			
Blood loss <100 vs. ≥100	0.264			
AUR on POD 2 yes vs. no	0.020	0.030	0.690	4.472
AUR on POD 4 yes vs. no	0.200			

LRP laparoscopic radical prostatectomy, *AUR* acute urinary retention, *POD* postoperative day

(first-day, last-day, maximum, or minimum), continence rates 6 and 9 months after LRP were significantly lower in group 1 (POD 2) than in group 2 (POD 4). In AUR cases, continence rates 3, 6, and 9 months after LRP were significantly lower in group 1 than in group 2. Moreover, a multivariate analysis identified AUR after catheter removal on POD 2 as the only predictive factor for incontinence 6 and 9 months after LRP. Meanwhile, AUR after catheter removal on POD 4 had no effect on the continence rate. Therefore, we consider it premature to remove the urinary catheter on POD 2 following LRP with a running VUA. To the best of our knowledge, our prospective study is the first to identify a relationship between the risk of incontinence and AUR following earlier catheter removal.

The duration of indwelling catheter use after RP, LRP, and RALP has progressively shortened; however, the optimal timing of removal has not yet been determined. Traditionally, urinary catheter removal after RP has been performed between 10 and 21 days postoperatively without any evidence [1–3]. However, some centers remove the urinary catheter between 5 and 12 days after RALP [17–19]. The advantages of early catheter removal include improved quality of life (QOL) and lower infection rate and bladder irritability symptoms [4, 11]. In one study, the majority of men who underwent RP indicated that the urinary catheter was more of a concern than postoperative pain [4]. Conversely, proponents of longer catheterization claim that early removal is associated with a risk of urinary extravasation, which, in turn, may lead to pelvic abscess, urinoma, urinary incontinence, or anastomotic stricture [20, 21]. AUR following urinary catheter removal on POD 2 was identified as the only predictive factor for incontinence after

LRP in our study. However, other studies demonstrated that early catheter removal was associated with a significantly higher continence rate after RP and LRP [22, 23]. In these studies, early catheter removal was defined as catheter removal on POD 4 or on or before POD 7, and no patients had catheters removed on POD 2. In the present study, all patients underwent early (POD 2 or POD 4) catheter removal, and any patient who underwent late catheter removal, such as after POD 7, was not included. However, to the best of our knowledge, no previous studies have compared the continence outcomes of urinary catheter removal on POD 2 with those of catheter removal after POD 2, such as POD 4. Thus, the present study evaluated the effects of the differential timing of early catheter removal.

Although catheter drainage to prevent urinary extravasation may reduce the risk of urinary incontinence, it is equally plausible that prolonged catheterization may contribute to urinary incontinence secondary to mechanical damage and inflammation of the urethral and bladder mucosa [22]. It is important to note that AUR and reinsertion of a catheter following earlier catheter removal (e.g., on POD 2) may have increased the risk of urinary incontinence by urinary extravasation and mechanical damage of the urethra. In our prospective study, AUR on POD 2 after catheter removal was the only predictive factor for incontinence after LRP. Therefore, our hypothesis that early catheter removal (≤7 days after surgery) is associated with good continence held true; however, POD 2 may be premature for catheter removal because of the risk of incontinence with AUR.

The evolution of minimally invasive techniques for the treatment of prostate cancer, such as LRP and RALP, has reduced postoperative pain and the duration of catheterization [11, 18, 24]. These improvements have been attributed to the development of intracorporeal suturing techniques with visualization of VUA. These technical advances have allowed us to challenge previous postoperative management plans. Removal of the urinary catheter on POD 4 has become routine in centers offering LRP [7, 11, 23]. Nadu et al. investigated a series of LRP cases using cystography and demonstrated that early urinary catheter removal (POD 2 and POD 4) was possible [11]. Eighty-five percent of men in that study exhibited no evidence of extravasation, and urinary catheters were successfully removed. This high success rate was attributed to the superior anastomosis achieved laparoscopically. However, that study did not include a subgroup analysis of urinary catheter removal on POD 2. The results of the present study showed that early catheter removal on POD 2 after LRP with a running VUA may increase the risk of incontinence.

AUR appears to be a risk after LRP and occurred in 21 (18.6 %) patients without clot formation in our series. Although all patients with AUR had their catheters reinserted without complications, a severe impact on continence was observed in group 1 (catheter removed on POD 2). The etiology of AUR after LRP is likely to be postoperative anastomotic edema, postoperative pain, or increased tone of the bladder neck smooth muscle [25]. Normal micturition is always re-established after several days of catheterization. Therefore, one explanation for the high rate of AUR with early catheter removal may be the presence of anastomotic edema. The incidence of AUR after early catheter removal was previously reported to be between 6.7 and 21.0 % [11, 25, 26].

Several studies have specifically investigated the incidence of anastomotic stricture after RP without early catheter removal, and reported rates ranging between 4.8 and 15 % [27–29]. Previous transurethral resection of the prostate, a history of smoking, and urinary extravasation have been associated with an increased rate of anastomotic stricture [28, 29]. Koch et al. showed that early catheter removal did not increase the incidence of anastomotic stricture over that of historical controls or previously reported rates [5]. In the present study, no patient had anastomotic stricture, which was better than previously reported findings. Therefore, the results of our study suggest that catheter removal on POD 2 or 4 did not promote stricture formation.

Urinary incontinence after RP has a significant impact on QOL and continues to be a major concern for patients [5]. Reported continence rates 1 year postoperatively ranged from 60 to 93 % after RP, from 66 to 95 % after LRP, and from 69 to 97 % after RARP [12, 30]. By defining continence as a pad-free status, the continence rate in the present study at 12 months was 83.7 % in group 2, which was within the average range [12]. Patients who had catheters removed on POD 4 showed the normal recovery of urinary continence.

Our study has a number of limitations. The overall sample size was small. We relied on patient reports of the degree of continence and use of protective pads. Therefore, urinary continence was not assessed using an objective test. Despite these limitations, we believe that our results indicate that early catheter removal on POD 2 increases the risk of incontinence with AUR and needs to be avoided in clinical practice.

Conclusions

In terms of the risk of urinary incontinence after LRP, in most patients, urinary catheter removal was safer on POD 4 than on POD 2.

Abbreviations

LRP: Laparoscopic radical prostatectomy; POD: Postoperative day; ULR: The urine loss ratio; AUR: Acute urinary retention; RP: Radical prostatectomy;

VUA: Vesicourethral anastomosis; RALP: Robot-assisted LRP; S.D.: Standard deviation; QOL: Quality of life.

Competing interests
The authors declare that they have no competing interests.

Authors' contributions
SH, TT, and MM formulated the database. MM performed the initial analyses and drafted the first manuscript. All authors assisted in the analysis and interpretation of data. RM, EK, and MO critically discussed the data and manuscript. AM conceived the study, participated in its design and coordination, and helped to draft the manuscript. All authors read and approved the final manuscript.

Acknowledgments
We thank Keisuke Shigeta for his work on language editing and manuscript revisions.

References
1. Shelfo SW, Obek C, Soloway MS. Update on bladder neck preservation during radical retropubic prostatectomy: impact on pathologic outcome, anastomotic strictures, and continence. Urology. 1998;51(1):73–8.
2. Murphy GP, Mettlin C, Menck H, Winchester DP, Davidson AM. National patterns of prostate cancer treatment by radical prostatectomy: results of a survey by the American College of Surgeons Commission on Cancer. J Urol. 1994;152(5 Pt 2):1817–9.
3. Steiner MS, Morton RA, Walsh PC. Impact of anatomical radical prostatectomy on urinary continence. J Urol. 1991;145(3):512–4. discussion 514–515.
4. Lepor H, Nieder AM, Fraiman MC. Early removal of urinary catheter after radical retropubic prostatectomy is both feasible and desirable. Urology. 2001;58(3):425–9.
5. Koch MO, Nayee AH, Sloan J, Gardner T, Wahle GR, Bihrle R, et al. Early catheter removal after radical retropubic prostatectomy: long-term followup. J Urol. 2003;169(6):2170–2.
6. Lau KO, Cheng C. Feasibility of early catheter removal after radical retropubic prostatectomy. Tech Urol. 2001;7(1):38–40.
7. Souto CA, Teloken C, Souto JC, Rhoden EL, Ting HY. Experience with early catheter removal after radical retropubic prostatectomy. J Urol. 2000;163(3):865–6.
8. Schuessler WW, Schulam PG, Clayman RV, Kavoussi LR. Laparoscopic radical prostatectomy: initial short-term experience. Urology. 1997;50(6):854–7.
9. Guillonneau B, Cathelineau X, Barret E, Rozet F, Vallancien G. Laparoscopic radical prostatectomy: technical and early oncological assessment of 40 operations. Eur Urol. 1999;36(1):14–20.
10. Hoznek A, Menard Y, Salomon L, Abbou CC. Update on laparoscopic and robotic radical prostatectomy. Curr Opin Urol. 2005;15(3):173–80.
11. Nadu A, Salomon L, Hoznek A, Olsson LE, Saint F, de La Taille A, et al. Early removal of the catheter after laparoscopic radical prostatectomy. J Urol. 2001;166(5):1662–4.
12. Ficarra V, Novara G, Artibani W, Cestari A, Galfano A, Graefen M, et al. Retropubic, laparoscopic, and robot-assisted radical prostatectomy: a systematic review and cumulative analysis of comparative studies. Eur Urol. 2009;55(5):1037–63.
13. Ates M, Teber D, Gozen AS, Tefekli A, Hruza M, Sugiono M, et al. A new postoperative predictor of time to urinary continence after laparoscopic radical prostatectomy: the urine loss ratio. Eur Urol. 2007;52(1):178–85.
14. Sato Y, Tanda H, Nakajima H, Nitta T, Akagashi K, Hanzawa T, et al. Simple and reliable predictor of urinary continence after radical prostatectomy: serial measurement of urine loss ratio after catheter removal. Int J Urol. 2014;21(7):647–51.
15. Van Kampen M, Geraerts I, De Weerdt W, Van Poppel H. An easy prediction of urinary incontinence duration after retropubic radical prostatectomy based on urine loss the first day after catheter withdrawal. J Urol. 2009;181(6):2641–6.
16. Rocco F, Carmignani L, Acquati P, Gadda F, Dell'Orto P, Rocco B, et al. Early continence recovery after open radical prostatectomy with restoration of the posterior aspect of the rhabdosphincter. Eur Urol. 2007;52(2):376–83.

17. Agarwal PK, Sammon J, Bhandari A, Dabaja A, Diaz M, Dusik-Fenton S, et al. Safety profile of robot-assisted radical prostatectomy: a standardized report of complications in 3317 patients. Eur Urol. 2011;59(5):684–98.

18. Coelho RF, Chauhan S, Orvieto MA, Sivaraman A, Palmer KJ, Coughlin G, et al. Influence of modified posterior reconstruction of the rhabdosphincter on early recovery of continence and anastomotic leakage rates after robot-assisted radical prostatectomy. Eur Urol. 2011;59(1):72–80.

19. Joshi N, de Blok W, van Muilekom E, van der Poel H. Impact of posterior musculofascial reconstruction on early continence after robot-assisted laparoscopic radical prostatectomy: results of a prospective parallel group trial. Eur Urol. 2010;58(1):84–9.

20. Dalton DP, Schaeffer AJ, Garnett JE, Grayhack JT. Radiographic assessment of the vesicourethral anastomosis directing early decatheterization following nerve-sparing radical retropubic prostatectomy. J Urol. 1989;141(1):79–81.

21. Leibovitch I, Rowland RG, Little Jr JS, Foster RS, Bihrle R, Donohue JP. Cystography after radical retropubic prostatectomy: clinical implications of abnormal findings. Urology. 1995;46(1):78–80.

22. Palisaar JR, Roghmann F, Brock M, Loppenberg B, Noldus J, von Bodman C: Predictors of short-term recovery of urinary continence after radical prostatectomy. World J Urol 2014. doi:10.1007/s00345-014-1340-3

23. Tiguert R, Rigaud J, Fradet Y. Safety and outcome of early catheter removal after radical retropubic prostatectomy. Urology. 2004;63(3):513–7.

24. Bhayani SB, Pavlovich CP, Hsu TS, Sullivan W, Su L. Prospective comparison of short-term convalescence: laparoscopic radical prostatectomy versus open radical retropubic prostatectomy. Urology. 2003;61(3):612–6.

25. Patel R, Lepor H. Removal of urinary catheter on postoperative day 3 or 4 after radical retropubic prostatectomy. Urology. 2003;61(1):156–60.

26. Noguchi M, Shimada A, Yahara J, Suekane S, Noda S. Early catheter removal 3 days after radical retropubic prostatectomy. Int J Urol. 2004;11(11):983–8.

27. Borboroglu PG, Sands JP, Roberts JL, Amling CL. Risk factors for vesicourethral anastomotic stricture after radical prostatectomy. Urology. 2000;56(1):96–100.

28. Park R, Martin S, Goldberg JD, Lepor H. Anastomotic strictures following radical prostatectomy: insights into incidence, effectiveness of intervention, effect on continence, and factors predisposing to occurrence. Urology. 2001;57(4):742–6.

29. Tomschi W, Suster G, Holtl W. Bladder neck strictures after radical retropubic prostatectomy: still an unsolved problem. Br J Urol. 1998;81(6):823–6.

30. Ficarra V, Novara G, Rosen RC, Artibani W, Carroll PR, Costello A, et al. Systematic review and meta-analysis of studies reporting urinary continence recovery after robot-assisted radical prostatectomy. Eur Urol. 2012;62(3):405–17.

Risk factors for biochemical recurrence after robotic assisted radical prostatectomy

Ryuta Tanimoto[*], Yomi Fashola, Kymora B Scotland, Anne E Calvaresi, Leonard G Gomella, Edouard J Trabulsi and Costas D Lallas

Abstract

Background: Radical prostatectomy is a standard surgical treatment of clinically localized prostate cancer. Margin status has been found to be an independent predictor of biochemical recurrence (BCR) after open radical prostatectomy in several large series but this is still controversy in Robotic Assisted Radical Prostatectomy (RARP) series. We therefore wanted to investigate the prognostic significance of positive surgical margin (PSM) and other pathological factors on BCR in patients treated with RARP by a single surgeon.

Methods: Prospectively collected data of 439 patients treated with RARP between October 2005 and June 2013 by a single surgeon at a single institution were analyzed. BCR was defined as follow-up PSA level > 0.2 ng/ml on two separate occasions or patients who had to undergo salvage therapy. Kaplan Meier curves and Log Rank test were used to compare the risk of BCR. Univariate and Multivariate Cox Regression analyses were performed to determine the prognostic impact of age, BMI, prostate weight, PSA prior to surgery, pathological T-stage, pathological Gleason sum, PSM and operative period.

Results: In this study period, 34 out of 439 had BCR, giving an overall BCR rate of 7.7% for this cohort. Overall 2- and 3-year BCR-free survival rates were 93% and 88%, respectively. Patients with a PSM had a 2-year BCR free survival of 88% compared to 94% in those with negative margins (p < .0001). On the multivariate analysis, PSM as well as pathological Gleason sum > = 8, PSA, pathological stage and operative period were significantly associated with BCR.

Conclusions: In our case series of RARP performed by a single surgeon, PSM as well as pathological Gleason sum, PSA, pathological stage and early operative period for this surgeon were the independent predictors of BCR.

Keywords: Biochemical recurrence, Biochemical recurrence free survival, Cox regression analysis, Positive surgical margin, Robotic assisted radical prostatectomy

Background

Radical retropubic prostatectomy (RRP) is a standard surgical treatment of clinically localized prostate cancer. Recently robotic-assisted radical prostatectomy (RARP) also has become very popular in the United States and Europe; it has been estimated that > 75% of radical prostatectomies are performed using the da Vinci platform (Intuitive Surgical, Inc., Sunnyvale, CA, USA) [1]. Systematic review of the literature revealed that RARP represented a safe procedure with better perioperative outcomes, such as reduced blood loss and postoperative hospital stay, when compared with open surgery [2,3]. Moreover, recent meta-analysis showed similar positive surgical margin (PSM) rates and biochemical recurrence (BCR) free survival estimates when comparing RARP with RRP and RARP with laparoscopic radical prostatectomy (LRP) [3]. At our institution, RARP was adopted in lieu of LRP in 2005 and our previous report also supported these findings [4].

Margin status is considered an independent predictor of BCR after open radical prostatectomy in several large

* Correspondence: tanimo10@gmail.com
Department of Urology, Kimmel Cancer Center, Thomas Jefferson University, 1025 Walnut St. Suite 1112, Philadelphia, PA 19107, USA

series [5-7]. This was also seen in some robotic prostatectomy series [8-11]. However, in the largest reported robotic series with a median follow-up of 36 months, margin status was not shown to be an independent BCR predictor [12].

The aim of this study was to assess the prognostic significance of PSM and other pathological factors on BCR in patients treated with RARP by a single surgeon.

Methods

A single institution retrospective review of RALP performed by a single surgeon between October 2005 and June 2013 was performed. This is a Thomas Jefferson University Institutional Review Board approved database (approval reference: 02.9000) in which data has been collected prospectively. The written informed consent for participation in the study was obtained from all patients. Patients were initially evaluated at a multidisciplinary clinic. Of 1062 consecutive patients who underwent RARP in our institution, a total of 561 patients were treated by a single surgeon (EJT) during this time. Following the exclusion of patients who did not have recorded PSA values postoperatively (n = 73) or had adjuvant radiation or hormonal treatment (n = 9), who had positive lymph node (n = 2), pT3b (n = 2), pT3a with positive surgical margin (n = 3), pT3a with tertiary GS 5 (n = 1) or high GS (4 + 5) with positive surgical margin (n = 1), the remaining 439 patients were evaluated in the present study. None of these patients had been administered hormones prior to surgery. All prostate specimens were submitted in their entirety and underwent standard whole mount step sectioned pathologic analysis in order to determine surgical Gleason score, pathological stage and margin status. The location of each positive margin on the prostatic specimen was examined. A confirmatory second level pathologic review with a genitourinary pathologist and the surgical team was performed weekly in a multidisciplinary genitourinary pathology conference. BCR was defined as follow-up PSA level > 0.2 ng/ml on two separate occasions or patients who had to undergo salvage therapy. Kaplan Meier curves and Log Rank Test were used to compare the risk of developing BCR. Univariate and Multivariate Cox Regression analyses were performed to determine the prognostic impact of pathological factors including age, BMI at surgery, pre-operative PSA (< 10 ng/ml versus > = 10 ng/ml), operative period (early operative period for this surgeon, 2005 – 2007 and later operative period 2008 – 2013), PSM, foci of PSM (unifocal versus multifocal versus none), pathological stage (T2 versus T3/4), pathological Gleason sum (<= 6 versus 7 versus > = 8), extracapsular extension (unifocal versus multifocal versus none), seminal vesicle involvement, perineural invasion, and prostate size as determined by weight in grams.

All procedures were performed by a single surgeon (EJT) using the da Vinci® Surgical System. Laparoscopic ports were placed using a 6-port transperitoneal approach. The seminal vesicles were approached posteriorly. Nerve sparing procedures were attempted for all patients with appropriate preoperative potency and acceptable oncologic risk. For the initial 50 RARP patients, obturator lymphadenectomy was performed if the preoperative Kattan nomogram [13] predicted greater than 1% risk of lymph node invasion. Subsequently, all patients were treated with obturator node dissection with high risk patients, as determined by the D'Amico criteria [14], receiving extended lymphadenectomy to include external iliac nodes.

Statistical analysis

All statistical analyses were two-tailed. Differences were considered significant if the p value was < 0.05. The statistical analysis was conducted with JMP version 9.0 (SAS Institute Inc, Cary, NC, USA).

Results

Out of 531 patients treated by a single surgeon, 439 were included in this study. The clinical and pathological characteristics of the 439 patients are listed in Table 1. Median patient age at prostatectomy was 59 years. Median PSA was 4.9 ng/ml (interquartile range, (IQR) 3.9 – 6.3). Overall, 422 patients (96%) underwent lymph node dissection with a median rate of 7 lymph nodes (IQR 4 – 12). Among those, 4 patients (0.9%) had at least 1 positive node. The median follow-up time was 16 months (IQR 6 – 34). In this study, 34 of the 439 follow-up patients (7.7%) experienced BCR. Among those, 31 (91%) BCR were due to elevated PSA recurrence and only 3 received salvage radiation therapy before a documented PSA increase. All 20 patients with secondary treatment had salvage radiation therapy with or without hormonal therapy. In all, 119 patients (27.1%) had PSM and among those, 102 (85.7%) were unifocal. The locations of PSM (Additional file 1: Table S1) were posterolateral (54.6%), bladder neck / base (14.3%) and apex (10.9%). The PSM rates were 20%, 49% and 50% in patients with stage pT2, pT3a and pT3b respectively. Unfortunately, we failed to identify improvements in the PSM over time (Additional file 2: Table S2).

Overall 2-, and 3-year BCR-free survival (BCRFS) rates were 93% and 88%, respectively (Figure 1a). Patients with a PSM had a 2-year BCRFS of 88% compared to 94% in those with negative margins (Figure 1b; p < 0.0001). The two year BCR free rate was 99%, 94% and 58% for patients with pathological Gleason sum < = 6, 7 and > = 8, respectively (Figure 1c; p < 0.0001); the same rate was 98% and 73% in patients with pT2 disease and with pT3/4 respectively (Figure 1d; p < 0.0001). Preoperative PSA > = 10

Table 1 Patient characteristics (n = 439)

		Median	IQR	BCR(+) Median	n = 34 IQR	BCR(−) Median	n = 405 IQR
Age	(years)	59	55-65	62	56-66	59	55-64
BMI	(kg/m²)	28.1	25.6-31.2	29.3	25.5-33.2	28	25.7-31.1
Preoperative PSA (ng/ml)		4.9	3.9-6.3	6.7	4.5-13.2	4.9	3.9-6.0
Follow up time (months)		16	6-34	33	3-49	15	6-33
		n	%	BCR(+)	n = 34	BCR(−)	n = 405
Clinical Stage							
	T1c	342	77.9%	22	64.7%	320	79.0%
	T2a	65	14.8%	5	14.7%	60	14.8%
	T2b	24	5.5%	5	14.7%	19	4.7%
	T2c	7	1.6%	2	5.9%	5	1.2%
	T3a	1	0.2%	0	0.0%	1	0.2%
Clinical Gleason							
	≤6	216	49.2%	8	23.5%	208	51.4%
	7	202	46.0%	21	61.8%	281	69.4%
	≥8	21	4.8%	5	14.7%	16	4.0%
Pathological Stage							
	T2a	50	11.4%	0	0.0%	50	12.3%
	T2b	7	1.6%	0	0.0%	7	1.7%
	T2c	280	63.8%	10	29.4%	270	66.7%
	T3a	75	17.1%	12	35.3%	63	15.6%
	T3b	24	5.5%	9	26.5%	15	3.7%
	T4	3	0.7%	3	8.8%	0	0.0%
Pathological Gleason							
	≤6	157	35.8%	0	0.0%	157	38.8%
	7	241	54.9%	6	17.6%	235	58.0%
	≥8	41	9.3%	28	82.4%	13	3.2%
Operative period							
	2005-2007	102	23.2%	14	41.2%	88	21.7%
	2008-2010	203	46.2%	13	38.2%	190	46.9%
	2011-2013	134	30.5%	4	11.8%	130	32.1%
Positive Surgical Margin		119	27.1%	20	58.8%		
BCR		34	7.7%	34	100.0%		
	PSA > 0.2	31	7.1%	31	91.2%		
	SalvageXRT	20	4.6%	20	58.8%		

(Figure 1e; p < 0.0001), and early operative period, 2005 – 2007 (Figure 1f; p = 0.0093), which was the period during which the first RARPs were performed by this surgeon, were also significantly associated with increased risk of BCR.

Table 2 summarizes data of the univariate and multivariate analyses for predictors of BCR. On univariate analysis, BMI, pathological Gleason sum > = 8, pathological stage, PSM, the foci of PSM, PSA and operative period were significantly related with BCR. Extracapsular extension (unifocal versus multifocal versus none), seminal vesicle involvement and perineural invasion were also related with BCR (p < 0.0001, p < 0.0001 and p = 0.0004, respectively; data not shown). On multivariable analysis, pathologic Gleason sum was the strongest predictor of BCR, with an HR of 6.76 (p = 0.0030) for Gleason > = 8 when compared to Gleason < = 6. The presence of PSM also represented independent predictors of BCR (HR 2.69; p = 0.0153) as well as PSA, pathological stage (HR 4.48; p = 0.0011) and early operative period (HR 0.38; p = 0.0113).

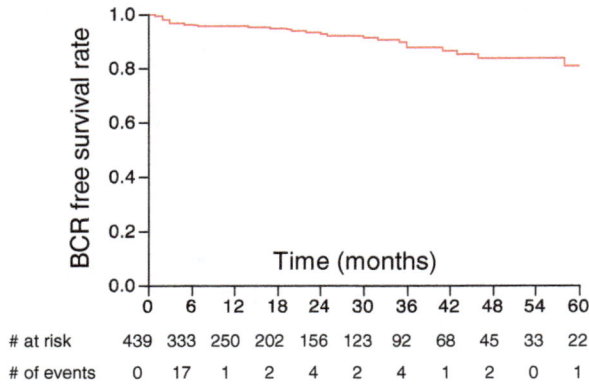

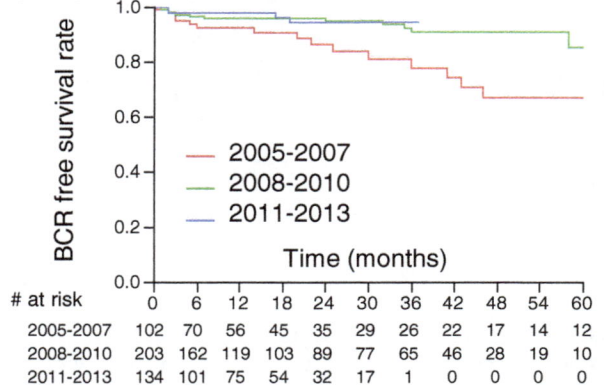

Figure 1 Kapalan-Meier curves. (a) overall, **(b)** Biochemical recurrence free survival (BCRFS) in patients with (red curve) and without positive surgical margins (blue curve). **(c)** BCRFS for pathological Gleason < =6(red curve), =7(green curve) and >=8(blue curve). **(d)** BCRFS for pathological stage pT2 (red curve), pT3-4 (blue curve). **(e)** BCRFS for preoperative PSA < 10 (red curve), preoperative PSA > =10. **(f)** BCRFS in patients operated in 2005–2007 (red curve), in 2008 - 2010(green curve), in 2011–2013 (blue curve).

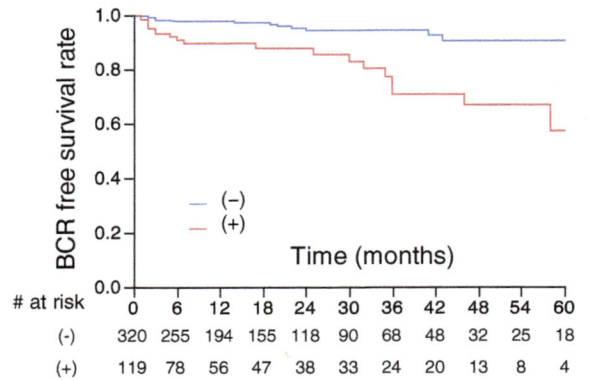

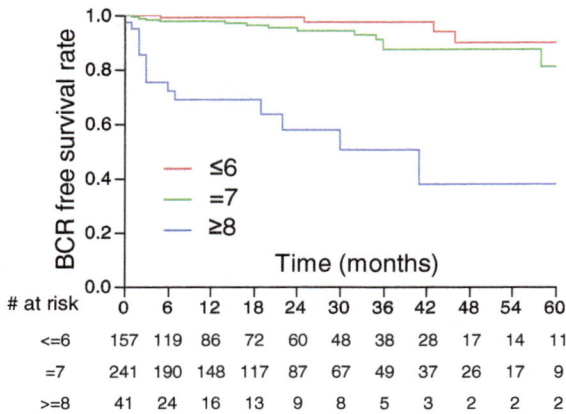

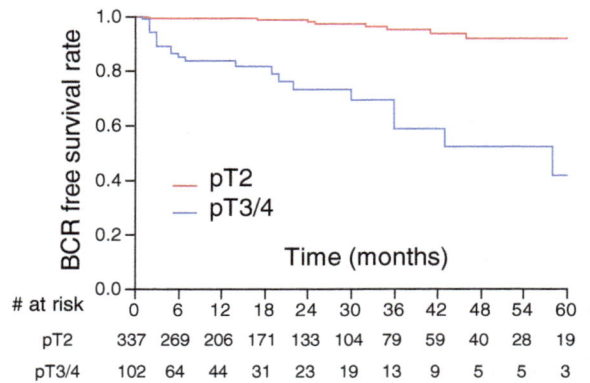

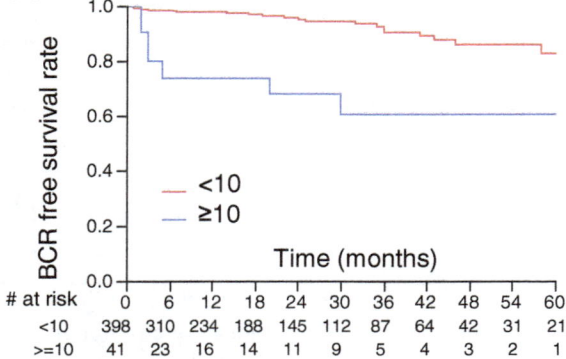

Table 2 Univariate and multivariate analyses of factors affecting BCR

	Univariate analysis			Multivariate analysis		
	Risk ratio	(95% CI)	p-value	Risk ratio	(95% CI)	p-value
Age	1.03	(0.98-1.09)	0.2279	0.98	(0.92-1.05)	0.6476
BMI	1.09	(1.02-1.17)	0.0158	0.97	(0.90-1.04)	0.3369
Prostate Weight (gm)	0.99	(0.96-1.01)	0.2851	-		
PSM	4.12	(2.09-8.34)	<0.0001	2.69	(1.21-6.14)	0.0153
PSM foci						
None	1.00			-		
Unifocal	3.49	(1.67-7.32)	0.0010	-		
Multifocal	9.23	(2.96-24.34)	0.0005	-		
Pathological Gleason						
≤6	1.00			1.00		
7	2.39	(0.86-8.42)	0.1001	1.78	(0.58-6.63)	0.3226
≥8	21.11	(7.71-73.90)	<0.0001	6.76	(1.87-29.21)	0.0030
Preoperative PSA						
<10	1.00			1.00		
≥10	6.66	(3.18-13.28)	<0.0001	2.53	(1.06-5.81)	0.0360
Pathological Stage						
pT2	1.00			1.00		
pT3-4	10.89	(5.33-23.98)	<0.0001	4.48	(1.83-11.30)	0.0011
Operative period						
Before 2007	1.00			1.00		
After 2008	0.36	(0.18-0.72)	0.0045	0.38	(0.18-0.80)	0.0113

BMI; body mass index, PSM; positive surgical margin.

Discussion

In our case series of RARP performed by a single surgeon, positive surgical margin as well as pathological Gleason sum, PSA, pathological stage and early operative period were the independent predictors of BCR.

Most RARP studies report short-term (< 12 months) follow-up outcomes, though 4 large studies recently reported BCR free survival (BCRFS) after RARP with a follow-up of more than 5 years [10,15-17]. The largest report of PSA outcomes in the RARP literature is from Menon et al. [16], who reported an overall BRFS of 86.4% for 1384 patients with a median follow-up of 60.2 months. Actual 3-and 5-yr BCRFS were 90.6% and 86.6%, respectively. On the other hand, Suardi et al. and Liss et al. reported 3- and 5-year BCRFS of 94%, 86% in 184 patients and 87.8%, 84.9% in 435 patients, respectively. In our study, mean follow-up was only 22 months and it is too early to define 5-year BCRFS, but the overall 2-year and 3-year BCRFS was 93% and 88%, respectively, which was comparable to previous reports.

The overall PSM rate in this series is 27.1% with a rate of 19.9% for pT2 tumors. This is comparable to other contemporaneous RARP series whose PSM rates were 6.5 - 29.5% overall and 2.5 - 22.7% in patients with stage

pT2 [8-11,16-26]. Regarding risk factors for BCR, all four large studies referenced above agreed that the pathological Gleason score was an independent factor, but two of them did not find that the presence of positive margins was significant on multivariate analysis. Menon et al. showed the significance of positive margin on BCR, although their previous series with follow-up of 36 months did not [12]. The reason for this may be that the actual BCR rate (2.4%) was too low to power the statistical significance in this cohort. Sooriakumaran et al. reported an RARP case series of 944 patients with median follow-up of 6.3 years, which showed that PSM status as well as preoperative PSA > 10, pathological Gleason sum > = 4 + 3, pathological T3 disease and lower surgeon case volume were all associated with increased risk of BCR on multivariable analysis.

Shikanov et al. reported not only the presence of PSM but also PSM length (> 3 mm) to be independently associated with BCR. Interestingly, patients with negative margins and those with a positive margin less than 1 mm had similar rates of biochemical recurrence [9]. This finding is in keeping with others and suggests PSM > 3 mm and multifocal positivity were associated with risk of BCR [27]. Moskovic et al. reported that high body mass index does not affect BCR following robotic assisted laparoscopic prostatectomy when BMI was stratified into 3 groups (> = 30, > = 25 and < 30, < 25), although there was a trend toward increased recurrence in the obese [28]. In the present study, higher BMI had higher BCR on univariate analysis, but not on multivariate analysis.

With regard to the effect of surgeon experience on BCR, Zorn et al. [29] demonstrated that the risk of PSA recurrence was quite stable over 700 cases when compared with 3 groups (cases 1–300, 301–500, and 501–700). Samadi et al. also assessed the effect of surgeon experience and technical modifications, which were categorized as initial, intermediate and current technique, on oncological outcome after RARP. Pathological T2 margin rates decreased continuously during the initial technique period, followed by a transient worsening of margin rates during the intermediate time period and a subsequent decrease during the period when the current technique was used, but no significant differences were noted in BCR rate between these groups. In both studies, follow-up duration was relatively short, and BCR-free survival analyses adjusted for covariates were not provided. In the present study, we adjusted BCR-free survival for the covariates including pathological factors with Cox Regression analysis. The early operative period, 2005–2007, which encompassed the first 100 cases, had a significantly higher rate of BCR compared to the late period, but there was no difference between 2008 – 2010 and 2011 – 2013. This suggested the risk of BCR was stable after 100 cases.

It is also important to remember that BCR does not necessarily lead to clinical recurrence or cancer specific mortality, and BCR without clinical progression might reflect the recurrence of indolent prostate cancer or the presence of benign prostatic tissue left behind after surgery [30]. Hence, it is necessary to follow up our cohort further and determine the impact of BCR on longer-term oncologic outcome.

Our study has some limitations. Many of the patients were from outside our geographic area and are followed locally. The median follow-up in these patients was 16 months, and so these results must be considered early. In addition, factors potentially correlating with BCR, such as length of PSM were not included in this analysis. The main strength of our study is that only patients treated by a single surgeon were selected for this analysis which was adjusted for the operative periods with the aim of decreasing the influence of surgeons' techniques on their outcomes.

Conclusions

In our case series of RARP performed by a single surgeon, positive surgical margins as well as pathologic Gleason sum, PSA, pathologic stage and early operative period were the independent predictors of BCR. Further follow-up is necessary to determine how this finding will translate into cancer-specific and overall survival outcome.

Abbreviations

BCR: Biochemical recurrence; RARP: Robotic Assisted Radical Prostatectomy; PSM: Positive surgical margin; PSA: Prostate specific antigen; BCRFS: Biochemical recurrence free survival; IQR: Interquartile range.

Competing interests

Drs. Ryuta Tanimoto, Yomi Fashola, Kymora B. Anne E. Calvaresi, CRNP, Scotland, Edouard J. Trabulsi, Costas D. Lallas declare no conflict of interest or financial ties. Dr. Leonard G. Gomella declares the following conflict of interest; a consultant to Astellas, Bayer, Dendreon and Janssen, and the research funding from Astellas and FSK.

Authors' contributions

RT, CDL, LGG and EJT designed the study. RT, AEC and YF wrote the manuscript and obtained infromation from charts. CDL and EJT performed the pathological review, RT performed the statistical analysis. RT, KBS, AEC, CDL and EJT reviewed and edited the manuscript. All authors read and approved the final manuscript.

Acknowledgements

The authors haven't received any source of funding.

References

1.   Mottrie A, De Naeyer G, Novara G, Ficarra V. Robotic radical prostatectomy: a critical analysis of the impact on cancer control. Curr Opin Urol. 2011;21(3):179–84.
2.   Gandaglia G, Sammon JD, Chang SL, Choueiri TK, Hu JC, Karakiewicz PI, et al. Comparative effectiveness of robot-assisted and open radical prostatectomy in the postdissemination era. J Clin Oncol. 2014;32(14):1419–26.
3.   Novara G, Ficarra V, Mocellin S, Ahlering TE, Carroll PR, Graefen M, et al. Systematic review and meta-analysis of studies reporting oncologic outcome after robot-assisted radical prostatectomy. Eur Urol. 2012;62(3):382–404.
4.   Trabulsi EJ, Zola JC, Gomella LG, Lallas CD. Transition from pure laparoscopic to robotic-assisted radical prostatectomy: a single surgeon institutional evolution. Urol Oncol. 2010;28(1):81–5.
5.   Eastham JA, Kuroiwa K, Ohori M, Serio AM, Gorbonos A, Maru N, et al. Prognostic significance of location of positive margins in radical prostatectomy specimens. Urology. 2007;70(5):965–9.
6.   Ochiai A, Sotelo T, Troncoso P, Bhadkamkar V, Babaian RJ. Natural history of biochemical progression after radical prostatectomy based on length of a positive margin. Urology. 2008;71(2):308–12.
7.   Swindle P, Eastham JA, Ohori M, Kattan MW, Wheeler T, Maru N, et al. Do margins matter? The prognostic significance of positive surgical margins in radical prostatectomy specimens. J Urol. 2008;179(5 Suppl):S47–51.
8.   Ginzburg S, Nevers T, Staff I, Tortora J, Champagne A, Kesler SS, et al. Prostate cancer biochemical recurrence rates after robotic-assisted laparoscopic radical prostatectomy. JSLS. 2012;16(3):443–50.
9.   Shikanov S, Song J, Royce C, Al-Ahmadie H, Zorn K, Steinberg G, et al. Length of positive surgical margin after radical prostatectomy as a predictor of biochemical recurrence. J Urol. 2009;182(1):139–44.

10. Sooriakumaran P, Haendler L, Nyberg T, Gronberg H, Nilsson A, Carlsson S, et al. Biochemical recurrence after robot-assisted radical prostatectomy in a European single-centre cohort with a minimum follow-up time of 5 years. Eur Urol. 2012;62(5):768–74.

11. Warner JN, Nunez RN, Mmeje CO, Colby TV, Ferrigni RG, Humphreys MR, et al. Impact of margin status at 37 months after robot assisted radical prostatectomy. Can J Urol. 2011;18(6):6043–9.

12. Menon M, Shrivastava A, Kaul S, Badani KK, Fumo M, Bhandari M, et al. Vattikuti Institute prostatectomy: contemporary technique and analysis of results. Eur Urol. 2007;51(3):648–57. discussion 657–648.

13. Kattan MW, Eastham JA, Stapleton AM, Wheeler TM, Scardino PT. A preoperative nomogram for disease recurrence following radical prostatectomy for prostate cancer. J Natl Cancer Inst. 1998;90(10):766–71.

14. D'Amico AV, Whittington R, Malkowicz SB, Schultz D, Blank K, Broderick GA, et al. Biochemical outcome after radical prostatectomy, external beam radiation therapy, or interstitial radiation therapy for clinically localized prostate cancer. JAMA. 1998;280(11):969–74.

15. Liss MA, Lusch A, Morales B, Beheshti N, Skarecky D, Narula N, et al. Robot-assisted radical prostatectomy: 5-year oncological and biochemical outcomes. J Urol. 2012;188(6):2205–10.

16. Menon M, Bhandari M, Gupta N, Lane Z, Peabody JO, Rogers CG, et al. Biochemical recurrence following robot-assisted radical prostatectomy: analysis of 1384 patients with a median 5-year follow-up. Eur Urol. 2010;58(6):838–46.

17. Suardi N, Ficarra V, Willemsen P, De Wil P, Gallina A, De Naeyer G, et al. Long-term biochemical recurrence rates after robot-assisted radical prostatectomy: analysis of a single-center series of patients with a minimum follow-up of 5 years. Urology. 2012;79(1):133–8.

18. Patel VR, Coelho RF, Rocco B, Orvieto M, Sivaraman A, Palmer KJ, et al. Positive surgical margins after robotic assisted radical prostatectomy: a multi-institutional study. J Urol. 2011;186(2):511–6.

19. Davis JW, Kamat A, Munsell M, Pettaway C, Pisters L, Matin S. Initial experience of teaching robot-assisted radical prostatectomy to surgeons-in-training: can training be evaluated and standardized? BJU Int. 2010;105(8):1148–54.

20. Tewari A, Rao S, Martinez-Salamanca JI, Leung R, Ramanathan R, Mandhani A, et al. Cancer control and the preservation of neurovascular tissue: how to meet competing goals during robotic radical prostatectomy. BJU Int. 2008;101(8):1013–8.

21. Ficarra V, Novara G, Secco S, D'Elia C, Boscolo-Berto R, Gardiman M, et al. Predictors of positive surgical margins after laparoscopic robot assisted radical prostatectomy. J Urol. 2009;182(6):2682–8.

22. Jaffe J, Castellucci S, Cathelineau X, Harmon J, Rozet F, Barret E, et al. Robot-assisted laparoscopic prostatectomy: a single-institutions learning curve. Urology. 2009;73(1):127–33.

23. Coelho RF, Chauhan S, Orvieto MA, Palmer KJ, Rocco B, Patel VR. Predictive factors for positive surgical margins and their locations after robot-assisted laparoscopic radical prostatectomy. Eur Urol. 2010;57(6):1022–9.

24. Lasser MS, Renzulli 2nd J, Turini 3rd GA, Haleblian G, Sax HC, Pareek G. An unbiased prospective report of perioperative complications of robot-assisted laparoscopic radical prostatectomy. Urology. 2010;75(5):1083–9.

25. Hong YM, Sutherland DE, Linder B, Engel JD. "Learning curve" may not be enough: assessing the oncological experience curve for robotic radical prostatectomy. J Endourol. 2010;24(3):473–7.

26. Carlucci JR, Nabizada-Pace F, Samadi DB. Robot-assisted laparoscopic radical prostatectomy: technique and outcomes of 700 cases. IJBS. 2009;5(3):201–8.

27. Sooriakumaran P, Ploumidis A, Nyberg T, Olsson M, Akre O, Haendler L, et al. The impact of length and location of positive margins in predicting biochemical recurrence after robotic-assisted radical prostatectomy with a minimum follow-up time of five years. BJU Int. 2013;115(1):106–13.

28. Moskovic DJ, Lavery HJ, Rehman J, Nabizada-Pace F, Brajtbord J, Samadi DB. High body mass index does not affect outcomes following robotic assisted laparoscopic prostatectomy. Can J Urol. 2010;17(4):5291–8.

29. Zorn KC, Wille MA, Thong AE, Katz MH, Shikanov SA, Razmaria A, et al. Continued improvement of perioperative, pathological and continence outcomes during 700 robot-assisted radical prostatectomies. Can J Urol. 2009;16(4):4742–9. discussion 4749.

30. Pound CR, Partin AW, Eisenberger MA, Chan DW, Pearson JD, Walsh PC. Natural history of progression after PSA elevation following radical prostatectomy. JAMA. 1999;281(17):1591–7.

A novel stepwise micro-TESE approach in non obstructive azoospermia

Giorgio Franco[1], Filomena Scarselli[2], Valentina Casciani[2], Cosimo De Nunzio[3], Donato Dente[4], Costantino Leonardo[1*], Pier Francesco Greco[2], Alessia Greco[2], Maria Giulia Minasi[2] and Ermanno Greco[2]

Abstract

Background: The purpose of the study was to investigate whether micro-TESE can improve sperm retrieval rate (SRR) compared to conventional single TESE biopsy on the same testicle or to contralateral multiple TESE, by employing a novel stepwise micro-TESE approach in a population of poor prognosis patients with non-obstructive azoospermia (NOA).

Methods: Sixty-four poor prognosis NOA men undergoing surgical testicular sperm retrieval for ICSI, from March 2007 to April 2013, were included in this study. Patients inclusion criteria were a) previous unsuccessful TESE, b) unfavorable histology (SCOS, MA, sclerahyalinosis), c) Klinefelter syndrome. We employed a stepwise micro-TESE consisting three-steps: 1) single conventional TESE biopsy; 2) micro-TESE on the same testis; 3) contralateral multiple TESE.

Results: SRR was 28.1 % (18/64). Sperm was obtained in both the initial single conventional TESE and in the following micro-TESE. The positive or negative sperm retrieval was further confirmed by a contralateral multiple TESE, when performed. No significant pre-operative predictors of sperm retrieval, including patients' age, previous negative TESE or serological markers (LH, FSH, inhibin B), were observed at univariate or multivariate analysis. Micro-TESE (step 2) did not improve sperm retrieval as compared to single TESE biopsy on the same testicle (step 1) or multiple contralateral TESE (step 3).

Conclusions: Stepwise micro-TESE could represent an optimal approach for sperm retrieval in NOA men. In our view, it should be offered to NOA patients in order to gradually increase surgical invasiveness, when necessary. Stepwise micro-TESE might also reduce the costs, time and efforts involved in surgery.

Keywords: Micro-TESE, TESE, Azoospermia, Sperm retrieval, ICSI

Background

Nonobstructive azoospermia (NOA) is a condition characterized by absence of sperm in the ejaculate due to impaired spermatogenesis. Nonobstructive azoospermia is reported in about 60 % of azoospermic patients and 15 % of all infertile men [1]. The histologic patterns associated with NOA include Sertoli cell-only syndrome (SCOS), maturation arrest (MA), hypospermatogenesis and sclera-hyalinosis. Nonobstructive azoospermic men could benefit from surgical sperm retrieval and assisted conception by intracytoplasmic sperm injection (ICSI). The goal of surgical sperm recovery is to retrieve an adequate number of sperm for ICSI.

Different approaches were used with the intention of increasing the chances of finding viable sperm in NOA patients and, at the same time, optimizing organ preservation [2–4]. The recent updated European Association of Urology (EAU) guidelines (2014) recommend testicular biopsy as the best procedure to provide a histological diagnosis and to find sperm. However, the same EAU guidelines are unclear as to the type of sperm retrieval procedure considered best and recommended for patients with NOA.

In 1999, Schlegel [5] reported a novel microsurgical method for testicular sperm extraction (microdissection

---

* Correspondence: costantino.leonardo@gmail.com
[1]Department Gynaecological-Obstetrical and Urological Sciences, Sapienza University, via del Policlinico n 155 cap, 00161 Rome, Italy
Full list of author information is available at the end of the article

TESE, or micro-TESE). The author introduced this technique with the aim of improving sperm recovery and reducing invasivity of TESE in patients with NOA.

During micro-TESE, with the use of an operating microscope, it is possible to identify and selectively extract larger seminiferous tubules which have higher probability of harboring spermatozoa.

A number of studies suggest that micro-TESE should become the standard in the management of men with NOA [5–9]. Micro-TESE appears to improve the frequency of successful sperm retrieval in NOA patients, despite the removal of dramatically less testicular tissue. Relevantly, the extraction of seminiferous tubules during micro-TESE does not compromise the subtunical blood vessels, therefore the testicular damage is reduced as compared to a standard TESE [5, 9–13]. Schlegel [5] reported an improvement of sperm retrieval from a rate of 45 % with conventional TESE to a rate of 63 % with micro-TESE. However, the literature reports acceptable recovery rates with different techniques including single TESE biopsy: 41.6–49.5 % [14, 15]; multiple conventional TESE: 52.5–56 % [16–18]; micro-TESE: 35–77 % [16, 19–24].

A conventional TESE biopsy with a single small incision is minimally invasive. A multiple conventional TESE with many superficial testicular incisions and tissue extractions is more invasive and can cause damage particularly to the testicular subtunical vessels. Micro-TESE could also entail some damage to testis: it requires an extended equatorial incision to expose the parenchyma. Some concern has recently been raised on the risk of hormonal impairment after micro-TESE due to testicular damage [12, 25, 26]. In addition, micro-TESE requires the need of specific surgical equipment and skills with increased costs and operative time.

Following our preliminary experience [27], in the present study we performed testicular sperm retrieval in NOA patients using a novel surgical approach consisting in steps of increasing invasiveness: we refer to this procedure as to "stepwise micro-TESE". Our aim was to evaluate the performance of TESE versus micro-TESE by comparing the two methods on the same testicles in terms of sperm retrieval. We also provide the clinical outcome after ICSI.

Methods

Study population

In the present study, from March 2007 to April 2013, 343 NOA patients were referred for sperm retrieval at our fertility clinic. Azoospermia was diagnosed when the absence of sperm was observed in two semen samples after 600 g centrifugation and screening at 400x magnification using an inverted microscope, according to the World Health Organization guidelines [28]. Surgical sperm retrieval was performed either by means of single or multiple conventional TESE or by micro-TESE. All the procedures were performed by a single expert surgeon (GF). In March 2007, it was decided that all future micro-TESE would have been performed with the new stepwise micro-TESE approach, consisting in a three-steps biopsy, as described later. Indications for stepwise micro-TESE were previous unsuccessful TESE/micro-TESE, unfavorable histology (complete SCOS or MA) and/or Klinefelter syndrome (KS).

Sixty-four patients received stepwise micro-TESE. Information collected included a clinical history and examination: patient's age was 35.4 ± 5.07; levels of serum FSH, luteinizing hormone (LH) and inhibin B were respectively 25.8 ± 12.45, 10.5 ± 6.57 and 19.7 ± 17.67. The etiology of azoospermia was defined for 38 patients whereas in the remaining 26 it was undefined: 25 were Klinefelter, 12 had a history of chriptorchidism and 1 with micro deletion of the AZFc. All patients were tested for Y-microdeletions. No patient with AZFa, AZFb, AZFab, AZFbc, AZFabc microdeletions were included in our stud group since it is our policy to discourage surgery (TESE or microTESE) in patients with these conditions due to the known no chance of success in sperm retrieval. Twenty-three out of the 64 patients with azoospermia had undergone previous unsuccessful sperm retrieval. Of the 64 patients, 2 (3.1 %) had a testicular volume >12 ml; 9 (14.1 %) had a volume between 6 and 12 ml, and 53 (82.82 %) had a severely reduced volume (<6 ml). No pre-operative hormonal treatment was planned in any patients; in particular, none of the KS men received testosterone replacement prior to surgery.

Surgical technique

The surgical procedure was performed under general anesthesia. After scrotal disinfection with iodopovidone and clorexidine digluconate, the spermatic cord and the scrotal skin were infiltrated with 8 ml of 7.5 mg/ml ropivacaine hydrochloride (Norepine, ASTA, Milan, Italy). The testicle on which the procedure was started was the one with larger volume or, in case no difference was evident between the two testicles, the procedure began on the right one, assuming that varicocele, if present, is on the left side. The scrotum was incised longitudinally for 2 cm on the median raphe and the testis was then delivered through the incision. The stepwise micro-TESE method consisted in three steps: for the initial TESE step, a small (5 mm) equatorial horizontal incision of the albuginea with extrusion of the testicular parenchima and scissors biopsy of approximately $5 \times 2 \times 3$ mm (Fig. 1a). The second step consisted in a micro-TESE: under an operative microscope (10-24X magnification;

Carl Zeiss, OPMI Surgical Microscope, Germany), an equatorial bilateral extension of the original incision was performed up to the hilum, with attention to preserving subtunical vessels. The testicle was then split open bluntly and tubules were retrieved with jewellers forceps from different sites of the two testicular sections (20 or more) aiming to locate and collect the larger ones with an increased chance of harboring spermatozoa (Fig. 1b); no attempt was made to retrieve tubules in the deep

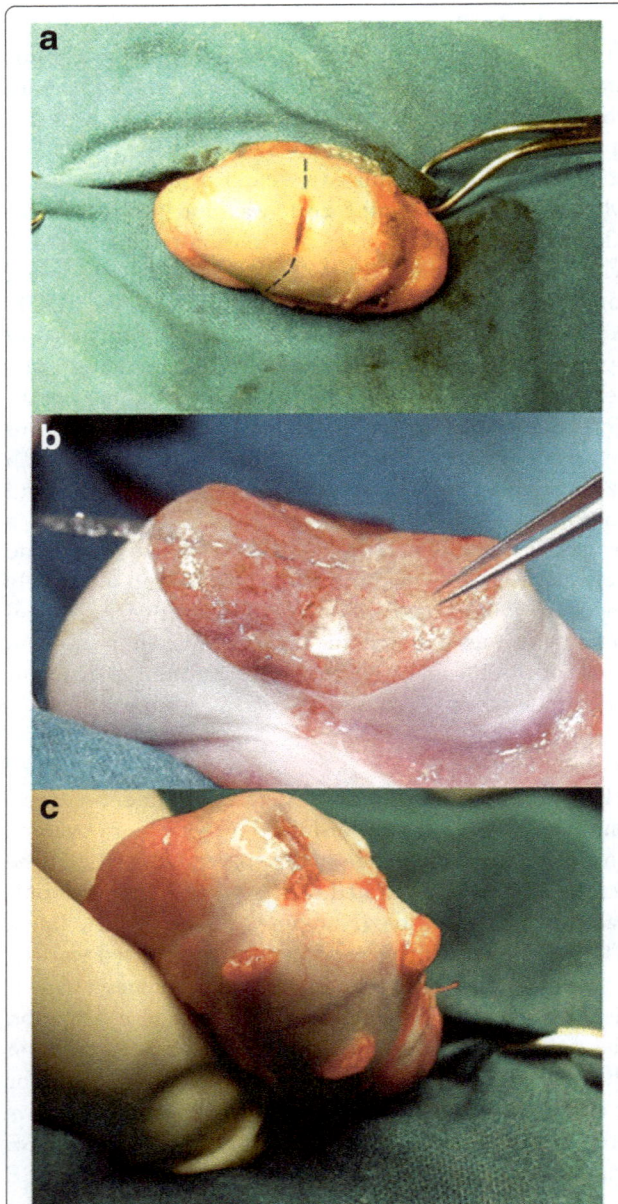

Fig. 1 Stepwise microTESE; **a** Conventional single TESE: the dotted line indicates the extension of the original incision in order to perform micro-TESE; **b** micro-TESE; **c** contralateral conventional multiple TESE

testicular parenchima [29]. At the end of the procedure, the albuginea incision was closed with a VICRYL 5/0 running suture. If no sperm was found so far, we proceeded with the third step: multiple conventional superficial biopsies (4–8 sampling) on the contralateral testicle (Fig. 1c). Each one of the multiple biopsies of the third step had identical procedure and sample size as described for the initial single TESE step. The surgical procedure was always performed by the same surgeon (GF) and the specimen processed by the same biological team.

For hystological examinations, a fragment of testicular parenchyma removed in the first TESE step was washed in buffered medium (Quinn's Advantages Medium with HEPES, SAGE, Cooper Surgical, Pasadena, USA) with 2.5 % Human Serum Albumin (HSA, Albutein, Alpha Therapeutic Milan, Italy), fixed in Bouin's solution (1 ml) and sent to the pathology laboratory. All histological examinations were performed by the same pathologist. The overall mean operating time was 1 h 30′ ± 30′. In our hands, mean operating time for micro-TESE is approximately 1 h 30′, while for single conventional TESE and for multiple TESE it is approximately 20′ and 45′ respectively.

The sequence of events during stepwise micro-TESE involves contemporarily the surgery room and the laboratory: starting from one testicle, the surgeon extracts the first tissue fragment (TESE) and places it in a Petri dish (containing 6–8 ml of buffered medium with HSA) which is immediately sent to the adjacent laboratory. Here, a biologist opens up the seminiferous tubules by mechanically dissecting the tissue with glass coverslides (wet preparation) as previously described [30]. The sperm search on the wet preparation is performed simultaneously by two biologists on two separate inverted microscopes (NIKON Eclipse S) at 400x magnification. After approximately 10–15 min, whether or not sperm are found in the wet preparation, the TESE sample is centrifuged (600G for 10 min). Part of the cell suspension is smeared and covered with mineral oil so that sperm search can continue on a more concentrated sample by one or more biologists simultaneously (for more severe cases even three or four biologists). If sperm is present, evaluation (motility, morphology) and quantification are provided. In parallel, after the initial tissue biopsy, the surgeon proceeds with micro-TESE. The microtubules extracted with micro-TESE are collected in a Petri dish and roughly shredded with coverslides as done for the initial TESE sample. If sperm are found in the two initial steps the contralateral biopsies are avoided. Sperm search in the smeared samples can last even for 4–6 h, long after the surgery procedure is concluded. If sperm is not found on the day of surgery, the search continues on the next days for 1–2 h on the remaining cell suspensions. When sperm is found, it is either used on fresh ICSI cycles or cryopreserved for future use [30]. The samples retrieved during the different steps of the procedure were always treated and frozen separately.

Statistical analysis

Statistical analysis was performed using the SPSS 12.0 software. Differences between groups of patients in medians for quantitative variables and differences in distributions for categorical variables were tested with the Kruskal-Wallis on way analysis of variance (ANOVA) and Chi-square test, respectively. Using multiple logistic regression with the enter method, variables evaluated in the univariate analysis were entered and investigated as predictors of sperm retrieval versus no sperm retrieval. The logistic regression analysis was carried out using data from patients for whom complete data were available. The variables considered for entry into the model included LH, FSH, Inhibin B, previous TESE (categorical variables). An alpha value of 5 % was considered as threshold for significance. Data are presented as median (range), mean ± standard deviation (SD). Odds ratios (OR) and 95 % confidence intervals (CI) were calculated for the parameters in each group, no sperm retrieval as reference group.

Results

In 18 out of 64 patients we were able to retrieve testicular spermatozoa (sperm retrieval rate, SRR = 28.1 %). No significant differences in terms of sperm retrieval were observed between TESE and micro-TESE [18/64 patients for TESE versus 18/64 for micro-TESE (Chi square test, $p = 1$)]. In all cases in which we retrieved sperm with micro-TESE we had previously retrieved sperm with the initial single TESE, either immediately in the wet preparation or with a longer search after centrifugation. On the other hand, when no sperm was found in the first procedure, none was found in the second micro-TESE nor in the contralateral testicle ($N = 46/64$).

Of the 18 patients with positive sperm retrieval, 11 received only the two initial steps on the first testicle sparing the contralateral biopsy due to the fact that sperm was immediately found in the first testis. In the other 7 patients, sperm was not immediately found in the first testis with the two initial procedures, therefore we proceeded anyway on the contralateral testicle: all of them eventually had positive sperm retrieval in both testis.

The hystological evaluation performed on the specimens obtained from our 64 patients was: 37/64 patients (57.8 %) SCOS, 15/64 (23.4 %) MA, and 12/64 (18.8 %) sclera-hyalinosis. The histological diagnosis of positive sperm retrieval patients was: 10 MA, 1 sclera-hyalinosis

and 7 SCOS. The histological diagnosis of negative sperm retrieval patients was: 5 MA, 11 had sclera-hyalinosis and 30 SCOS (Table 4). A significant (Chi square test, $p = 0.001$) higher sperm retrieval was obtained in patients with MA (10/15 = 67 % positive versus 5/15 = 33 % negative) when compared to patients with SCOS (7/37 = 18.9 % positive versus 30/37 = 81.1 % negative) and sclera-hyalinosis (1/12 = 0.8 % positive versus 11/12 = 99.2 % negative, Table 1). However, due to the small numbers of patients in each class, the statistical analysis has a reduced power.

The mean age of 18 men with positive sperm retrieval was 34.2 ± 7.16; mean FSH level was 25.9 ± 15.10, mean LH level was 12.5 ± 9.40 and mean inhibin B level was 14.9 ± 5.63. On the other hand, in the 46 with negative sperm retrieval, mean age was 35.9 ± 3.94. Average levels of FSH, LH and inhibin B were 25.7 ± 11.60, 9.7 ± 4.88 and 20.0 ± 18.86, respectively. No significant differences for each of these variables were observed between patients with positive and negative sperm retrieval (Table 2). Twenty-three patients had previously undergone a TESE elsewhere, and for 6 of them stepwise micro-TESE resulted in a positive sperm retrieval (26 %). On the other hand, of the 41 patients who had not previously undergone a TESE elsewhere, 12 had positive sperm retrieval with step-wise micro-TESE (29 %; Chi square test, NS; Table 3). With a multiple logistic regression the predictive value of serological markers (FSH, LH and inhibin B) and of a previous unsuccessful TESE was investigated (Table 4). No significant pre-operative predictors of sperm retrieval, including previous TESE or serological markers, were observed at univariate or multivariate analysis.

Stepwise micro-TESE was always optimally tolerated by patients with minimal post-operative pain and no major complications. Fifteen out of the 18 patients with positive sperm retrieval had sperm cryopreservation whereas 3 of them underwent an ICSI cycle with fresh sperm. Our results in terms of fertilization and live birth rate are comparable with those in the literature. Overall, 2 patients (1 KS with AZFc deletion and 1 SCOS) had unsuccessful fertilization both with cryopreserved sperm. Four patients had embryo transfer with negative

Table 1 Histological diagnosis of patients with positive or negative sperm retrieval after stepwise micro-TESE. Significantly higher sperm retrieval was obtained in patients with MA when compared to patients with SCOS and sclera-hyalinosis

Histology	Positive sperm retrieval	Negative sperm retrieval	Chi square
MA (15 cases)	10/15 (67 %)	5/15 (33 %)	$P = 0.001$
SCO (37 cases)	7/37 (18.9 %)	30/37 (81.1 %)	
Sclera-hyalinosis (12 cases)	1/12 (0.8 %)	11/12 (99.2 %)	

Table 2 Mean Age and preoperative variables (FSH, LH and inhibin B) in patients with positive or negative sperm retrieval after stepwise micro-TESE: none of these variables was predictive of sperm retrieval

	Positive	Negative	p
N	18	46	
Mean age	34.2 ± 7.16	35.9 ± 3.94	0.191
FSH	25.9 ± 15.10	25.7 ± 11.60	0.525
LH	12.5 ± 9.40	9.7 ± 4.88	0.586
Inhibin B	14.9 ± 5.63	20.0 ± 18.86	0.887

Table 4 Multiple logistic regression with the enter method. Variables evaluated in the univariate analyses were entered and investigated as predictors of sperm retrieval versus no sperm retrieval

	OR	95.0 % C.I.		P
FSH	0.979	0.863	1.112	0.749
LH	1.035	0.829	1.293	0.760
Inhibin B	0.944	0.787	1.132	0.532
Previous TESE	0.257	0.014	4.584	0.356

beta-HCG (1 MA and 1 SCOS with cryopreserved sperm; 2 MA with fresh sperm). One SCOS patient had positive beta-HCG with cryopreserved sperm but no heartbeat was observed. One MA patient underwent an ICSI cycle with fresh sperm resulting in abortion at 8 weeks of gestation. Finally 3 ICSI cycles (all MA with cryopreserved sperm) ended with 4 babies delivered: 1 twin (1 female and 1 male) and 2 singleton (2 males) pregnancies (live-birth rate 27.2 % = 3/11 ICSI cycles).

Discussion

In this study, a novel stepwise micro-TESE technique was performed on 64 patients with severe NOA undergoing testicular sperm extraction. First, a single TESE sample was taken from one testicle and, after this, a micro-TESE was performed extending the same testicular incision. The third step consisted in contralateral conventional multiple biopsies in case of negative sperm retrieval on the first testis. The rationale behind our study design was to explore the possibility of a gradual sperm retrieval approach aiming to minimize invasiveness, and to compare the efficiency of micro-TESE with conventional TESE. In our fertility center, surgery proceeds in parallel with sperm search in the laboratory and we are used to move to the contralateral testis in all cases of negative sperm retrieval, in order to maximize the chance of success. The contralateral multiple TESE served also as an additional control that micro-TESE was correctly performed in the first testis. Unexpectedly, no differences were seen in SRR among the initial TESE, the following micro-TESE and the final contralateral multiple TESE.

Conventional multiple TESE consists in random incisions which may result in atrophy and devascularization of the surrounding testicular tissue. This effect, together

Table 3 Sperm retrieval rate was similar in the groups of patients who underwent or not a previous unsuccesful TESE

	Previous TESE	No previous TESE	Chi square
Positive sperm retrieval	6/23 (26 %)	12/41 (29 %)	P = 0.552

with the intratesticular bleeding and scar formation, can easily damage the spermatogenetic pathway and hormone production [8]. Micro-TESE with microtubules extraction from superficial sites of the section is less invasive than conventional multiple TESE [5]. This method, thanks to the optical magnification, allows a sparing of subtunical albuginea and intratesticular vessels with a minimal excision of testicular parenchyma. In fact, single seminiferous tubules can be collected without impairing the surrounding tissues. In the literature, there are many reports indicating micro-TESE as a more efficient method to retrieve spermatozoa with reasonable scarce invasiveness when compared to multiple biopsies. Tsujimura and colleagues [13] reported a SRR of 45 % obtained with salvage micro-TESE performed after previous failed conventional TESE. Overall, the reported rates of successful sperm retrieval with micro-TESE varies between 47 and 66 % [7, 8, 12, 31, 32]. However, in our view, it is reasonable to believe that many of these successful micro-TESE cases might have benefited from a less invasive approach of sperm retrieval. In these studies, micro-TESE was apparently offered to all NOA patients, even those with good prognosis. For instance, the operated population often included NOA patients with the histologic pattern of hypospermatogenesis, although it is well known that SRR in this situation is very high with any sperm retrieval technique [33].

We operate in a private fertility center where micro-TESE, due to its higher costs (approximately 50 % higher than for conventional TESE) is offered only to NOA patients with severe clinical diagnosis and prognosis (complete SCOS or MA, KS, previous unsuccessful TESE). This might be an explanation why our overall SRR of 28.1 % (18/64) is low when compared to those reported in the literature. However, it should be noticed that in other reports, when looking only to NOA subpopulations with severe prognosis, a similarly low SRR was reported, as described in a detailed review from Ghalayini et al. [24].

In contrast with what expected, our micro-dissection step did not improve the chance of finding sperm: the SRR obtained with micro-TESE or with the initial single conventional TESE coincided. Moreover, the multiple TESE performed on the contralateral testicle always confirmed the outcome obtained on the first testicle, either successful or not.

A possible reason for our micro-TESE not improving SRR could be that our tubule collection method during micro-TESE remained superficial. Ramasamy and colleagues [29] have recently reported their technique of micro-TESE starting with a superficial extraction of tubules followed by a deeper and more extensive search below the superficial section. This second step improved the SRR by 18.4 % [29]. It is reasonable to assume that by extending our tubules collection to the deeper part of the testis, our SRR could be improved as well. However, one must take into account that an extensive procedure might entail additional damage and significantly prolong surgical time [34].

In another study from Marconi and colleagues [32], four surgical methods were compared, namely unifocal conventional TESE, unifocal micro-TESE, trifocal conventional TESE and trifocal conventional TESE plus micro-TESE. Consistently with our results, no difference was observed between micro-TESE and trifocal conventional TESE. Only the combination of trifocal conventional TESE plus unifocal micro-TESE significantly increased the SRR when compared to unifocal conventional TESE.

A surgical approach similar to ours has been applied by Turunc and colleagues [31]. The authors performed exclusively micro-TESE in a subgroup of severe NOA patients with testicular atrophy, obtaining a SRR of approximately 20 %. Another larger group of patients with a less severe prognosis, underwent firstly a trifocal conventional TESE. Only when no sperm was found, micro-TESE was performed by joining the three original incisions, therefore increasing the SRR from about 34 % up to 51 %. Anyway, it has to be pointed out that the majority of successes were obtained with the initial conventional TESE. These data support our belief that micro-TESE should not be offered indiscriminately to all NOA patients but a gradual approach should be warranted.

A large proportion of our population was represented by men with KS (25/64 = 39.1 %). In our view this condition is one of the most severe forms of NOA [30]. Of these 25 patients, 6 had positive sperm retrieval (24 %). Theoretically, micro-TESE should be an ideal approach for men with KS who are characterized by small testes, extensive sclera-hyalinosis and scattered areas of remaining tubules. In this situation, the magnification system used during micro-TESE helps in identifying the tubules among the sclerotic tissue. The SRR of KS man in the present series resulted considerably low when compared to other published studies, including one from our group (ref. 30). A possible explanation is that, in the present study group,

the mean age of KS patients (35.5 ± 5.18) was substantially higher than that reported in other studies [30, 35, 36]. It is in fact well known how sclera-hyalinosis increases and spermatogenesis declines with age in KS patients.

The histology in our patient's population was represented by SCOS (57.8 %), MA (23.4 %) and sclera-hyalinosis (18.8 %). The condition of hypospermatogenis, a less severe form of NOA, was not represented among our 64 patients. Interestingly, we observed a significantly higher SRR in patients with MA (Table 1) when compared to the other histological diagnosis, although our sample size is limited to obtain definitive conclusions. On the contrary, sclera-hyalinosis appeared to be related to a scarce chance of retrieving sperm. The literature is still controversial in terms of the prognostic value of testicular histology. Some authors report a higher success rate of micro-TESE in case of SCOS [21, 29]. This could be reasonably due to an incomplete SCOS, a condition in which larger microtubules with spermatogenesis can be easily identified with the optical magnification among those with only Sertoli cells. The histological diagnosis of our patients population can explain our low SRR in the present series: most of our patients had and unfavorable histology of SCOS (57.8 %) and sclera-hyalinosis (18.8 %); only a smaller proportion had MA (23.4 %) and nearly all of them had positive SRR (10/15).

In our experience, no significant pre-operative predictors of sperm retrieval, including previous TESE or serological markers, were observed at univariate or multivariate analysis (Tables 2, 3 and 4). Particularly, in our study, levels of FSH, LH, inhibin B were not predictive of sperm retrieval, consistently to the results reported elsewhere [37, 38]. In contrast, other groups reported a positive predictive power of some pre-operative variables, such as FSH (39; 17) and inhibin B [39, 40]. Furthermore, in the subgroup of patients who had undergone a previous negative TESE elsewhere ($N = 23$, SRR = 26 %), the SRR did not differ from the subgroup of patients who had not received a previous negative TESE ($N = 41$, SRR = 29 %, Table 3).

Conclusions

Our study indicate that 1) in patients with poor prognosis NOA even micro-TESE did not improve the chance of retrieving sperm; 2) in all patients with successful sperm retrieval, the initial, less invasive single conventional biopsy would have been enough to obtain sperm; 3) micro-TESE was always optimally tolerated by patients and left minimal if no scars; 4) due to the priority that should be always given to organ preservation, we believe that the gradual approach of stepwise micro-TESE could be ideal for testicular sperm retrieval in all NOA men. In this way costs, time and efforts involved in the surgery procedure would be drastically reduced.

Abbreviations

AZF: azoospermia factor; beta-HCG: beta human chorionic gonadotropin; EAU: European Association of Urology; FSH: follicle stimulation hormone; HSA: Human Serum Albumin; ICSI: intracytoplasmic sperm injection; KS: Klinefelter syndrome; LH: luteinizing hormone; MA: maturation arrest; micro-TESE: microdissection testicular sperm extraction; NOA: non-obstructive azoospermia; SCOS: Sertoli cell-only syndrome; SRR: sperm retrieval rate; TESE: testicular sperm extraction.

Competing interest

The authors declare that they have no competing interests.

Authors' contributions

GF and EG conceived the study concept and design. FS and VC carried out acquisition of data and drafting the manuscript. CDD and CL carried out analysis and interpretation of the data. DD and MGM carried out drafting of the manuscript. PFG and AG carried out Critical revision of the manuscript. CDD and CL carried out statistical analysis. All Authors read and approve the final version of the manuscript.

Acknowledgments

The authors would like to thank to Dr Mario Terrible, PhD, for his precious help during data acquisition evaluation and discussion.

Funding

Not applicable.

Author details

[1]Department Gynaecological-Obstetrical and Urological Sciences, Sapienza University, via del Policlinico n 155 cap, 00161 Rome, Italy. [2]Centre for Reproductive Medicine, European Hospital, Rome, Italy. [3]Department Urology, Sant' Andrea Hospital, Sapienza University, Rome, Italy. [4]Robotic Urology Department, Policlinico Abano Terme, Padova, Italy.

References

1. Dabaja AA, Schlegel PN. Microdissection testicular sperm extraction: an update. Asian J Androl. 2013;15:35–9.
2. Oliveira Filho AB, Souza RS, Azeredo-Oliveira MT, Peruquetti RL, Cedenho AP. Microdissection testicular sperm extraction causes spermatogenic alterations in the contralateral testis. Genet Mol Res. 2010;9:1405–13.
3. Glina S, Soares JB, Antunes Jr N, Galuppo AG, Paz LB, Wonchockier R. Testicular histopathological diagnosis as a predictive factor for retrieving spermatozoa for ICSI in non-obstructive azoospermic patients. Int Braz J Urol. 2005;31:338–41.
4. Van Peperstraten A, Proctor ML, Johnson NP, Philipson G. Techniques for surgical retrieval of sperm prior to intracytoplsmic sperm injecyion (ICSI) for azoospermia. Cochrane Database Syst Rev. 2008;(2):CD002807.
5. Schlegel PN. Testicular sperm extraction: microdissection improves sperm yield with minimal tissue excision. Hum Reprod. 1999;14:131–5.
6. Silber SJ. Microsurgical TESE and the distribution of spermatogenesis in non-obstructive azoospermia. Hum Reprod. 2000;15:2278–84.
7. Amer M, Ateyah A, Hany R, Zohdy W. Prospective comparative study between microsurgical and conventional testicular sperm extraction in non-obstructive azoospermia: follow-up by serial ultrasound examinations. Hum Reprod. 2000;15:653–6.
8. Ramasamy R, Yagan N, Schlegel PN. Structural and functional changes to the testis after conventional versus microdissection testicular sperm extraction. Urology. 2005;65:1190–4.
9. Ramasamy R, Ricci JA, Palermo GD, Gosden LV, Rosenwaks Z, Schlegel PN. Successful fertility treatment for Klinefelter's syndrome. J Urol. 2009;182:1108–13.
10. Okada H, Dobashi M, Yamazaki T, Hara I, Fujisawa M, Arakawa S, et al. Conventional versus microdissection testicular sperm extraction for nonobstructive azoospermia. J Urol. 2002;168:1063–7.
11. Okubo K, Ogura K, Ichioka K, Terada N, Matsuta Y, Yoshimura K, et al. Testicular sperm extraction for non-obstructive azoospermia: results with conventional and microsurgical techniques. Hinyokika Kiyo. 2002;48:275–80.
12. Tsujimura A, Matsumiya K, Miyagawa Y, Tohda A, Miura H, Nishimura K, et al. Conventional multiple or microdissection testicular sperm extraction: a comparative study. Hum Reprod. 2002;17:2924–9.
13. Tsujimura A, Miyagawa Y, Takao T, Takada S, Koga M, Takeyama M, et al. Salvage microdissection testicular sperm extraction after failed conventional testicular sperm extraction in patients with nonobstructive azoospermia. J Urol. 2006;175:1446–9.
14. Vernaeve V, Verheyen G, Goossens A, Van Steirteghem A, Devroey P, Tournaye H. How successful is repeat testicular sperm extraction in patients with azoospermia? Hum Reprod. 2006;21:1551–4.
15. Donoso P, Tournaye H, Devroey P. Which is the best sperm retrieval technique for non-obstructive azoospermia? A systematic review. Hum Reprod Update. 2007;13:539–49.
16. Colpi GM, Piediferro G, Nerva F, Giacchetta D, Colpi EM, Piatti E. Sperm retrieval for intra-cytoplasmic sperm injection in non-obstructive azoospermia. Minerva Urol Nefrol. 2005;57:99–107.
17. Colpi GM, Colpi EM, Piediferro G, Giacchetta D, Gazzano G, Castiglioni FM, et al. Microsurgical TESE versus conventional TESE for ICSI in non-obstructive azoospermia: a randomized controlled study. Reprod Biomed Online. 2009;18:315–9.
18. Bromage SJ, Falconer DA, Lieberman BA, Sangar V, Payne SR. Sperm retrieval rates in subgroups of primary azoospermic males. Eur Urol. 2007;51:534–9.
19. El-Haggar S, Mostafa T, Abdel Nasser T, Hany R, Abdel HA. Fine needle aspiration vs. mTESE in non-obstructive azoospermia. Int J Androl. 2008;31:595–601.
20. Talas H, Yaman O, Aydos K. Outcome of repeated micro-surgical testicular sperm extraction in patients with non-obstructive azoospermia. Asian J Androl. 2007;9:668–73.
21. Esteves SC, Verza S, Prudencio C, Seol B. Sperm retrieval rate (SRR) in nonobstructive azoospermia (NOA) are related to testicular histopathology results but not to the etiology of azoospermia. Fertil Steril. 2010;94:S132.
22. Esteves SC, Miyaoka R, Agarwal A. Surgical treatment of male infertility in the era of intracytoplasmic sperm injection - new insights. Clinics. 2011;66:1463–77.
23. Ravizzini P, Carizza C, Abdelmassih V, Abdelmassih S, Azevedo M, Abdelmassih R. Microdissection testicular sperm extraction and IVF-ICSI outcome in nonobstructive azoospermia. Andrologia. 2008;40:219–26.
24. Ghalayini IF, Al-Ghazo MA, Hani OB, Al-Azab R, Bani-Hani I, Zayed F, et al. Clinical comparison of conventional testicular sperm extraction and microdissection techniques for non-obstructive azoospermia. J Clin Med Res. 2011;19:124–31.
25. Takada S, Tsujimura A, Ueda T, Matsuoka Y, Takao T, Miyagawa Y, et al. Androgen decline in patients with nonobstructive azoospemia after microdissection testicular sperm extraction. Urology. 2008;72:114–8.
26. Tsujimura A. Microdissection testicular sperm extraction: prediction, outcome, and complications. Int J Urol. 2007;14:883–9.
27. Franco G. Sperm retrieval in the azoospermic patient. In: Greco E, editor. Male infertility and ART. Firenze: Pacini Editore Press; 2008. p. 50–6.
28. World Health Organization. WHO Laboratory manual for the examination and processing of human semen and Sperm-Cervical Mucus and interaction. Cambridge: WHO; 2010.
29. Ramasamy R, Reifsnyder JE, Husseini J, Eid PA, Bryson C, Schlegel PN. Localization of sperm during microdissection testicular sperm extraction in men with nonobstructive azoospermia. J Urol. 2013;189:643–6.
30. Greco E, Scarselli F, Minasi MG, Casciani V, Zavaglia D, Dente D, et al. Birth of 16 healthy children after ICSI in cases of nonmosaic Klinefelter syndrome. Hum Reprod. 2013;28:1155–60.
31. Turunc T, Gul U, Haydardedeoglu B, Bal N, Kuzgunbay B, Peskircioglu L, et al. Conventional testicular sperm extraction combined with the microdissection

technique in nonobstructive azoospermic patients: a prospective comparative study. Fertil Steril. 2010;94:2157–60.

32. Marconi M, Keudel A, Diemer T, Bergmann M, Steger K, Schuppe HC, et al. Combined trifocal and microsurgical testicular sperm extraction is the best technique for testicular sperm retrieval in "low-chance" nonobstructive azoospermia. Eur Urol. 2012;62:713–9.

33. Tournaye H, Liu J, Nagy PZ, Camus M, Goossens A, Silber S, et al. Correlation between testicular histology and outcome after intracytoplasmic sperm injection using testicular spermatozoa. Hum Reprod. 1996;11:127–32.

34. Ramasamy R, Fisher ES, Ricci JA, Leung RA, Schlegel PN. Duration of microdissection testicular sperm extraction procedures: relationship to sperm retrieval success. J Urol. 2011;185:1394–7.

35. Plotton I, Giscard d'Estaing S, Cuzin B, Brosse A, Benchaib M, Lornage J, et al. Preliminary results of a prospective study of testicular sperm extraction in young versus adult patients with nonmosaic 47, XXY Klinefelter syndrome. J Clin Endocrinol Metab. 2015;100(3):961–7.

36. Sabbaghian M, Modarresi T, Hosseinifar H, Hosseini J, Farrahi F, Dadkhah F, et al. Comparison of sperm retrieval and intracytoplasmic sperm injection outcome in patients with and without Klinefelter syndrome. Urology. 2014;83(1):107–10.

37. Raheem A, Garaffa G, Rushwan N, De Luca F, Zacharakis E, Abdel Raheem T, et al. Testicular histopathology as a predictor of a positive sperm retrieval in men with non-obstructive azoospermia. BJU Int. 2013;111:492–9.

38. Gul U, Turunc T, Haydardedeoglu B, Yaycioglu O, Kuzgunbay B, Ozkardes H. Sperm retrieval and live birth rates in presumed Sertoli-cell-only syndrome in testis biopsy: a single centre experience. Andrology. 2013;1:47–51.

39. Bohring C, Schroeder-Printzen I, Weidner W, Krause W. Serum levels of inhibin B and follicle-stimulating hormone may predict successful sperm retrieval in men with azoospermia who are undergoing testicular sperm extraction. Fertil Steril. 2002;78:1195–8.

40. Brugo-Olmedo S, De Vincentiis S, Calamera JC, Urrutia F, Nodar F, Acosta AA. Serum inhibin B may be a reliable marker of the presence of testicular spermatozoa in patients with nonobstructive azoospermia. Fertil Steril. 2001;76:1124–9.

Sensitivity of initial biopsy or transurethral resection of bladder tumor(s) for detecting histological variants on radical cystectomy

Peng Ge[1,2†], Zi-Cheng Wang[1,2†], Xi Yu[1,2], Jian Lin[1,2*] and Qun He[1,2*]

Abstract

Background: To investigate the efficacy of initial biopsy or transurethral resection of bladder tumor for detecting histological variants on radical cystectomy and to assess the prognostic significance of variant histology on urothelial carcinoma outcomes after radical cystectomy.

Methods: Clinical and histopathological characteristics of 147 patients with variant histology who underwent radical cystectomy for urothelial carcinoma between 2006 and 2012 were assessed. Sensitivity was calculated as the proportion of radical cystectomy specimens with a particular variant that also presented the variant in the biopsy or transurethral resection specimen. The Kaplan-Meier method and multivariate Cox proportional hazard regression analysis were used to estimate cancer-specific survival.

Results: Of the 147 patients, 116 (79 %) were diagnosed with a single variant histology, and 31 (21 %) had multiple patterns. Squamous differentiation (31 %) was the most common single variant histology, followed by glandular differentiation (28 %). Except for small cell variant (100 %), the sensitivity of biopsy and transurethral resection was most effective for the diagnosis of squamous differentiation, 19 % vs. 40 % respectively, followed by glandular differentiation, 11 % vs. 21 % respectively. A total of 6 % and 49 % patients could be variant-free partially due to biopsy or complete resection(s) respectively. Presence of variant differentiation in urothelial carcinoma at cystectomy was significantly associated with inferior survival both in univariate analysis ($P = 0.005$) and multivariate analysis (HR4.48, 95 % CI:1.03-19.53).

Conclusions: Overall sensitivity of biopsy or transurethral resection to detect variant differentiation on cystectomy is relatively low. Patients with variant differentiation on cystectomy specimens have inferior survival.

Keywords: Urothelial carcinoma, Variant histologic differentiation, Cystectomy, Pathology, Prognosis

Background

More than 90 % of bladder cancers are urothelial carcinomas. Urothelial carcinoma of the bladder (UCB) has a propensity to undergo divergent or variant differentiation, resulting in a wide spectrum of subtypes [1–3]. Thirteen morphotypes were discussed in the 2004 *World Health Organization Classification of Tumours of the Urinary Tract* [4]. Since then, several new divergent subtypes have been described [2, 5].

Generally, about 7 to 81 % of bladder UCBs have some type of variant differentiation [3, 6–8]. The recognition of histological variants in UCB is of significance to both pathologists and clinicians because (a) some variants may affect prognostic consequences, (b) some may need different modalities compared with those used in conventional UCB, and (c) knowledge of the histological variants may be crucial to avoid diagnostic misinterpretations [5]. That applies, for example, to tumors consisting of plasmocytoid or micropapillary components. UCB patients with plasmocytoid histology may lead to diagnosis delays and inappropriate therapies because of absence of gross hematuria and the lack of visible tumor at cystoscopy [9, 10]. Given that micropapillary carcinoma is

* Correspondence: linjianbj@163.com; bdyyqhe@sina.com
†Equal contributors
[1]Department of Urology, Peking University First Hospital and Institute of Urology, Peking University, Beijing 100034, China
[2]National Research Center for Genitourinary Oncology, Beijing 100034, China

less sensitive to immunotherapy or chemotherapy compared to traditional UCB, one leading group has suggested early cystectomy should be taken into consideration in the clinical management of those patients with micropapillary histology for pTa and pT1 tumors [5, 11]. Hence, early detection of variant differentiation is crucial.

However, the diagnosis of UCB variants may be challenging. A common feature of the variant patterns is that the frequency with which they are diagnosed is influenced by many factors: the extensiveness of the tumor pathologically sampled, the proportion of the divergent element of the whole tumor, the attentiveness of the pathologist detecting small foci of the respective pattern, the severity of artifact caused by tangential sectioning, cautery and mechanical injury, etc. [3–5, 12].

This study was aimed at investigating the sensitivity of biopsy and/or transurethral resection of bladder tumor (TURBT) for detecting the histological differentiation on radical cystectomy (RC). We also assess the prognostic significance of variant histology in UCB at cystectomy.

Methods
Patient population and pathologic evaluation
This was a retrospective, single-institution study approved by Peking University First Hospital review board (No. 2014692). We retrospectively reviewed all the pathology reports available at our institution with informed consent for each UCB patient treated with RC from the time of first visit to the time of RC. The variant histology in this study are those recognized by 2004 WHO Classification of Tumors and the literature [4, 5]. Four highly experienced pathologists specializing in urologic pathology were involved in reviewing these cases. Pathological grade and stage were assigned according to the recommendations, respectively [4, 13]. Any problematic cases were re-reviewed by a dedicated urologic pathologist (author QH) to verify the initial diagnoses. Any amount of variant differentiation was reported.

Inclusion criteria: (a) From the time of first visit to the time of RC, all the treatments were done at our hospital; first visit was defined as patients had never received biopsy or underwent biopsy for only once at other institutions before coming to our hospital and the pathological sections of biopsy were re-reviewed by the pathologists at our medical center; (b) Detailed medical record information was available. Exclusion criteria: (a) Patients received TURBT(s) or partial cystectomy at other institutions before initiation of therapy at our institution; (b) Patients presented extravesical malignant primary tumors before RC; (c) Patients underwent biopsy or TURBT without subsequent RC as well as any with pure nonurothelial morphology [1].

Between 2006 and 2012, a total of 620 consecutive patients were treated with RC for UCB at Peking University First Hospital. Ultimately, 147 patients who met all the above-described criteria with a diagnosis of variant differentiation in pure or mixed form after RC, the matched preceding biopsy or TURBT(s), were included in this study. Among those patients, 63 who underwent biopsy only once without TURBT were included in the analysis of biopsy sensitivity, while the remaining 84 who underwent TURBT at least once were used to calculate the sensitivity of TURBT. For study purposes TURBT was defined as resection of all visible tumor while biopsy partial sampling [1].

Follow-up
Follow-up was performed generally quarterly for the first year, semiannually for the next 2 years and annually thereafter with laboratory and imaging studies unless otherwise clinically indicated. Outcomes of interest was cancer-specific survival (CSS). CSS duration was calculated from date of cystectomy to death due to bladder cancer; surviving patients were censored at last follow-up [14, 15].

Statistical analysis
Sensitivity was calculated as the proportion of RC specimens with a particular variant that also had the variant in the biopsy or last TURBT (LTURBT) specimen [1]. The Kaplan–Meier method was used to graphically display survivor functions. Multivariate Cox proportional hazards models were used to estimate independent relationships between categorical variables that were univariably prognostic for CSS. The assumptions of proportional hazards with respect to the log-hazard were checked using the Schoenfeld residual test and no major model violations were observed. All analyses were performed using SAS version 9.2 (SAS Institute, Cary, NC, USA) and/or SPSS version 20.0 (IBM Corp, Armonk, NY, USA). Two-sided $P \leq 0.050$ was considered statistically significant.

Results
Histologic spectrum of variant differentiation
Of the 147 patients, 116 (79 %) were diagnosed with a single variant histology, whereas the remaining 31 (21 %) had multiple patterns of variant histologic components on RC, the matched preceding biopsy or TURBT(s). In decreasing order of frequency, the spectrum of divergent differentiation included: squamous (31 %), glandular (28 %), sarcomatoid (12 %), small cell (2 %), clear cell (2 %), microcystic (2 %), lymphoepithelioma-like (1 %), and undifferentiated (1 %).

Sensitivity of biopsy or TURBT for detecting histological variants on RC
The sensitivity of biopsy and LTURBT to detect a certain variant varied (Table 1). Except for small cell variant (100 %), the sensitivity of biopsy and LTURBT was most effective for the diagnosis of squamous differentiation,

Table 1 The sensitivity of biopsy and LTURBT for detecting variant differentiation

Variant	No. biopsy	RC	% sensitivity	No. LTURBT[a]	RC	% sensitivity
Squamous	8	28	19	26	20	40
Glandular	4	27	11	18	19	21
Sarcomatoid	0	19	0	14	11	9
Small cell	1	1	100	1	3	0
Lymphoepithelioma-like	0	3	0	0	0	0
Plasmacytoid	0	1	0	0	1	0
Clear cell	0	2	0	0	3	0
Nested	0	0	0	1	0	0
Microcystic	0	3	0	1	1	0
Undifferentiated	0	1	0	0	0	0

[a]Last transurethral resection of bladder tumor precystectomy

19 % vs. 40 % respectively, followed by glandular differentiation, 11 % vs. 21 % respectively. Sarcomatoid variant with a sensitivity of 9 % was only detected on LTURBT. Surprisingly, it seemed to be invalid for biopsy or LTURBT to detect lymphoepithelioma-like (0 %), plasmacytoid (0 %), clear cell (0 %), nested (0 %), and undifferentiated variant (0 %).

Forty-five patients (31 %) exhibited variant(s) only on biopsy or TURBT(s), including 4 cases for biopsy, and 41 cases for TURBT(s). In other words, this suggested that the efficacy of biopsy and TURBT(s) upon removing the variant components during the disease course was 6 % (4 of 64) and 49 % (41 of 84) respectively partially due to extensive sampling and complete resection. There were 71 patients who underwent TURBT only once and 13 underwent TURBT at least twice (varying from twice to six times) during the time of first visit to the time of RC. For those who underwent TURBT only once, 34 (48 %) were found free of variant complements on RC. Interestingly, for patients who underwent TURBT at least twice, 5 patients were diagnosed with different variant histologic subtypes on RC, the matched preceding biopsy or TURBT (Table 2).

Cancer-specific survival

Follow-up information was available for 139 patients (94.6 %); 28 patients died of bladder cancer during follow-up. The mean age of the 139 patients was 66 years (SD:11.1). The median follow-up was 31 months (range 2–90). Of those, 95 UCB patients were identified with variant differentiation on RC specimens. Fig. 1 shows that variant differentiation on RC was statistically significantly associated with inferior survival ($P = 0.005$). Similarly, multivariate analyses after being adjusted for the effects of pathologic stage demonstrated that presence of variant differentiation in urothelial carcinoma at cystectomy was independently associated with cancer-specific mortality (HR4.48, 95 % CI:1.03-19.53).

Discussion

In this current study, we investigated the sensitivity of biopsy and/or TURBT for detecting the histological differentiation on RC and assessed the prognostic significance of variant histology on urothelial carcinoma outcomes after RC. Our results indicate that overall sensitivity of biopsy or TURBT to detect variant differentiation on RC is relatively low. Presence of variant differentiation in urothelial carcinoma at cystectomy portends inferior survival.

Table 2 Variants detected on TURBT and RC of patients who underwent TURBT at least twice (n = 13)

Patient ID	No. TURBT[a]	No. variant[b]	RC[c]	Variant (TURBT/No.TURBT)[d]
1	6	1	Glandular	Sarcomatoid (6/6)
2	5	1	UC[e]	Clear cell (1/5)
3	4	1	Glandular	Glandular (4/4)
4	4	2	UC	Squamous (2/4), Nested (4/4)
5	3	1	Sarcomatoid	Glandular (3/3)
6	2	1	Glandular	Squamous (2/2)
7	2	1	Squamous	Squamous (2/2)
8	2	2	Squamous	Squamous (1/2), Squamous (2/2)
9	2	1	UC	Squamous (1/2)
10	2	1	UC	Small cell (2/2)
11	2	1	UC	Squamous (1/2)
12	2	1	UC	Sarcomatoid (1/2)
13	2	1	UC	Squamous (1/2)

All the specimens were re-reviewed by a dedicated pathologist QH
[a]The total number of TURBT
[b]The total number of TURBT with a diagnosis of variant differentiation
[c]The diagnosis of radical cystectomy specimen
[d]TURBT/No.TURBT = The ordinal number of TURBT with a diagnosis of variant differentiation / The total number of TURBT
[e]Urothelial carcinoma without variant differentiation

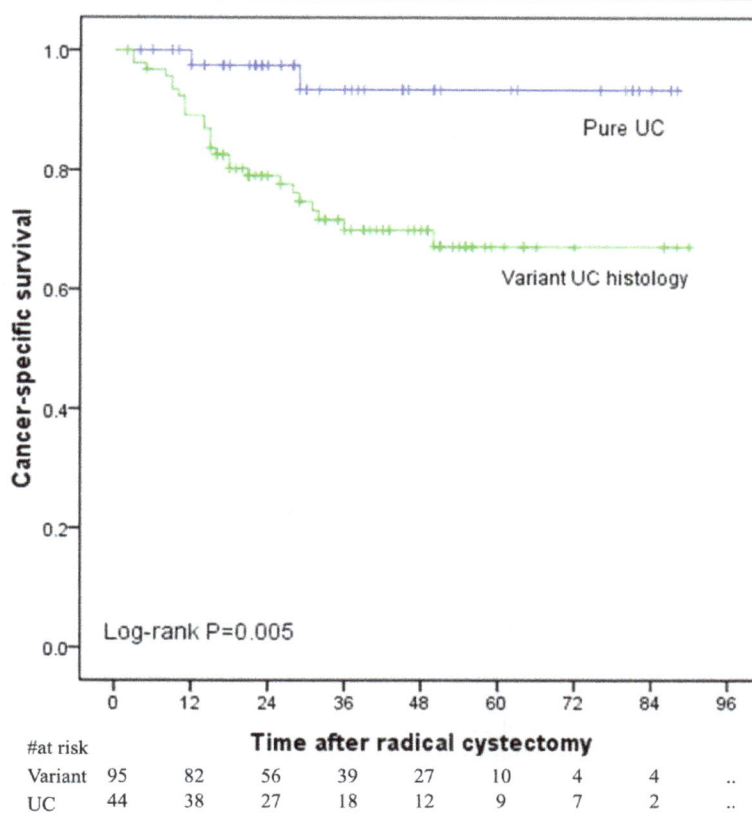

Fig. 1 Kaplan-Meier plot displays estimated cancer-specific survival in 139 patients treated with radical cystectomy, stratified by pure vs. variant differentiation in urothelial carcinoma at cystectomy (UC, urothelial carcinoma)

It is not an uncommon phenomenon that UCB has a great propensity to undergo variant differentiation. In accordance with previous studies [3, 15], the most prevalent mixed differentiation in this current series was squamous, accounting for 31 % of all cases. Squamous differentiation, characterized by the presence of intercellular bridges, keratin pearls or keratinization, has an unfavorable response to radiation and chemotherapy compared with pure UCB [5]. Previous studies have shown that its frequency runs parallel with grade and stage [16, 17]. Glandular differentiation, as the second common variant, is exemplified by the presence of true glandular spaces within the tumor, presented in 28 % of all cases [4]. After squamous and glandular subtypes, there is sarcomatoid differentiation, which is featured by biphasic malignant neoplasms with the evidence of expressing epithelial and mesenchymal markers, accounting for 12 % of all cases. In a sarcomatoid carcinoma, molecular evidence strongly argues for a monoclonal origin of both epithelial and mesenchymal components [18, 19]. Additionally, history of previous radiation or cyclophosphamide can be a valuable clue in ascertaining the diagnosis [4]. Other unusual architectural patterns (small cell, lymphoepithelioma-like, clear cell, microcystic,

undifferentiated) of UCB only accounted for a little proportion of the whole, namely 8 %. Those variants, compared with squamous and glandular differentiation, are more complicated for the pathologist to reach a direct diagnosis and can sometimes mimic reactive processes, benign lesions or metastasis of other tumors. For instance, lymphoepithelioma-like carcinoma, for which the sine que non feature is the presence of a pronounced lymphoid infiltrate, may be partially or substantially obscured by a variable desmoplastic response, a brisk inflammatory infiltrate and even a prominent chronic inflammatory cell infiltrate [5].

Although some studies have contributed to raising the awareness of these entities and improved diagnosis, the diagnosis of UCB variants may still be challenging for (a) the limitation of biopsy samples and transurethral resectates available to the pathologist, (b) the artifact caused by tangential sectioning, cautery and mechanical injury, and (c) even more importantly the difficulty of discriminating over selected mimics [3–5, 12]. In this study, the most sensitive variants detected by biopsy and LTURBT are squamous and glandular subtypes. This finding corroborates a previous study in which Ahmed et al. reported that the sensitivity of TURBT to detect squamous and glandular variant was 53 % and 25 % respectively [1]. Similar to the squamous differentiation, the sensitivity of LTURBT to detect glandular variant is nearly twice as that of biopsy. Compared to other variants, the sensitivity of biopsy and LTURBT to detect squamous and glandular differentiation was relatively higher. For most variants, Table 1 suggests an unfavorable sensitivity. However, considering their nature of rarity, more studies based on multi-center and/or international collaboration with large sample size are warranted to further validate these conclusions.

It is well known that sensitivity lies in correct diagnoses. In order to make a correct diagnosis, several points should be noted. First, recognition of the immunochemical profile is quite important for pathologists to distinguish certain variants from the confounding variables. Mahul et al. [5] summarized the immunohistochemical markers associated with urothelial differentiation in detail. Second, morphology should be made the best advantage. One case in point is that immunohistochemistry is less significant compared with morphology in discrimination nested variant over florid von Brunn's nests, as the reliable immunohistochemical cut-point is difficult to be determined [12]. Besides, in some cases, clinicopathological correlation is helpful in excluding an extravesical primary tumor [5]. Recently, Hughes et al. [20] have reported the effect of Fourier transform infrared (FTIR) microspectroscopy to diagnose some selected variants, which might open a new door for variant diagnosis.

In this study, we found that 49 % patients who underwent TURBT at least once were not diagnosed with variants on RC specimens. That is to say, approximately 50 % of the patients could be in variant-free condition partially due to complete resection(s). Dissimilarly, Ahmed et al. reported that 6 % (9/159) patients demonstrated variant(s) only on precystectomy biopsy or TURBT [1]. The factors that could influence the variant diagnosis could also explain the discrepant results between the two studies. Interestingly, among the 13 patients who underwent TURBT at least twice, 12 of them presented variants detected in some but not in all TURBTs (Table 2). Similarly, Matthew et al. found that some patients had a different or additional mixed histologic type on cystectomy than they did on transurethral resection of bladder tumor [21]. This raises several practical questions encountered in clinical work. First, for those who are diagnosed with different variant differentiation at biopsy, TURBT(s) or RC, what treatment algorithms should be applied in clinical management? Besides, for those who are diagnosed with variant differentiation at biopsy/TURBT and without variant subtype diagnosis on RC, should we adopt the same follow-up strategies used on the UCB patients without a diagnosis of variant differentiation during the disease course? Further investigations are needed to validate the paradigms.

Despite a number of individual studies have evaluated the impact of histological variants on prognosis of patients with UCB, this question remains in debate [14, 22]. We also evaluated the impact of variant differentiation on clinical outcomes. Of the 139 patients with available follow-up information, 95 UCB patients were identified with variant differentiation on RC specimens. Patients with variant differentiation on RC specimen have inferior survival both in univariate analysis ($P = 0.005$) and multivariate analysis (HR4.48, 95 % CI:1.03–19.53). Of note, our data were limited by an overall shorter median follow-up time of 31 months and small sample size. The statistical power was weakened by very few recurrent and death events. More investigations with a large number of patients, with a longer follow-up time and with a centralized pathologic re-review are warranted to validate these conclusions. Ultimately, our understanding of urinary bladder cancer biology should not be limited to histologic variants. The underlying genetic and molecular drivers of tumor induction, promotion, and progression and as well as makers of chemosensitivity also need to be investigated [14].

Our study is not devoid of potential limitations that need to be addressed. First and foremost are the limitations inherent to its retrospective nature. Besides, the follow-up time and sample size were the limitations of this study.

Conclusions
Overall sensitivity of biopsy or TURBT to detect variant differentiation on RC was relatively low. Nearly 50 % of the patients could be variant free partially due to complete resection(s). Patients with variant differentiation on RC specimen have inferior survival. Further studies on the approach to early detection of variant differentiation and the management tactics for the UCB patient presenting different variant differentiation at biopsy, TURBT or RC, may be facilitated.

Abbreviations
UCB: Urothelial carcinoma of the bladder; TURBT: Transurethral resection of bladder tumor; RC: Radical cystectomy; CSS: Cancer-specific survival; LTURBT: Last transurethral resection of bladder tumor.

Competing interests
The authors declare that they have no competing interests.

Authors' contributions
PG and ZCW contributed equally to this work and they designed the study, obtained data, performed the statistical analysis, wrote the manuscript and interpreted the data. XY participated in the conception and design of the study and acquisition of data. JL and QH participated in the conception and design of the study and interpretation of the data and reviewed and edited the manuscript. All authors read and approved the final manuscript.

Acknowledgements
The authors are thankful for the Wu Jieping Medical Foundation (No. WJP-LC-12036). The authors declare that the sponsor had no role in the study design, data collection, data analyses, data interpretation, or writing of the manuscript.

References

1. Abd EA, Watts KE, Elson P, Fergany A, Hansel DE. The sensitivity of initial transurethral resection or biopsy of bladder tumor(s) for detecting bladder cancer variants on radical cystectomy. J Urol. 2013;189(4):1263–7.

2. Samaratunga H, Delahunt B. Recently described and unusual variants of urothelial carcinoma of the urinary bladder. Pathology. 2012;44(5):407–18.

3. Shah RB, Montgomery JS, Montie JE, Kunju LP. Variant (divergent) histologic differentiation in urothelial carcinoma is under-recognized in community practice: Impact of mandatory central pathology review at a large referral hospital. Urol Oncol 2013;31(8):1650-5.

4. Eble JN, Sauter G, Epstein JI, Sesterhenn IA. Pathology and Genetics of Tumors of the Urinary System and Male Genital Organs. Lyon: IARC. 2004;90–109.

5. Amin MB. Histological variants of urothelial carcinoma: diagnostic, therapeutic and prognostic implications. Mod Pathol. 2009;22 Suppl 2:S96–S118.

6. Domanowska E, Jozwicki W, Domaniewski J, Golda R, Skok Z, Wisniewska H, et al. Muscle-invasive urothelial cell carcinoma of the human bladder: multidirectional differentiation and ability to metastasize. Hum Pathol. 2007;38(5):741–6.

7. Jozwicki W, Domaniewski J, Skok Z, Wolski Z, Domanowska E, Jozwicka G. Usefulness of histologic homogeneity estimation of muscle-invasive urinary bladder cancer in an individual prognosis: a mapping study. Urology. 2005;66(5):1122–6.

8. Billis A, Schenka AA, Ramos CC, Carneiro LT, Araujo V. Squamous and/or glandular differentiation in urothelial carcinoma: prevalence and significance in transurethral resections of the bladder. Int Urol Nephrol. 2001;33(4):631–3.

9. Fritsche HM, Burger M, Denzinger S, Legal W, Goebell PJ, Hartmann A. Plasmacytoid urothelial carcinoma of the bladder: histological and clinical features of 5 cases. J Urol. 2008;180(5):1923–7.

10. Boyle H, Flechon A, Droz JP. Treatment of uncommon malignant tumours of the bladder. Curr Opin Urol. 2011;21(5):309–14.

11. Kamat AM, Gee JR, Dinney CP, Grossman HB, Swanson DA, Millikan RE, et al. The case for early cystectomy in the treatment of nonmuscle invasive micropapillary bladder carcinoma. J Urol. 2006;175(3 Pt 1):881–5.

12. Shanks JH, Iczkowski KA. Divergent differentiation in urothelial carcinoma and other bladder cancer subtypes with selected mimics. Histopathology. 2009;54(7):885–900.

13. Greene FL, Page DL, Fleming ID, Balch CM, Fritz AG. AJCC cancer staging manual. 6th ed. New York: Springer; 2002. p. 335–40.

14. Xylinas E, Rink M, Robinson BD, Lotan Y, Babjuk M, Brisuda A, et al. Impact of histological variants on oncological outcomes of patients with urothelial carcinoma of the bladder treated with radical cystectomy. Eur J Cancer. 2013;49(8):1889–97.

15. Mitra AP, Bartsch CC, Bartsch GJ, Miranda G, Skinner EC, Daneshmand S. Does presence of squamous and glandular differentiation in urothelial carcinoma of the bladder at cystectomy portend poor prognosis? An intensive case–control analysis. Urol Oncol. 2014;32(2):117–27.

16. Martin JE, Jenkins BJ, Zuk RJ, Blandy JP, Baithun SI. Clinical importance of squamous metaplasia in invasive transitional cell carcinoma of the bladder. J Clin Pathol. 1989;42(3):250–3.

17. Black PC, Brown GA, Dinney CP. The impact of variant histology on the outcome of bladder cancer treated with curative intent. Urol Oncol. 2009;27(1):3–7.

18. Sung MT, Wang M, MacLennan GT, Eble JN, Tan PH, Lopez-Beltran A, et al. Histogenesis of sarcomatoid urothelial carcinoma of the urinary bladder: evidence for a common clonal origin with divergent differentiation. J Pathol. 2007;211(4):420–30.

19. Lopez-Beltran A, Requena MJ, Cheng L, Montironi R. Pathological variants of invasive bladder cancer according to their suggested clinical significance. Bju Int. 2008;101(3):275–81.

20. Hughes C, Iqbal-Wahid J, Brown M, Shanks JH, Eustace A, Denley H, et al. FTIR microspectroscopy of selected rare diverse sub-variants of carcinoma of the urinary bladder. J Biophotonics. 2013;6(1):73–87.

21. Wasco MJ, Daignault S, Zhang Y, Kunju LP, Kinnaman M, Braun T, et al. Urothelial carcinoma with divergent histologic differentiation (mixed histologic features) predicts the presence of locally advanced bladder cancer when detected at transurethral resection. Urology. 2007;70(1):69–74.

22. Erdemir F, Tunc M, Ozcan F, Parlaktas BS, Uluocak N, Kilicaslan I, et al. The effect of squamous and/or glandular differentiation on recurrence, progression and survival in urothelial carcinoma of bladder. Int Urol Nephrol. 2007;39(3):803–7.

Diagnostic and treatment factors associated with poor survival from prostate cancer are differentially distributed between regional and metropolitan Victoria, Australia

Rasa Ruseckaite[1*], Fanny Sampurno[1], Jeremy Millar[1,2], Mark Frydenberg[3] and Sue Evans[1]

Abstract

Background: Men diagnosed with prostate cancer (PCa) in specific regional areas in Victoria, Australia have a poorer five-year survival rate compared to men living elsewhere in Victoria. This study aims to describe patterns-of- presentation and -care for men diagnosed with PCa in a specific regional Victorian area, and compare the outcomes with other Victorian regions.

Methods: Information on consecutive men diagnosed between 2008 and 2013 was extracted from the Prostate Cancer Outcomes Registry-Victoria. Descriptive analyses summarized diagnostic and treatment patterns of the 7,204 men with PCa in the selected region ($n = 373$), metropolitan Melbourne ($n = 2,565$) and remaining areas of Victoria ($n = 4,266$) to compare risk factors, treatments and time-taken-to-treatment.

Results: Men with PCa in the selected region were more likely to be diagnosed at older age (aged 68.6 vs 66 years in the rest of Victoria), and incidentally rather than through case-finding PSA blood tests. They were more likely to be presented with higher NCCN risk of the disease (High: 26 %, 24 % and 20.3 %; Very high/Metastasis: 11.8 %, 5.2 % and 5.7 % in the study region, metropolitan Melbourne and elsewhere in Victoria, respectively).

Men in the selected region were also more likely to have a longer time from diagnosis to treatment (on average 15–30 days longer when compared to the rest of Victoria).

Conclusions: Poorer outcomes of men with PCa in this specific region might be explained by multiple factors, including clinical-, patient-, and health-system-related. This range of explanatory factors, occurring at multiple points along the pathway of diagnosis and detection, suggests that interventions to improve outcomes for PCa in regional areas such as this need to be systematic. Interventions specifically addressing any one factor in isolation are unlikely to have much effect.

Keywords: Prostate cancer, Regional, Clinical registry, Patterns-of-care

Abbreviations: ADT, Androgen deprivation therapy; AS, Active surveillance; BT, Brachytherapy; DHHS, Department of health and human services; EBRT, External beam radiation therapy; GP, General practitioner; HDR, High-dose rate brachytherapy; ICS, Integrated cancer service; IQR, Interquartile range; LDR, Low-dose rate brachytherapy; NCCN, National
(Continued on next page)

* Correspondence: rasa.ruseckaite@monash.edu
[1]Department of Epidemiology and Preventive Medicine, School of Public Health and Preventive Medicine, Faculty of Medicine Nursing and Health Sciences, Monash University, Melbourne, Australia
Full list of author information is available at the end of the article

(Continued from previous page)
comprehensive cancer network; OR, Odds ratio; PCa, Prostate cancer; PCOR-Vic, Prostate cancer outcomes registry – Victoria; PSA, Prostate-specific antigen; SEIFA, Socio-economic index of advantage and disadvantage; TRUS, Transrectal ultrasonography of the prostate; TURP, Transurethral resection of the prostate; WW, Watchful waiting

Background

Australia and New Zealand have among the highest incidence of prostate cancer (PCa) in the world with a combined age-standardised incidence rate of 104.4 cases per 100,000 [1]. Previous studies demonstrated statistically significant and increasing mortality excess for PCa in regional and rural areas in Australia and New Zealand [2, 3]. Haynes et al. [4] investigated cancer survival in New Zealand and showed that survival from PCa was poor in men living distantly from primary care and cancer centres. Geographic patterns of PCa mortality and variations in access to medical care were also examined in the US by Jemal et al. and Singh et al. [5, 6]. These studies showed that men in non-metropolitan counties generally had higher death rates and incidence of late-stage disease and lower prevalence of prostate-specific antigen (PSA) screening than in metropolitan areas. Rural and urban inequalities and increased PCa mortality were explained by the variation in screening, management of the disease and access to medical services and primary care [7, 8].

There is disparity between PCa survival in regional areas compared with metropolitan areas across Australia (5-year relative survival = 87.7 % vs 91.4 %, $p < 0.001$) [9]. According to the Victorian Cancer Registry (VCR) data, [10] the relative survival for one regional geographic region in Victoria, defined by a Government cancer health service boundary (an Integrated Cancer Service [ICS] area) five years after the diagnosis was approximately by 7 % lower than in metropolitan Melbourne (93 %, 95 % CI 92–93 %) and amongst the lowest in regional Victoria.

Potential causes for worse outcomes in this particular ICS could include epidemiological errors (i.e. wrong classification and coding of the disease); differences in the makeup of the population (i.e. more men with PCa risk factors living in this area); differences in disease at diagnosis (i.e. men are diagnosed with more advanced disease); differences in access to treatment (i.e. less men have curative treatment); and differences in patterns of treatment (i.e. some forms of treatment not available). The aim of this study was to evaluate factors associated with poorer survival outcomes in one regional Victorian ICS and compare the outcomes with other Victorian regions.

Methods

Study region

The selected regional ICS (further referred to as "a study region") covers over 18 % of Victoria's total landmass. In 2011, the region's estimated resident population was 270,512 and represented ~5 % of Victoria's total population [11]. By 2026, its population is projected to increase by 21 % compared with an overall state average increase of 23 %. This region comprises of 16 health services.

Victorian prostate cancer registry

The Victorian Prostate Cancer Registry (now termed the Prostate Cancer Outcomes Registry-Victoria, PCOR-Vic) was established in 2009 as a rapid case-ascertainment registry to monitor patterns- and quality- of-care for Victorian men diagnosed with PCa. The registry collects data on PCa cases from 38 metropolitan and regional public and private hospitals in Victoria. Based on the latest update from Victorian Cancer Registry [12], these sites account for about 70 % of incidence PCa cases in that State, and more than 10,000 men have been accrued. Registry recruitment is linked with mandatory notification of cancer status to the population-based Victorian Cancer Registry. Details of the registry, including methods for data collection, are described elsewhere [13].

Inclusion and exclusion criteria

Men from the PCOR-Vic were included in the study if they had been diagnosed with a pathological diagnosis of PCa between August 2008 and July 2013 and were notified to the registry after the date on which the relevant hospital began contributing data. An explanatory statement, available in 12 common languages, was sent to men who were eligible to participate in the study about 9 months after they had been diagnosed. The statement invited them to participate in the PCOR-VIC and provided an opt-out option. Consent was obtained from clinicians to include all their patients into the registry. Patients were ineligible if their diagnosing or treating doctor informed the registry that they were not capable of providing consent.

Recruitment and data collection

An explanatory statement and accompanying letter was sent to men who were eligible to participate in the study. A waiver of consent was provided to enable collection of diagnostic and treatment details on all men with PCa, who (1) died before consent could be sought; and (2) were diagnosed via a transurethral resection of the prostate (TURP) and in whom their treating clinician has requested not to contact the patient. Men were able to opt out of the registry at any time. Histopathological data were captured through hospital information systems and pathology reports. Clinical information was collected from medical records by trained data collectors. Treatments provided within 12 months of diagnosis were included in the analysis. More detailed information about the steps of data collection is provided elsewhere [13].

Statistical analysis

The National Comprehensive Cancer Network (NCCN) risk criteria for disease progression were used to classify patients into low-, intermediate- and high-risk disease (Table 1) [14].

Where the clinical T category was not recorded, if the Gleason score was ≤6 and the PSA concentration was <10 ng/mL, the patient was deemed to be at low risk for disease progression. In our study for data analysis purposes PSA levels were grouped into five categories: (1) <1 ng/mL, (2) 1–4 ng/mL, (3) 4.01–10 ng/mL, (4) 10.01–20 ng/mL, and (5) >20 ng/mL. Four Gleason score categories were used in this study: (1) score <7, (2) score = 7 (3 + 4), (3) score = 7 (4 + 3), and (4) ≥8.

Treatments provided within 12 months of diagnosis were included in the analysis. The following treatment categories were used: (1) Surgery (radical prostatectomy), (2) External Beam Radiotherapy Therapy and/or high dose radiation (EBRT/EBRT + HDR), (3) EBRT + Surgery, (4) Low dose radiation (LDR), (5) HDR, (6) Brachytherapy, dose unknown (BT-Unknown), (7) Androgen Deprivation Therapy (ADT), (8) Chemotherapy, (9) Active Surveillance (AS), Watchful Waiting (WW) and (10) Others (i.e. high intensity focused ultrasound etc.). For those patients whose treatment information was not recorded, treatment type was coded as "unknown". Active treatment was defined as any Surgery, EBRT, BT, HDR, LDR, ADT or other treatment, but excluded no active treatment option. Note that we could not reliably differentiate watchful waiting from active surveillance, and thus we have called them "no active treatment". Where treatment information was missing

(i.e. the treatment field in the registry was left blank) it was coded as 'unknown' rather than no active treatment. More detailed information about the treatment types is provided elsewhere [13].

Distance to primary treatment facility was calculated using the patient's residential address postcode and the hospital location on Whereis®. The Whereis® is one of Australia's most popular free navigation applications, which provides maps and coordinates of Australian cities, towns and travel destinations with driving directions and traveller information [15].

Descriptive statistics summarized these variables in men from the study region, metropolitan Melbourne and the rest of Victoria. Analyses of variance and X^2 tests for independence were used to examine demographic, diagnostic and treatment characteristics and their differences. Kruskal–Wallis and Mann–Whitney U tests were used to compare time and distance to treatment amongst the groups. Post-hoc tests were used to evaluate pairwise differences between categories for each group of patients. Type 1 errors were controlled using the Bonferroni approach, setting the level of significance to $P = 0.0033$.

A binary logistic regression analysis was performed to assess the impact of a number of factors (both individually and together) on the likelihood of men being offered an active treatment (i.e. no AS/WW) in the selected region. In the present study, the model predicted active treatment (i.e. "active treatment" outcome was set as 1, and all other treatments as 0) from demographic characteristics and diagnostic characteristics. All individual factors and their interactions that were significantly predictive, were added to the multivariate model. Univariate analysis (step 1) for all variables and their interactions was conducted to identify significant individual predictors, which yielded six significant potential factors and interactions that might be associated with men receiving active treatment of the disease. The six category variables were then added into a multivariate model (step 2).

Stata/IC 12.1 (StataCorp, TX, USA) was used for all analyses.

Table 1 Risk adjustment model adopted among men with PCa from clinical registries in Victoria

Variable	NCCN
Low	Clinical T1–T2a stage AND GS 2–6 AND PSA level <10 ng/mL
Intermediate	Clinical T2b–T2c stage OR GS = 7 OR PSA level 10–20 ng/mL
High	Clinical T3a stage OR GS 8–10 OR PSA level >20 ng/mL
Very high (locally advanced)	Clinical T3b–T4 Any T, N1
Metastatic	Any T, Any N, M1

NCCN, National Comprehensive Cancer Network; GS, Gleason Score; PSA, Prostate Specific Antigen

Results

A total of 10,827 men with PCa were notified to the PCOR-Vic between August 2008 and July 2013. Of these, 3,610 (33.3 %) cases were excluded from the data analysis as their diagnosis was confirmed before the commencement of the study and 13 (0.12 %) patients opted out. The records of 7,204 eligible and consented men diagnosed in three regional and one metropolitan ICS were included in the analysis. 373 (5.2 %) of these men were diagnosed in the study region, 2,565 (35.6 %) were from metropolitan Melbourne and the remaining

4,266 (59.2 %) patients were diagnosed elsewhere in Victoria.

Demographic and diagnostic characteristics

The average and median age of PCa men in the study region was significantly higher when compared to other Victorian men (Table 2). The median (IQR) age at diagnosis of men in the study region was 68.4 (45–92.5) years compared to 66 (38–96) in Melbourne and 66 (39–95) in the rest of Victoria.

Men diagnosed in the region had lower rates of socio-economic advantage using Socio-Economic Advantage and Disadvantage (SEIFA) categories [16], with more than half the men (54 %) in the study region from the no more than the 4th decile of SEIFA scores whereas, for example, in the men from metropolitan regions more than half (54 %) were in the *highest* two deciles, with fully 25 % in the highest decile of SEIFA scores. The SEIFA score is a composite of a number of average measures within an area including equivalent household income, occupancy type, level of educational attainment, level of employment/unemployment, occupational skill level, crowding, car ownership, marital status, housing and income support.

In addition the vast majority (87.4 %) of men in the study region was treated in public hospitals, which was different from metropolitan Melbourne and the rest of Victoria; men in the study region were more than four times less likely to be treated in a private hospital than men in metropolitan Victoria or other regional areas in Victoria.

The vast majority of men in the study region were diagnosed via TRUS; although a significantly higher percentage of new diagnoses was detected via TURP when compared to metropolitan Melbourne or other Victorian regions (20.7 %, 16.2 % and 6.8 % respectively).

When compared to the other regions, the study region also presented with a higher proportion of men with elevated levels of PSA (>20 ng/mL) at diagnosis (19.3 %, 11.7 % and 10 % respectively). Men in the study region were also more likely to be diagnosed with a higher Gleason score (8–10) than those diagnosed elsewhere in Victoria (27.6 %, 22.5 % and 18.3 % respectively) and presented with higher NCCN risk of the disease (High: 26 %, 24 % and 20.3 %; Very high/Metastasis: 11.8 %, 5.2 % and 5.7 % in the study region, metropolitan Melbourne and elsewhere in Victoria, respectively).

Treatment characteristics

Treatment modalities, time to the initial treatment and travel distance are summarized in the Table 3. A significantly lower proportion of men with a low risk disease (19.2 %) in the study region were treated with a radical prostatectomy when compared to metropolitan Melbourne (29.7 %) and

the rest of Victoria (43.9 %). Men in this area had to travel a longer distance (median [IQR] of 31.6 [18.9-69.3] km) to their health services provider, compared to those treated in metropolitan Melbourne (11.8 [6.2-25.9] km), or the rest of Victoria (21.6 [9.1-55.5] km).

By comparing men in the same "risk group" across regions, we can to some extent adjust for difference in management patterns overall that might be influenced by the more advanced higher grade disease seen in the region, by comparing more "like with like". In the risk group in which attempts at curative treatment are most clearly indicated, the intermediate risk group, men had different management patterns. There were a significantly lower proportion of men in the study region - nearly half as frequent - who undertook a prostatectomy [(27.4 vs 51.0 % vs 58.5 %). EBRT treatment as also at least a third less frequent (10.4 % vs 15.1 % vs 18.3 %) when compared to metropolitan Melbourne or the rest of Victoria, even within this identical intermediate risk group. As a consequence, there was also a significantly higher proportion of men (more than twice as likely) did not receive active treatment in this particular region (31.9 % vs 15.1 % vs 10.7 %). For these men, the median [IQR] amount of time between diagnosis and treatment in the study region was notably longer: 101 (56–191) vs 71.5 (44–119) vs 61 (39–103) days in metropolitan Melbourne and the rest of Victoria respectively. Men with intermediate risk PCa in the study region also needed to travel more than four times longer distances to their treating institution (56.4 [23.1-114.9] km) than those in metropolitan Victoria.

In a high-risk cancer group, 13.4 % of men undertook a prostatectomy in the study region, significantly less (less than half as common) than in metropolitan Melbourne (27.3 %) or in the rest of Victoria (36.1 %). There men were more than twice as likely to be treated with androgen deprivation (ADT), 35.1 %, compared to 14.9 % in metropolitan Melbourne and 9.1 % in the rest of Victoria. A median [IQR] amount of time between diagnosis and treatment was 57 [34–90] days, significantly longer than in metropolitan Melbourne (49.5 [31–84.25] days) or in the rest of Victoria (43 [27–65] days). Men in the selected ICS travelled a median [IQR] of 42.3 [19–82.7] km, almost four-time further than those treated in metropolitan Melbourne (11.7 [6.2-25.7] km), or twice as far as in the rest of Victoria (20.8 [9.8-61.3] km).

In a very high/metastatic risk group patterns-of- care were similar as in other groups, with more patients in the study region (52.3 %) being treated with ADT when compared to 30.8 % in metropolitan Melbourne, or 34.3 % in the rest of Victoria. The median [IQR] amount of time to the first treatment in the study region was 27 [6–67.5] days, 27 [9–58.5] in metropolitan Melbourne and 19.5 [7–50] elsewhere. Men needed to travel the

Table 2 Demographic and clinical characteristics of men with PCa in the study region, metropolitan Melbourne and the rest of Victoria

	Study region, n (%)	Metropolitan, n (%)	Rest of Victoria, n (%)	p
Included into the study	373 (5.2 %)	2,565 (35.6 %)	4,266 (59.2 %)	0.000
Age groups				0.000
< 55	24 (6.4 %)	293 (11.4 %)	549 (12.9 %)	
56–65	117 (31.4 %)	896 (34.9 %)	1,551 (36.4 %)	
65–75	145 (38.9 %)	909 (35.4 %)	1,632 (38.3 %)	
> 76	87 (23.3 %)	467 (18.2 %)	534 (12.5 %)	
Age (mean, SD)	68.6 (8.9)	66.7 (9.3)	65.5 (8.8)	0.000
SEIFA				0.000
Lowest 10 % (0–10 %)	70 (18.9 %)	93 (3.6 %)	217 (5.1 %)	
Lowest 11–20 %	57 (15.4 %)	68 (2.7 %)	197 (4.6 %)	
Lowest 21–30 %	9 (2.4 %)	77 (3.0 %)	232 (5.5 %)	
Lowest 31–40 %	64 (17.3 %)	127 (5.0 %)	392 (9.2 %)	
Lowest 41–50 %	113 (29.9 %)	160 (6.2 %)	293 (6.9 %)	
Highest 51–60 %	32 (8.6 %)	119 (4.6 %)	291 (6.8 %)	
Highest 61–70 %	18 (4.9 %)	208 (8.1 %)	496 (11.7 %)	
Highest 71–80 %	8 (2.2 %)	325 (12.7 %)	546 (12.8 %)	
Highest 81–90 %	1 (0.3 %)	747 (29.0 %)	907 (21.2 %)	
Highest 10 % (91–100 %)	1 (0.3 %)	641 (25.0 %)	695 (16.2 %)	
Type of hospital				0.000
Private	47 (12.6 %)	1,390 (54.2 %)	2,822 (66.2 %)	
Public	326 (87.4 %)	1,175 (45.8 %)	1,444 (33.8 %)	
Method of diagnosis				0.000
TRUS	285 (76.4 %)	2,081 (81.1 %)	3,919 (91.9 %)	
TURP	77 (20.7 %)	416 (16.2 %)	291 (6.8 %)	
Other	11 (2.9 %)	68 (2.7 %)	56 (1.3 %)	
PSA (ng/mL)				0.000
< 4	45 (12.1 %)	427 (16.6 %)	688 (16.1 %)	
4.01–10	176 (47.2 %)	1,337 (52.1 %)	2,408 (56.4 %)	
10.01–20	74 (19.8 %)	395 (15.4 %)	679 (15.9 %)	
> 20.01	72 (19.3 %)	301 (11.7 %)	426 (10.0 %)	
Unknown	6 (1.6 %)	105 (4.1 %)	65 (1.5 %)	
Gleason score				0.000
< 7	155 (41.6 %)	851 (33.2 %)	1,641 (38.5 %)	
7 (3 + 4)	69 (18.6 %)	736 (28.7 %)	1,306 (30.6 %)	
7 (4 + 3)	41 (10.9 %)	394 (15.4 %)	535 (12.6 %)	
≥ 8	103 (27.6 %)	577 (22.5 %)	782 (18.3 %)	
Unknown	5 (1.3 %)	7 (0.3 %)	2 (0.0 %)	
NCCN risk group				0.000
Low	73 (19.6 %)	478 (18.6 %)	911 (21.4 %)	
Intermediate	113 (30.3 %)	1,064 (41.5 %)	1,887 (44.2 %)	
High	97 (26.0 %)	616 (24.0 %)	867 (20.3 %)	
Very high/Metastatic	44 (11.8 %)	133 (5.2 %)	245 (5.7 %)	
Unknown	46 (12.3 %)	274 (10.7 %)	356 (8.3 %)	

Table 3 Treatment modalities, stratified by NCCN risk group, of men with PCa in the study region, metropolitan Melbourne and the rest of Victoria

NNCCN Risk group	Low*			Intermediate*			High*			Very high/Metastatic*		
	Study region, n (%)	Metropolitan, n (%)	Rest of Victoria, n (%)	Study region, n (%)	Metropolitan, n (%)	Rest of Victoria, n (%)	Study region, n (%)	Metropolitan, n (%)	Rest of Victoria, n (%)	Study region, n (%)	Metropolitan, n (%)	Rest of Victoria, n (%)
No treatment /AS/WW	46 (63.0 %)	244 (51.0 %)	337 (37.0 %)	36 (31.9 %)	161 (15.1 %)	201 (10.7 %)	8 (8.2 %)	45 (7.3 %)	44 (5.1 %)	1 (2.3 %)	4 (3.0 %)	3 (1.2 %)
Surgery (Prostatectomy)	14 (19.2 %)	142 (29.7 %)	400 (43.9 %)	31 (27.4 %)	543 (51.0 %)	1,104 (58.5 %)	13 (13.4 %)	168 (27.3 %)	313 (36.1 %)	2 (4.5 %)	9 (6.8 %)	21 (8.6 %)
EBRT/EBRT +HDR	5 (6.8 %)	33 (6.9 %)	56 (6.1 %)	23 (10.4 %)	161 (15.1 %)	345 (18.3 %)	35 (36.1 %)	233 (37.8 %)	311 (35.9 %)	11 (25.0 %)	60 (45.1 %)	109 (44.5 %)
EBRT + Surgery	1 (1.4 %)	5 (1.0 %)	26 (2.9 %)	3 (2.7 %)	78 (7.3 %)	108 (5.7 %)	5 (5.2 %)	60 (9.7 %)	96 (11.1 %)	0 (0.0 %)	6 (4.5 %)	9 (3.7 %)
LDR	5 (6.8 %)	22 (4.6 %)	69 (7.6 %)	7 (6.2 %)	53 (5.0 %)	68 (3.6 %)	0 (0.0 %)	0 (0.0 %)	1 (0.1 %)	1 (2.3 %)	0 (0.0 %)	0 (0.0 %)
HDR	0 (0.0 %)	0 (0.0 %)	1 (0.1 %)	1 (0.9 %)	6 (0.6 %)	3 (0.2 %)	0 (0.0 %)	1 (0.2 %)	1 (0.1 %)	1 (2.3 %)	0 (0.0 %)	1 (0.4 %)
BT-Unknown	1 (1.4 %)	8 (1.7 %)	5 (0.5 %)	0 (0.0 %)	8 (0.8 %)	6 (0.3 %)	0 (0.0 %)	1 (0.2 %)	2 (0.2 %)	0 (0.0 %)	0 (0.0 %)	0 (0.0 %)
ADT	0 (0.0 %)	3 (0.6 %)	2 (0.2 %)	9 (8.0 %)	13 (1.2 %)	23 (1.2 %)	34 (35.1 %)	92 (14.9 %)	79 (9.1 %)	23 (52.3 %)	41 (30.8 %)	84 (34.3 %)
Chemotherapy	0 (0.0 %)	0 (0.0 %)	0 (0.0 %)	0 (0.0 %)	0 (0.0 %)	0 (0.0 %)	1 (1.0 %)	1 (0.2 %)	1 (0.1 %)	4 (9.1 %)	5 (3.8 %)	13 (5.3 %)
Other	0 (0.0 %)	5 (1.0 %)	4 (0.4 %)	0 (0.0 %)	6 (0.6 %)	2 (0.1 %)	0 (0.0 %)	0 (0.0 %)	1 (0.1 %)	0 (0.0 %)	1 (0.8 %)	0 (0.0 %)
Not known	1 (1.4 %)	16 (3.3 %)	11 (1.2 %)	3 (2.7 %)	35 (3.3 %)	27 (1.4 %)	1 (1.0 %)	15 (2.4 %)	18 (2.1 %)	1 (2.3 %)	7 (5.3 %)	5 (2.0 %)
Total	73 (100 %)	478 (100 %)	911 (100 %)	113 (100 %)	1,064 (100 %)	1,887 (100 %)	97 (100 %)	616 (100 %)	867 (100 %)	44 (100 %)	133 (100 %)	245 (100 %)
Median (IQR) days to initial treatment	N/A	N/A	N/A	101 (56–191)	71.5 (44–119)	61 (39–103)	57 (34–90)	49.5 (31–84.25)	43 (27–65)	27 (6–67.5)	27 (9–58.5)	19.5 (7–50)
Median (IQR) km to treating hospital	31.6 (18.9-69.3)	11.8 (6.2-25.9)	21.6 (9.1-55.5)	56.4 (23.1-114.9)	13.1 (7.2-27.4)	20.7 (10-51.4)	42.3 (19-82.7)	11.7 (6.2-25.7)	20.8 (9.8-61.3)	39.4 (19.2-80.7)	11.4 (5.5-24.7)	25.6 (11.2-71.6)

*$p < 0.05$

median [IQR] distance of 39.4 [19.2-80.8] km to their treatment institution, longer than in metropolitan Melbourne (11.4 [5.5-24.7] km) or in the rest of Victoria (25.6 [11.2-71.6] km).

Regression analysis of factors determining treatment type
Table 4 summarizes the contributions of factors in the univariate and multivariate model to men receiving active treatment.

A full multivariate model containing all six category variables was statistically significant, $\chi^2(17,\ N = 6,528) = 1491,869\ p < 0.05$ indicating ability to distinguish between men with PCa who had active treatment ($N = 5,751$) vs those with no active treatment. The model explained between 21 % (Cox and Snell R Square) and 34 % (Nagelkerke R Square) of the variance in treatment type.

When compared to the selected region, men diagnosed in metropolitan areas had nearly twice the odds of receiving active treatment (OR = 1.89, 95 % CI, 1.35-2.64), and those in the rest of Victoria were even at higher odds, OR = 2.59, 95 % CI, 1.86-3.61). Men older than 75 years of age were nearly 90 % less likely to receive active treatment, compared to younger men of 55 years or less, OR = 0.13, (95 % CI, 0.09-0.17). Men with PCa were also more likely to receive an active treatment in public hospitals, OR = 1.44, (95 % CI, 1.22-1.69).

Those men whose diagnosis was detected via TURP were less likely to receive an active treatment, OR = 0.22, (95 % CI, 0.17-0.28) than men diagnosed via TRUS. When combined with other factors, higher NCCN Risk levels were also associated with an increased likelihood of men receiving an active treatment. For example, men

Table 4 Significant factors associated with the likelihood of active treatment in men with PCa (NS – Not Significant)

Factors	Univariate model		Multivariate model	
	Odds Ratio	CI at 95 %	Odds Ratio	CI at 95 %
Region				
Selected Region (Ref)	1		1	
Metropolitan	1.53	1.21-1.94	1.89	1.35-2.64
Rest of Victoria	2.21	1.74-2.78	2.59	1.86-3.61
Age				
< 55 (Ref)	1		1	
56-65	0.76	0.61-0.94	0.62	0.47-0.80
65-75	0.75	0.61-0.93	0.41	0.31-0.53
> 76	0.41	0.33-0.52	0.13	0.09-0.17
Type of hospital				
Private (Ref)	1		1	
Public	1.52	1.34-1.72	1.44	1.22-1.69
Method of diagnosis				
TRUS (Ref)	1		1	
TURP	0.17	0.15-0.20	0.22	0.17-0.28
Other	1.44	0.85-2.44	0.79	0.35-1.76
NCCN Risk				
Low (Ref)	1		1	
Intermediate	5.03	4.34-5.84	6.12	5.16-7.25
High	11.48	9.12-14.45	27.69	20.81-36.87
V.high/Metastatic	38.85	19.15-78.82	138.39	65.32-293.22
Region × NCCN Risk				
Selected Region × Low (Ref)	1		NS	NS
Metropolitan × Intermediate	3.61	2.97-4.38	NS	NS
Metropolitan × High	8.16	5.94-11.23	NS	NS
Metropolitan × V.high/Metastatic	20.75	7.64-56.42	NS	NS
Rest of Victoria × Intermediate	5.39	4.53-6.43	NS	NS
Rest of Victoria × High	12.04	8.75-16.55	NS	NS
Rest of Victoria × V.high/Metastatic	51.92	16.56-162.79	NS	NS

with v.high/metastatic disease had extremely high odds of receiving active treatment than men diagnosed with low risk disease, OR = 138.39, (95 % CI, 65.32-293.22).

Univariate model also revealed, that compared to men in the selected region diagnosed with low risk disease, those in the other areas, and at higher risk of the disease were more likely to receive an active treatment.

Discussion

Higher death rates from prostate (and other) cancers occur in patients from non-metropolitan regions. The population-based PCOR-Vic has enabled more precise identification of the underlying factors in one selected ICS in regional Victoria. We found that men in the study region were startlingly lower in measures of socio-economic advantage. They were older. A higher percentage of newly PCa cases in the study region (almost a fifth) were detected during TURP, a procedure performed to alleviate symptoms of urinary obstruction and not done primarily usually because PCa. Although TURP is generally not used to detect PCa anymore, as it makes a poor tool for early cancer detection [17], it used to be a common mean of detection of PCa before PSA screening was introduced.

We also found that men in the study region presented with a significantly higher level of PSA levels and Gleason score at diagnoses when compared to other Victorian regions, which supports previous research findings that men in rural and regional areas are more likely to have elevated PSA and Gleason score [18–21]. Overall, men in the study region presented for treatment at a more advanced disease stage when compared to the rest of Victoria, similarly to the findings reported by Baade and Coory, [2, 3] showing that men living in regional areas tend to be diagnosed at advanced stages of the disease. A possible reason for higher rates of a more advanced disease in the study region could possibly be due to issues of high PSA testing rates in metropolitan areas [2, 18].

Men in the study region, in the low and intermediate disease groups, were significantly less likely to undergo active treatment. There is emerging evidence that many men with early stage disease are appropriately managed with AS rather than having active invasive treatment [22, 23]. Yet, since the rates of no treatment are higher than the rates of no treatment in metropolitan Victoria, particularly in the intermediate risk group (where AS would not usually be recommended), it may be that higher rates of non-treatment represent a significant proportion of men diagnosed in the region are not having treatment as would be appropriate, rather than being placed on systematic program of active follow-up and surveillance as would be done if they were on AS. Variability in treatment patterns in different regions could also potentially reflect the managing clinicians' treatment preferences, perhaps different in the region than other parts of Victoria, since this factor is known to be a strong determinant of the treatment received [24, 25].

There was a notable time delay between diagnosis and treatment in men with intermediate/very high risk disease in the study region when compared to the rest of Victoria. While reasons for such delay are unknown - the findings may reflect a preference by their treating doctor to manage the disease conservatively or that men themselves are more reluctant to take up the option for active treatment than in other areas of Victoria - delays of more than 30–60 days can adversely affect pathological outcomes in men in these risk groups treated with radical prostatectomy [26].

Men in the study region also travelled much longer distances for their treatment, which could have influenced their choice of treatment and determined their health outcomes. Previous studies showed that prognosis and outcomes from PCa are known to be worse for men living in rural areas and needing to travel longer distances to their treatment providers [4, 27]. Longer time and distance required to travel could act as an economic and financial barrier in men's treatment choice, which may potentially explain why, compared with metropolitan regions, there are more men in the study region with high risk disease but who did not receive active treatment. The disadvantaged socio-economic category for many men in the region could be imagined to worsen barriers caused by distance.

As suggested by Ng et al. [28], the reasons for such discrepancies as we noted in treatment and outcomes between metropolitan and regional areas could possibly be explained by clinical-, patient-, and health-system-related factors. Potential patient-related barriers to PCa care could include not consulting a general practitioner (GP) in a timely manner [29], a lack of desire for treatment due to a 'I will be OK' attitude, or financial/time barriers if the care is only available outside the patient's regional area, thus requiring considerable time and travel expenses [15]. Urban–rural disparities in PCa incidence and mortality may arise from differences in demographic and socioeconomic characteristics of these two groups that may influence access to and utilization of diagnostic and treatment services [30].

It is not surprising that men in regional areas in Australia face distinct health issues because of their location, work, and lifestyle. There is evidence that these men are more likely to experience chronic health conditions and have more risk factors for serious disease than their metropolitan counterparts. For example, epidemiological studies of Begg and Beard have demonstrated that rural dwellers are more likely than metropolitan dwellers to report daily smoking and risky drinking behavior, [31, 32] are less likely to possess an adequate level of health literacy and have higher mortality rates from injury, cardiovascular disease and diabetes [33].

The other potential reason could be a limitation on GPs referral choice, and issues concerning the quality of care due to potential for impediments to professional development of regional doctors and specialists [28]. It may be that specialists, diagnostic equipment and other medical technology, and operating rooms are much more restricted in the regional areas. Internationally, patients with cancer are increasingly being managed by multidisciplinary teams, allowing the use of varying professional skills with numerous benefits for the patient [34] and this approach is promoted by the Victorian Department of Health and Human Services. A lack of uro-oncology multidisciplinary meetings in the selected study region could also be associated with poorer outcomes in men with PCa [16].

The Australian and Victoria Governments as well as community groups have been determined to allocate resources to reduce inequity in health outcome [35]. This highlights the importance of our work. Our study has demonstrated that there are interlinked chain of factors that are associated with the poorer outcomes: the men are older, they are startlingly more likely to be in disadvantaged socio-economic groups, the live much further away from specialist health care providers, they are much more likely to be diagnosed "by accident", as it were, and then they wait much longer for treatment. They have more advanced and more aggressive disease when they do get diagnosed; but even adjusting for this, they are much more likely not to receive any attempt at curative treatment, and much more likely to be treated in a public hospital. The health services in the region have fewer services available for the care of men with PCa. Hitherto, work has established the disparities in outcome in regional areas, but the causes were mostly supposition in the absence of data. Registries provide the data on the factors associated with these outcomes.

The major strength of this study is the use of clinical registry data, containing a detailed diagnosis and treatment information of the patients with PCa. The PCOR-Vic enables rapid and reliable ascertainment of patterns of care and quality of life data of men diagnosed with PCa and reports back to treating clinicians in regional and metropolitan Victoria [13]. However, some limitations to this study also need to be noted. Firstly, there were a relatively small number of PCa men in the study region. Another important limitation is that we did not seek to identify reasons why men received no treatment within 12 months of diagnosis in the study region. It may be that they were receiving AS, had decided not to pursue active curative treatment, were awaiting therapy on the basis of their PSA level taken at 12 months, or

were inadequately managed. Finally, we were unable to investigate other factors, such as obesity, smoking habits or alcohol consumption in the study region as the registry does not collect such information.

This study has identified a number of key areas of difference in the study region. Identifying these differences allows logical plans for where the effort needs to be made to enable improvement, and where more information is needed. The findings of this study have been shared with health service providers and policy-makers in the study region. They have an on-going strategy to address many of the key points identified, to better provide health care services for men diagnosed with PCa in the region. A project is underway to better understand factors associated with why men are presenting with more advanced PCa disease than in other areas of Victoria. This multifaceted project will involve patients living in the region and their GPs. It is important that we understand reasons for this so that interventions can be targeted to areas of greatest need.

Conclusions

The PCOR-Vic has enabled for the first time clarity around the factors associated with PCa in an Australian regional location, documenting many structure, process or outcome measurements where the location performs worse than other metropolitan or regional areas in Victoria. It suggests plans to improve outcomes need to be made on a systematic basis. Registries such as the PCOR-Vic provide vital on-going insight on how resources are best allocated to improve the lot of men diagnosed with PCa.

Acknowledgements
The authors gratefully acknowledge the funders, and would also like to thank Mr Ian Nethercote and Big Barbie Bash for their support and assistance.

Funding
Data contributing to this project was funded by Cancer Australia (ID 1010384), the Victorian Department of Health and Human Services and Movember Foundation. During the time of the study RR was supported by the Movember Foundation. SE received a Monash Partners Academic Fellowship.

Authors' contributions
RR wrote the manuscript and performed statistical analysis of the data. FS contributed to the data analysis and interpretation of the results. JM and MF participated in the design of the study and provided substantial conceptual advice. SE conceived the study, contributed to the data collection and was principal investigators of the study. All authors critically revised the manuscript and gave their final approval before submission.

Competing interests
The authors declare that they have no competing interests.

Author details
[1]Department of Epidemiology and Preventive Medicine, School of Public Health and Preventive Medicine, Faculty of Medicine Nursing and Health Sciences, Monash University, Melbourne, Australia. [2]Alfred Health Radiation Oncology, Melbourne, Australia. [3]Department of Surgery, Monash Medical Centre, Melbourne, Australia.

References

1. Center M, Jemal A, Lortet-Tieulent J, Ward E, Ferlay J, Brawley O et al. International variation in prostate cancer incidence and mortality rates. Eur Urol. 2012;61(6):doi: 10.1016/j.eururo.2012.02.054. Epub Mar 8.

2. Thomas AA, Pearce A, Sharp L, Gardiner RA, Chambers S, Aitken J, Molcho M, Baade P. Socioeconomic disadvantage but not remoteness affects short-term survival in prostate cancer: A population-based study using competing risks. Asia Pac J Clin Oncol. 2016. doi: 10.1111/ajco.12570.

3. Coory MD, Baade PD. Urban–rural differences in prostate cancer mortality, radical prostatectomy and prostate-specific antigen testing in Australia. Med J Aust. 2005;182(3):112–5.

4. Jones AP, Haynes R, Sauerzapf V, Crawford SM, Zhao H, Forman D. Travel time to hospital and treatment for breast, colon, rectum, lung, ovary and prostate cancer. Eur J Cancer. 2008;44(7):992–9. doi:10.1016/j.ejca.2008.02.001.

5. Jemal A, Ward E, Wu X, Martin HJ, McLaughlin CC, Thun MJ. Geographic patterns of prostate cancer mortality and variations in access to medical care in the United States. Cancer Epidemiol Biomarkers Prev. 2005;14(3):590–5. doi:10.1158/1055-9965.epi-04-0522.

6. Singh GK, Williams SD, Siahpush M, Mulhollen A. Socioeconomic, Rural–urban, and Racial Inequalities in US Cancer Mortality: Part I-All Cancers and Lung Cancer and Part II-Colorectal, Prostate, Breast, and Cervical Cancers. J Cancer Epidemiol. 2011;2011:107497. doi:10.1155/2011/107497.

7. Smailyte G, Kurtinaitis J. Cancer mortality differences among urban and rural residents in Lithuania. BMC Public Health. 2008;8:56. doi:10.1186/1471-2458-8-56.

8. Stamatiou K, Skolarikos A. Rural residence and prostate cancer screening with prostate-specific antigen. Rural Remote Health. 2009;9(2):1227.

9. Baade PD, Youlden DR, Coory MD, Gardiner RA, Chambers SK. Urban–rural differences in prostate cancer outcomes in Australia: what has changed? Med J Aust. 2011;194(6):293–6.

10. Cancer Council of Victoria. Cancer Survival Victoria. Cancer Council Victoria; 2011. http://www.cancervic.org.au/.

11. ABS. Australian Bureau of Statistics. 2015.

12. Punnen S, Cowan JE, Chan JM, Carroll PR, Cooperberg MR. Long-term Health-related Quality of Life After Primary Treatment for Localized Prostate Cancer: Results from the CaPSURE Registry. Eur Urol. 2014. doi:10.1016/j.eururo.2014.08.074.

13. Evans S, Millar J, Wood J, Davis I, Bolton D, Giles G, et al. The prostate cancer registry: monitoring paterns and quality of care for men diagnosed with prostate cancer. BJUI. 2012;111:e158–66.

14. National Comprehensive Cancer Network. NCCN clinical practice guidelines in oncology: prostate cancer [subscription only]. In: http://www.nccn.org/professionals/physician_gls/pdf/prostate.pdf. Accessed Nov 2014.

15. Rankin SL, Hughes-Anderson W, House AK, Heath DI, Aitken RJ, House J. Costs of accessing surgical specialists by rural and remote residents. ANZ J Surg. 2001;71(9):544–7.

16. Rao K, Manya K, Azad A, Lawrentschuk N, Bolton D, Davis ID, et al. Uro-oncology multidisciplinary meetings at an Australian tertiary referral centre–impact on clinical decision-making and implications for patient inclusion. BJU Int. 2014;114 Suppl 1:50–4. doi:10.1111/bju.12764.

17. Zigeuner R, Schips L, Lipsky K, Auprich M, Salfellner M, Rehak P, et al. Detection of prostate cancer by TURP or open surgery in patients with previously negative transrectal prostate biopsies. Urology. 2003;62(5):883–7.

18. Baldwin LM, Andrilla CH, Porter MP, Rosenblatt RA, Patel S, Doescher MP. Treatment of early-stage prostate cancer among rural and urban patients. Cancer. 2013;119(16):3067–75. doi:10.1002/cncr.28037.

19. Grivas N, Hastazeris K, Kafarakis V, Tsimaris I, Xousianitis Z, Makatsori A, et al. Prostate cancer epidemiology in a rural area of North Western Greece. Asian Pac J Cancer Prev. 2012;13(3):999–1002.

20. Obertova Z, Hodgson F, Scott-Jones J, Brown C, Lawrenson R. Rural–urban Differences in Prostate-Specific Antigen (PSA) Screening and Its Outcomes in New Zealand. J Rural Health. 2015. doi:10.1111/jrh.12127.

21. Steenland K, Goodman M, Liff J, Diiorio C, Butler S, Roberts P, et al. The effect of race and rural residence on prostate cancer treatment choice among men in Georgia. Urology. 2011;77(3):581–7. doi:10.1016/j.urology.2010.10.020.

22. Bul M, Zhu X, Valdagni R, Pickles T, Kakehi Y, Rannikko A, et al. Active surveillance for low-risk prostate cancer worldwide: the PRIAS study. Eur Urol. 2013;63(4):597–603. doi:10.1016/j.eururo.2012.11.005.

23. Cheng JY. The Prostate Cancer Intervention Versus Observation Trial (PIVOT) in Perspective. J Clin Med Res. 2013;5(4):266–8. doi:10.4021/jocmr1395w.

24. Hu JC, Gu X, Lipsitz SR, Barry MJ, D'Amico AV, Weinberg AC, et al. Comparative effectiveness of minimally invasive vs open radical prostatectomy. Jama. 2009;302(14):1557–64. doi:10.1001/jama.2009.1451.

25. Fowler Jr FJ, McNaughton Collins M, Albertsen PC, Zietman A, Elliott DB, Barry MJ. Comparison of recommendations by urologists and radiation oncologists for treatment of clinically localized prostate cancer. Jama. 2000; 283(24):3217–22.

26. Berg WT, Danzig MR, Pak JS, Korets R, RoyChoudhury A, Hruby G, et al. Delay from biopsy to radical prostatectomy influences the rate of adverse pathologic outcomes. Prostate. 2015;75(10):1085–91. doi:10.1002/pros.22992.

27. McCombie SP, Hawks C, Emery JD, Hayne D. A 'One Stop' Prostate Clinic for rural and remote men: a report on the first 200 patients. BJU Int. 2015. doi:10.1111/bju.13100.

28. Ng JQ, Hall SE, Holman CD, Semmens JB. Inequalities in rural health care: differences in surgical intervention between metropolitan and rural Western Australia. ANZ J Surg. 2005;75(5):265–9. doi:10.1111/j.1445-2197.2005.03375.x.

29. Turrell G, Oldenburg BF, Harris E, Jolley DJ, Kimman ML. Socioeconomic disadvantage and use of general practitioners in rural and remote Australia. Med J Aust. 2003;179(6):325–6.

30. Obertova Z, Brown C, Holmes M, Lawrenson R. Prostate cancer incidence and mortality in rural men–a systematic review of the literature. Rural Remote Health. 2012;12(2):2039.

31. Beard J, Tomaska N, Earnest A, Summerhayes R, Morgan G. Influence of socioeconomic and cultural factors on rural health. Austral J Rural Health. 2009;17(1):10–5.

32. Begg S, Vos T, Barker B, Stevenson C, Stanley L, Lopez A. The burden of disease and injury in Australia 2003. AIHW: Canberra; 2007.

33. Australian Institute of Health and Welfare. A snapshot of men's health in regional and remote Australia. Canberra: AIHW2010 Contract No.: at. no. PHE 120.

34. Carter S, Garside P, Black A. Multidisciplinary team working, clinical networks, and chambers; opportunities to work differently in the NHS. Qual Saf Health Care. 2003;12 Suppl 1:i25–8.

35. Boxall A. What are we doing to ensure the sustainability of the health system? Department of Parliamentary Services. Parliamentary Library. Canberra. 2011. 2015. http://www.aph.gov.au/library/pubs/rp/2011-12/12rp04.pdf.

Predicting 90-day and long-term mortality in octogenarians undergoing radical cystectomy

Michael Froehner[1]*, Rainer Koch[2], Matthias Hübler[3], Ulrike Heberling[1], Vladimir Novotny[1], Stefan Zastrow[1], Oliver W. Hakenberg[4] and Manfred P. Wirth[1]

Abstract

Background: Radical cystectomy bears a considerable perioperative mortality risk particularly in elderly patients. In this study, we searched for predictors of perioperative and long-term competing (non-bladder cancer) mortality in elderly patients selected for radical cystectomy.

Methods: We stratified 1184 consecutive patients who underwent radical cystectomy for high risk superficial or muscle-invasive urothelial or undifferentiated carcinoma of bladder into two groups (age < 80 years versus 80 years or older). Multivariable and cox proportional hazards models were used for data analysis.

Results: Whereas Charlson score and the American Society of Anesthesiologists (ASA) physical status classification (but not age) were independent predictors of 90-day mortality in younger patients, only age predicted 90-day mortality in patients aged 80 years or older (odds ratio per year 1.24, $p = 0.0422$). Unlike in their younger counterparts, neither age nor Charlson score or ASA classification were predictors of long-term competing mortality in patients aged 80 years or older (hazard ratios 1.07-1.10, p values 0.21-0.77).

Conclusions: This data suggest that extrapolations of perioperative mortality or long-term mortality risks of younger patients to octogenarians selected for radical cystectomy should be used with caution. Concerning 90-day mortality, chronological age provided prognostic information whereas comorbidity did not.

Keywords: Bladder cancer, Radical cystectomy, 90-day mortality, Competing mortality, Comorbidity, Age

Background

Radical cystectomy bears a considerable perioperative mortality risk particularly in elderly patients [1–5]. Robot-assisted surgery has been evaluated as a novel technique in order to decrease adverse outcome in elderly patients [6]. Currently, there is, however, still insufficient evidence to prefer any approach to radical cystectomy [7]. Elderly patients tend to be treated less aggressively although they may benefit from such treatment similarly as their younger counterparts [8, 9]. Since patients with a long remaining life expectancy and a low risk of perioperative mortality are more likely to benefit from radical surgery, identifying those patients could improve disease management. Until now, few tools are available in order to estimate the postoperative and long-term competing mortality risks in octogenarian candidates for radical cystectomy [1–5, 7–9].

Methods

Study sample

We studied a sample of 1184 consecutive patients who underwent radical cystectomy for high risk superficial or muscle-invasive urothelial or undifferentiated carcinoma of bladder at our institution between 1993 and 2015. Institutional review board approval was obtained (EK84032009). The patients were stratified into two groups by an a priori chosen cutoff (age < 80 years versus 80 years or older). Demographic data is given in Table 1.

* Correspondence: Michael.Froehner@uniklinikum-dresden.de
[1]Department of Urology, University Hospital Carl Gustav Carus, Technische Universität Dresden, Fetscherstrasse 74, D-01307 Dresden, Germany
Full list of author information is available at the end of the article

Table 1 Demographic data of the study population in all patients, patients aged 80 years or older and patients younger than 80 years. Comorbidity profile and tumor-related parameters as well as 90-day mortality and 5-year bladder cancer specific and competing mortality rates were less favorable in patients aged 80 years or older compared with their younger counterparts

Parameter	Whole sample	< 80 years	80 years or older	p
Sample size	1184	1061	123	–
Mean follow-up (censored patients)	7.4 years	7.6 years	3.8 years	–
Median follow-up (censored patients)	6.2 years	6.5 years	2.5 years	–
Mean age	68.7 years	67.1 years	82.6 years	–
Bladder confined disease	684 (58%)	629 (59%)	55 (45%)	0.0020
Extravesical extension	500 (42%)	432 (41%)	68 (55%)	0.0020
Positive lymph nodes	308 (26%)	272 (26%)	36 (29%)	0.38
Extravesical extension or positive lymph nodes	576 (49%)	500 (47%)	76 (62%)	0.0021
Bladder confined disease and negative lymph nodes	608 (51%)	561 (53%)	47 (38%)	0.0021
ASA classes 3-4	493 (42%)	421 (40%)	72 (59%)	< 0.0001
Charlson score 2 or higher	449 (38%)	383 (36%)	66 (54%)	0.0001
Mean Charlson score	1.57	1.50	2.18	< 0.0001
Median Charlson score	1.00	1.00	2.00	–
CCS class 2 or higher	131 (11%)	109 (10%)	22 (18%)	0.0108
NYHA class 2 or higher	211 (18%)	177 (17%)	34 (28%)	0.0026
Female patients	255 (22%)	206 (19%)	49 (40%)	< 0.0001
Any neoadjuvant chemotherapy	55 (5%)	53 (5%)	2 (2%)	0.09
Adjuvant cisplatin-based chemotherapy	258 (22%)	257 (24%)	1 (1%)	< 0.0001
Current smokers	327 (28%)	315 (30%)	12 (10%)	< 0.0001
University degree/master craftsman	274 (23%)	250 (24%)	24 (20%)	0.31
Mean body mass index	27.0 kg/m^2	27.0 kg/m^2	26.7 kg/m^2	0.26
Median body mass index	26.7 kg/m^2	26.7 kg/m^2	26.4 kg/m^2	–
Continent diversion	390 (33%)	388 (37%)	2 (2%)	< 0.0001
Number of removed lymph nodes (if recorded)	18.4	18.8	15.2	< 0.0001
History of myocardial infarction	86 (7%)	72 (7%)	14 (11%)	0.06
Diabetes mellitus	288 (24%)	250 (24%)	38 (31%)	0.07
Lung disease	218 (18%)	196 (18%)	22 (18%)	0.87
Cerebrovascular disease	65 (5%)	56 (5%)	9 (7%)	0.35
Peripheral vascular disease	129 (11%)	111 (10%)	18 (15%)	0.16
Deaths from non-cancer causes	205	170	35	–
Deaths from bladder cancer	372	325	47	–
Deaths from second cancer	66	64	2	–
Deaths from unknown causes	7	5	2	–
90-day mortality	4.2%	3.7%	8.9%	< 0.0001
5-year bladder cancer-specific mortality	30.3%	28.9%	44.3%	0.0038
5-year competing (non-bladder cancer) mortality	14.1%	12.5%	28.7%	0.0005

CCS Classification of angina pectoris of the Canadian Cardiovascular Society [21]; *NYHA* Classification of cardiac insufficiency of the New York Heart Association [22]; *ASA* American Society Association physical status classification [11]

Variables and data collection

Beside age as a continuous variable, numeric comorbidity (measured by the Charlson score [10]) and the clinical impression of the patient (measured by the American Society of Anesthesiologists (ASA) physical status classification [11]) (Table 2) and - concerning long-term competing (non-bladder cancer) mortality - a variety of single conditions were analyzed as possible predictors of outcome (Table 3). Comorbidity data was obtained from premedication records and discharge documents. Follow-up

Table 2 A: Optimal multivariable logit models predicting 90-day mortality and B: Optimal multivariable proportional hazard models predicting non-bladder cancer (competing) mortality with 95% confidence intervals and *p* values in all patients, patients aged 80 years or older and patients younger than 80 years including the variables age, Charlson score and ASA classification

	Whole sample		< 80 years		80+ years	
A: Endpoint 90-day mortality						
Parameter	OR (95% CI)	*p*	OR (95% CI)	*p*	OR (95% CI)	*p*
Age (continuous variable, per year)	1.05 (1.01-1.09)	0.0106	n. s.*		1.24 (1.01-1.51)	0.0422
Charlson-Score (continuous variable, per point)	1.16 (1.02- 1.31)	0.0197	1.22 (1.07-1.39)	0.0029	n. s.**	
ASA classes 3-4 (versus classes 1-2)	6.95 (2.80-17.2)	< 0.0001	9.28 (3.11-27.8)	< 0.0001	n. s.**	
B: Endpoint non-bladder-cancer (competing) mortality						
Parameter	HR (95% CI)	*p*	HR (95% CI)	*p*	HR (95% CI)	*p*
Age (continuous variable, per year)	1.04 (1.02-1.05)	< 0.0001	1.04 (1.02-1.06)	< 0.0001	n. s.***	
Charlson-Score (continuous variable, per point)	1.17 (1.02-1.24)	< 0.0001	1.18 (1.11-1.26)	< 0.0001	n. s.***	
ASA classes 3-4 (versus classes 1-2)	1.59 (1.21-2.08)	0.0008	1.67 (1.25-2.25)	0.0006	n. s.***	

ASA American Society Association physical status classification [11]; *OR* Odds ratio; *HR* Hazard ratio; *CI* Confidence interval; *n. s.* Not significant. *Full model: age: OR 1.04 (0.99-1.09), p = 0.14, Charlson score: OR 1.21 (1.06-1.38), *p* = 0.0050, ASA classes 3-4: OR 8.48 (2.83-25.40), p = 0.0001. **Full model: age: OR 1.18 (0.97-1.48), *p* = 0.10, Charlson score: OR 0.90 (0.61-1.34), *p* = 0.60, ASA classes 3-4: OR 3.45 (0.66-17.95), *p* = 0.14. ***Full model: age: HR 1.08 (0.96-1.22), *p* = 0.21, Charlson score: HR 1.07 (0.96-1.27), *p* = 0.41, ASA classes 3-4: HR 1.10 (0.58-2.09), *p* = 0.77

Table 3 Optimal multivariable proportional hazard models with 95% confidence intervals and p values for competing risks predicting competing in all patients, patients aged 80 years or older and patients younger than 80 years, respectively investigating single conditions as possible predictors of competing mortality. Only single conditions occurring in at least 5 patients were included in the analysis

	Whole sample		< 80 years		80+ years	
Parameter	HR (95% CI)	*p*	HR (95% CI)	p	HR (95% CI)	*p*
Age (continuous variable, per year)	1.05 (1.03-1.06)	< 0.0001	1.06 (1.04-1.08)	< 0.0001		
Angina pectoris (CCS classes 2-4 versus 0-1)			1.89 (1.37-2.61)	0.0001		
Hypertension (versus none)						
History of thromboembolism (versus none)						
Myocardial infarction (versus none)	1.74 (1.21-2.51)	0.0029			2.20 (1.05-4.62)	0.0357
Cardiac insufficiency (NYHA classes 2-4 versus 0-1)						
Peripheral vascular disease (versus none)						
Cerebrovascular disease (versus none)						
Chronic lung disease (versus none)	1.41 (1.06-1.88)	0.0167				
Ulcer disease (versus none)						
Diabetes mellitus (versus none)	1.45 (1.12-1.88)	0.0051	1.37 (1.04-1.82)	0.0261		
Connective tissue disease (versus none)						
Hemiplegia (versus none)						
Moderate or severe renal disease (versus none)						
Solid tumor, leukemia or lymphoma (versus none)						
Liver disease (versus none)			2.38 (1.25-4.54)	0.0081		
Dementia (versus none)						
Current smoker (versus ex–/non-smokers[a])	1.58 (1.21-2.07)	0.0008	1.75 (1.34-2.30)	< 0.0001		
Body mass index < 25 kg/m² (versus 25+ kg/m²)						
ASA class 3-4 (versus classes 1-2)	1.68 (1.30-2.18)	< 0.0001	1.77 (1.34-2.34)	< 0.0001		
Male sex (versus female)			1.75 (1.18-2.62)	0.0052		

CCS Classification of angina pectoris of the Canadian Cardiovascular Society [21]; *NYHA* Classification of cardiac insufficiency of the New York Heart Association [22]; *ASA* American Society Association physical status classification [11]; *HR* Hazard ratio; *CI* Confidence interval; [a]or unknown smoking status

data were collected from urologists, general practitioners, the patients and their relatives, health insurance companies, local authorities and the local tumor register. All patients were observed for at least 90 days after surgery. Bladder cancer was considered the cause of death when uncontrolled disease progression was present at the time of death. Deaths from causes other than bladder cancer or unknown causes ($n = 7$) were considered deaths from competing causes. 90-day mortality (from all causes) and competing (non-bladder cancer) mortality were the study endpoints.

Statistical analyses

Concerning 90-day mortality, complete information for each patient (yes or no) was available. Multivariable logit models were used for the identification of predictors of 90-day mortality. Non-bladder cancer (competing) mortality was calculated from incomplete observations with censoring (and of observation in patients still alive) and competing (deaths from bladder cancer) events. Proportional hazard models for competing risks were used for the identification of predictors of non-bladder cancer (competing) mortality. Because of the limited number of events available for 90-day mortality, we dispensed from an analysis of multiple single conditions for this endpoint as done with long-term non-bladder cancer (competing) mortality (Table 3). The analyses were done with the Statistical Analysis Systems V9.4 statistical package (SAS Institute, Cary, NC).

Results

Tumor-associated parameters (proportion of extravesical extension or positive lymph nodes), 5-year bladder cancer-specific mortality, 90-day mortality and non-bladder cancer (competing) mortality were less favorable in the octogenarian subgroup (Table 1). Octogenarians were more frequently female, less frequently current smokers, had a higher burden of comorbidity and did only rarely receive adjuvant and neoadjuvant chemotherapy (Table 1). Cumulative mortality curves from bladder cancer and from causes other than bladder cancer (competing causes) are shown in Fig. 1. Both types of mortality were higher in octogenarians compared with their younger counterparts (Fig. 1).

Whereas in younger patients the comorbidity measures Charlson score and ASA classification (but not age) were independent predictors of 90-day mortality, in those aged 80 years or older only chronological age was an independent predictor of 90-day mortality (Table 2). Remarkably, despite the range restriction of this variable in patients aged 80 years or older, chronological age became only an independent predictor of 90-day mortality after inclusion of this subgroup (Table 2).

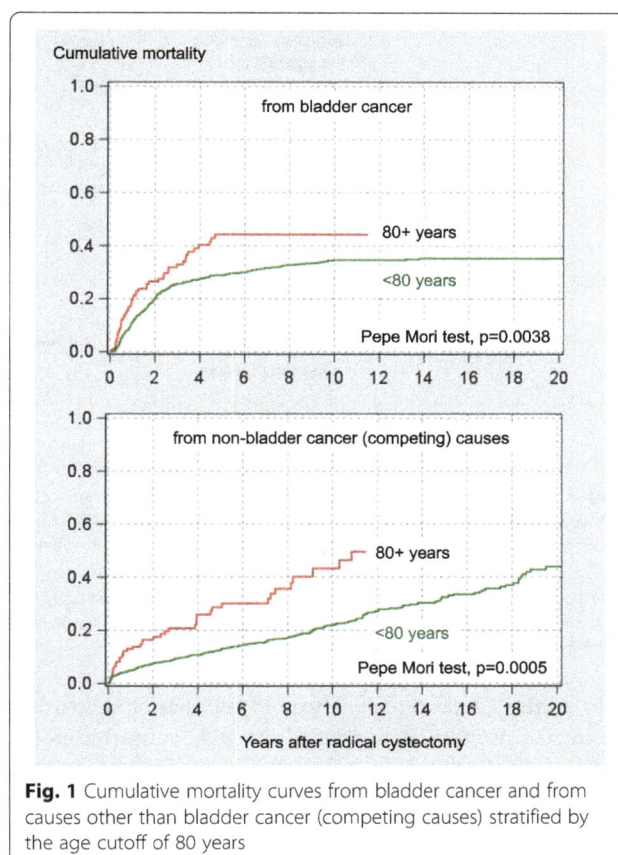

Fig. 1 Cumulative mortality curves from bladder cancer and from causes other than bladder cancer (competing causes) stratified by the age cutoff of 80 years

Whereas in younger patients age, Charlson score and ASA classification were independent predictors of long-term competing mortality with p values < 0.001, all three parameters were far apart from the significance level in patients aged 80 years or older (Table 2). In contrast, in younger patients, the ASA classification was of distinct and probably clinically meaningful impact on 90-day and long-term competing mortality after radical cystectomy in younger patients (Tables 2 and 3, Fig. 2). When single conditions were analyzed, in patients younger than 80 years a complex model containing age and six comorbidity-related variables predicted long-term competing mortality whereas in their older counterparts only one variable (history of myocardial infarction) was a significant predictor (Table 3).

Discussion

This study suggests that extrapolations of 90-day mortality or long-term competing mortality risks of younger patients to octogenarians selected for radical cystectomy should be used with caution. Concerning 90-day mortality, in octogenarians selected for radical cystectomy chronological age could have greater impact than numeric comorbidity. In the full model predicting 90-day mortality in patients aged 80 years or older, the odds

Stratification according to the age-adjusted Charlson score	90-day mortality	5-year competing mortality
≤ median (4 points)	1.0% (0.5-2.3) → ASA 1-2 → 0.2% (0.0-1.5); → ASA 3-4 → 1.7% (0.5-4.2)	4.8% (3.0-6.6) → ASA 1-2 → 3.2% (1.6-5.0); → ASA 3-4 → 11.4% (4.9-17.9)
> median (4 points)	6.7% (4.8-9.4) → ASA 1-2 → 1.7% (0.5-5.2); → ASA 3-4 → 9.6% (6.8-13.5)	21.7% (17.8-25.6) → ASA 1-2 → 9.3% (4.8-13.9); → ASA 3-4 → 28.7% (23.3-34.0)

Fig. 2 Impact of the stratification of patients younger than 80 years by the ASA classification on 90-day mortality and 5-year competing (non-bladder cancer) mortality rates after primary stratification by the age-adjusted Charlson score [16] (in brackets: 95% confidence intervals). Within the same risk group indicated by the age-adjusted Charlson score, the 90-day mortality differed by the factor 5-8 and 5-year competing mortality differed approximately by the factor 3 between patients with an ASA class 1-2 versus those with a ASA class 3-4. Such large differences are probably relevant for clinical decision making. For age-adjustment of the Charlson score, 1 point is added for an age of 50-59 years, 2 points for an age of 60-69 years, 3 points for an age of 70-79 years, 4 points for an age of 80-89 years and 5 points for an age of 90-99 years [16]

ratio of the Charlson score was lower than 1 indicating the loss of prognostic impact of numeric comorbidity (in contrast to findings in other types of cancer surgery [12]), whereas the ASA class with an odds ratio of 3.45 (95% confidence interval 0.66-17.95) sustained some of its prognostic impact visible in younger patients (Table 2). It is conceivable that with a larger sample size this classification might reach the significance level in the elderly subgroup as well.

Comorbidity has been found associated with perioperative death 90-day mortality and 5-year mortality after radical cystectomy [13, 14]. Nomograms have been developed and validated predicting all-cause mortality including variables related to age and comorbidity measured by the Charlson score [15].

In the current study, in patients younger than 80 years, particularly the ASA classification was of distinct and probably clinically meaningful impact on 90-day and long-term competing mortality after radical cystectomy in younger patients (Fig. 2). Whereas the 2017 guidelines of the American Urological Association (AUA) dispensed from detailed recommendations on comorbidity classifications [2], the current guidelines of the European Association of Urology (EAU) discouraged using the ASA classification as comorbidity measure in candidates for radical cystectomy [7]. The huge differences in 90-day and 5-year competing mortality observed after stratification by the ASA classification after previous stratification by the age-adjusted Charlson score [16] (the tool that is recommended by the EAU guidelines for comorbidity assessment [7]) in patients younger than 80 years suggest that the guideline's discouragement of using the ASA classification should be revised for this subset of patients.

Compared with patients who were 70-79 years of age, octogenarians undergoing radical cystectomy had similar complication rates but increased mortality [17] underlining the need for an identification of vulnerable elderly patients prior to surgery. Furthermore, with a median of 23 months (95% confidence interval 20-27 months), in a recent large multicenter study, the overall survival rate has been reported to be relatively short octogenarians undergoing radical cystectomy [18]. In the current study, with a median of about 30 months, overall survival was something longer (Fig. 1). In a large octogenarian muscle-invasive bladder cancer sample including various types of management, in contrast to the current study comorbidity measured by the Charlson score was an independent predictor of overall mortality with a moderate association with mortality [18]. The inclusion of more impaired patients (only 26% underwent radical cystectomy [18]), an under-recording of less severe conditions in a multicenter cancer registry [18] and a larger sample size may be discussed as possible explanations for these differing findings.

It is conceivable that self-selection by accumulation of minor forms of chronic -diseases during the long life span and the elimination of severe life-threatening forms by premature mortality might diminish the prognostic significance of individual comorbid conditions in octogenarians. In geriatric patients undergoing emergency general surgery, in contrast to age and ASA classification frailty assessed by the Rockwood frailty index predicted postoperative and major complications [19]. Although it would be of interest, few data is available on the role of frailty assessment in elderly candidates for radical cystectomy until now [5].

This study has several limitations. The number of patients aged 80 years or older was limited. Concerning 90-day mortality, the number of events in this subgroup did not allow an analysis with a multitude of variables. Possibly, a multicenter approach including a huge number of octogenarians with well documented clinical data would be promising in order to identify factors other than age and comorbidity that could be associated with outcome in elderly candidates for radical cystectomy [20]. This study was focused on mortality; minor degree complications were not taken into consideration. 90-day mortality in octogenarians undergoing radical cystectomy is higher outside of academic centers [4]. It is possible that different results could be obtained outside an academic setting. Finally, it should be kept in mind that this analysis was based on patients selected for radical cystectomy; the results may not necessarily be extrapolated to a less strictly selected sample of elderly patients.

Conclusions

This data suggest that extrapolations of perioperative mortality or long-term mortality risks of younger patients to octogenarians selected for radical cystectomy should be used with caution. Cystectomy should not be denied in octogenarians by numeric comorbidity. Concerning 90-day mortality, in octogenarians selected for radical cystectomy chronological age could have greater impact than numeric comorbidity.

Abbreviations
ASA: American Society Association physical status classification; CCS: Classification of angina pectoris of the Canadian Cardiovascular Society; CI: confidence interval; HR: Hazard ratio; NYHA: Classification of cardiac insufficiency of the New York Heart Association; OR: Odds ratio

Acknowledgements
The authors thank Dipl.-Med. C. Werner, Regionales Klinisches Krebsregister Dresden (Regional Clinical Cancer Registry Dresden) for providing follow-up data.

Authors' contributions
MF, RK and MPW were responsible for the concept and framework of the paper. MF, RK, MH, UH, VN, SZ, OWH and MPW participated in collecting and evaluating the data. MF wrote the paper. MF, RK, MH and MPW were largely responsible for the drafting and final editing. All authors read and approved the final manuscript.

Competing interests
Competing financial interests: The authors declare that they have no competing interests..

Author details
[1]Department of Urology, University Hospital Carl Gustav Carus, Technische Universität Dresden, Fetscherstrasse 74, D-01307 Dresden, Germany.

[2]Department of Medical Statistics and Biometry, University Hospital Carl Gustav Carus, Technische Universität Dresden, Fetscherstrasse 74, D-01307 Dresden, Germany. [3]Department of Anesthesiology, University Hospital Carl Gustav Carus, Technische Universität Dresden, Fetscherstrasse 74, D-01307 Dresden, Germany. [4]Department of Urology, University of Rostock, Ernst-Heydemann-Strasse 6, D-18055 Rostock, Germany.

References
1. Ha MS, Chang IH. Significance of age and comorbidity as prognostic indicators for patients with bladder cancer. Asian J Androl. 2010;12:766–74.
2. Chang SS, Bochner BH, Chou R, Dreicer R, Kamat AM, Learner SP, et al. Treatment of non-metastatic mucle-invasive bladder cancer: AUA/ASTRO/SUO guideline. J Urol. 2017;198:552–9.
3. Hounsome LS, Verne J, McGrath JS, Gillatt DA. Trends in operative caseload and mortality rates after radical cystectomy for bladder cancer in England for 1998-2010. Eur Urol. 2015;67:1056–62.
4. Zakaria AS, Santos F, Tanguay S, Kassouf W, Aprikian AG. Radical cystectomy in patients over 80 years old in Quebec: a population-based study of outcomes. J Surg Oncol. 2015;111:917–22.
5. Fonteyne V, Ost P, Bellmunt J, Droz JP, Mongiat-Artus P, Inman B, et al. Curative treatment for muscle invasive bladder cancer in elderly patients: A systematic review. Eur Urol. 2017;73(1):40–50 [Epub ahead of print].
6. De Groote R, Gandaglia G, Geurts N, Goossens M, Pauwels E, D'Hondt F, et al. Robot-assisted radical cystectomy for bladder cancer in octogenarians. J Endourol. 2016;30:792–8.
7. Witjes AJ, Lebret T, Compérat EM, Cowan NC, De Santis M, Bruins HM, et al. Updated 2016 EAU guidelines on muscle-invasive and metastatic bladder cancer. Eur Urol. 2017;71:462–75.
8. Donat SM, Siegrist T, Cronin A, Savage C, Milowsky MI, Herr HW. Radical cystectomy in octogenarians--does morbidity outweigh the potential survival benefits? J Urol. 2010;183:2171–7.
9. Hollenbeck BK, Miller DC, Taub D, Dunn RL, Underwood W 3rd, Montie JE, et al. Aggressive treatment for bladder cancer is associated with improved overall survival among patients 80 years old or older. Urology. 2004;64:292–7.
10. Charlson ME, Pompei P, Ales KL, MacKenzie CR. A new method of classifying prognostic comorbidity in longitudinal studies: development and validation. J Chronic Dis. 1987;40:373–83.
11. American Society of Anesthesiologists: American Society of Anesthesiologists physical status classification system. Available at website http://www.asahq.org/resources/clinical-information/asa-physical-status-classification-system (Accessed 31 Oct 2017).
12. Chang CM, Yin WY, Wei CK, Wu CC, Su YC, Yu CH, et al. Adjusted age-adjusted Charlson comorbidity index score as a risk measure of perioperative mortality before cancer surgery. PLoS One. 2016;11:e0148076.
13. Boorjian SA, Kim SP, Tollefson MK, Carrasco A, Cheville JC, Thompson RH, et al. Comparative performance of comorbidity indices for estimating perioperative and 5-year all cause mortality following radical cystectomy for bladder cancer. J Urol. 2013;190:55–60.
14. Aziz A, May M, Burger M, Palisaar RJ, Trinh QD, Fritsche HM, et al. Prediction of 90-day mortality after radical cystectomy for bladder cancer in a prospective European multicenter cohort. Eur Urol. 2014;66:156–63.
15. Williams SB, Huo J, Chu Y, Baillargeon JG, Daskivich T, Kuo YF, et al. Cancer and all-cause mortality in bladder cancer patients undergoing radical cystectomy: development and validation of a nomogram for treatment decision-making. Urology. 2017;110:76–83.
16. Charlson M, Szatrowski TP, Peterson J, Gold J. Validation of a combined comorbidity index. J Clin Epidemiol. 1994;47:1245–51.
17. Haden TD, Prunty MC, Jones AB, Deroche CB, Murray KS, Pokala N. Comparative perioperative outcomes in septuagenarians and octogenarians undergoing radical cystectomy for bladder cancer - do outcomes differ? Eur Urol Focus. 2017. https://doi.org/10.1016/j.euf.2017.08.005 [Epub ahead of print].
18. Fischer-Valuck BW, Rao YJ, Rudra S, Przybysz D, Germino E, Samson P, et al. Treatment patterns and overall survival outcomes of octogenarians with muscle invasive cancer of the bladder: an analysis of the National Cancer Database. J Urol. 2018;199:416–23.
19. Joseph B, Zangbar B, Pandit V, Fain M, Mohler MJ, Kulvatunyou N, et al. Emergency general surgery in the elderly: Too old or too frail? J Am Coll Surg. 2016;222:805–13.

20. Schiffmann J, Gandaglia G, Larcher A, Sun M, Tian Z, Shariat SF, et al. Contemporary 90-day mortality rates after radical cystectomy in the elderly. Eur J Surg Oncol. 2014;40:1738–45.
21. Canadian Cardiovascular Society. Canadian cardiovascular society grading of angina pectoris. Website: http://www.ccs.ca/images/Guidelines/Guidelines_POS_Library/Ang_Gui_1976.pdf. Accessed 31 Oct 2017.
22. The Criteria Committee of the New York Heart Association. Nomenclature and criteria for diagnosis of diseases of the heart and great vessels. 9th ed. Boston: Little, Brown & Co; 1994. p. 253–6.

Multi-tract percutaneous nephrolithotomy combined with EMS lithotripsy for bilateral complex renal stones

Taisheng Liang[1], Chenming Zhao[2], Gang Wu[1], Botao Tang[1], Xiangdong Luo[1], Shangguang Lu[1], Yu Dong[1] and Huan Yang[2*]

Abstract

Background: The treatment of bilateral complex renal stones is a tough challenge for urologists. This study aimed to evaluate the efficiency and safety of bilateral ultrasonography-guided multi-tract percutaneous nephrolithotomy (PCNL) combined with EMS lithotripsy for the treatment of such cases.

Methods: Twenty-seven patients suffering from bilateral complex renal calculi underwent t bilateral multi-tract PCNL. The PCNL began with the establishment of percutaneous nephrostomy access, which was achieved under ultrasound guidance followed by stone fragment and removal by EMS lithotripsy. The same processes were then performed on the ipsilateral and contralateral renal units until the operation terminated. Sheaths left in situ to provide the tracts for the two-stage and the three-stage PCNL procedures. Peri- and postoperative clinical data were collected and analysed.

Results: Renal stones of both sides were completely cleared within three PCNL sessions in 24 cases. Among them, four, thirteen, and seven cases underwent single, second-stage and third-stage procedures, respectively. The total stone-free rate was 88.9%. Three patients failed to receive complete stone clearance. Mean operation time was 78.7 (26–124) min, the mean estimated blood loss was 97.3 (30–250) ml, and the mean length of hospital stay was 18 (10–31) days. No patient required blood transfusion and postoperative fever occurred in 6 cases. Within the follow-up period, stone recurrence occurred in 6 patients.

Conclusions: Ultrasonography-guided multi-tract PCNL using EMS is an efficient method for the treatment of complex renal calculi. According to our experience, it is safe to make multiple tracts on both sides simultaneously.

Keywords: Bilateral complex renal stones, Multi-tract, PCNL

Background

Complex renal stones usually refer to staghorn calculi, multiple stones or those associated with anatomical or functional abnormalities. Due to the complicated etiological factors, large stone burdens, high operation risks and high recurrence, it is always a challenge for surgeons to treat such stones, especially those occur in bilateral kidneys. Since Fernström first described percutaneous nephrolithotomy (PCNL) under radiological control in 1976, it has been the standard method for the treatment of large renal stones [1]. Complex stones often require multiple nephrostomy tracts, long operating time, and repeated procedures, which are associated with more access-related complications such as bleeding, infection and deterioration in renal function. Nevertheless, according to the current guidelines, PCNL is still the first-line choice for the management of large or staghorn renal stones [2, 3]. Owning to developments in the technique, it is possible to safely perform multi-tract PCNL on bilateral kidneys at one time. Over the past 4 years, we performed 27 bilateral multi-tract PCNL procedures for the treatment of complex renal stones; therefore, we evaluated the safety and efficacy of this approach.

Methods

Between October 2011 and November 2015, 27 patients (12 males and 15 females) with bilateral complex stones

---

* Correspondence: yhpz123@163.com
[2]Department of Urology, Tongji Hospital, Tongji Medical College, Huazhong University of Science and Technology, Wuhan, China
Full list of author information is available at the end of the article

were admitted to our department. The mean age was 47.8 (41–63) years. All patients had history of renal stones ranging between 6 and 17 years. Eight patients had been treated by operations, five on one side, and three on both sides. All stones were detected by abdominal computerized tomography (CT), and plain film of kidney-ureter-bladder (KUB) as bilateral staghorn or multiple stones. The stone size varied from 2.5 to 8.6 cm. Three cases were associated with moderate to severe unilateral hydronephrosis and nine cases with moderate to severe bilateral hydronephrosis. Urological anatomical abnormalities were observed in five patients: three with ureter pelvic junction obstruction (UPJO) and two with duplex renal pelvis.

PCNL procedures and other aspects of patient treatment mentioned were standard practice. The PCNL procedures were performed under general epidural anaesthesia. A 6-Fr external ureteral catheter was inserted retrograde into the renal pelvis in a lithotomy position for retrograde saline injection if intraoperative artificial hydronephrosis was needed. Then, the patient was placed into the prone position with the renal region elevated. The appropriate percutaneous puncture was achieved under the guidance of ultrasonography (FCUBE9, Korea) using an 18-gauge needle (Urovison, Germany). The first tract was the one that led straight to the maximal stone burden, but stayed away from renal columns, usually through the posterior intermediate calyx. Afterward, the guidewire was inserted into the pelvis or addressed to the target stone. Guided by the wire, tract dilation was accomplished by polytetrafluoroethylene dilators (Urovison, Germany) to 24 Fr. Due to the rigid characteristics of these stones, we applied the pneumatic and ultrasonic endoscopic lithotripter (Electro Medical Systems/EMS-IV) to fragment and remove them. After the stones within the field of vision through the first tract were cleared, the second or third tract was established in the same way to reach those stones in other calyxes. After lithotripsy processes, a 6-Fr double-J stent installed antegrade in the ureter remained for 4 weeks. The operations were terminated by the placement of a 20-Fr nephrostomy tube in each tract. One example of establishment of multiple tracts is shown in Fig. 1. At 5–7 days after PCNL, all patients underwent an X-ray of the KUB to evaluate the residual stones. If necessary, a two-stage or three-stage PCNL operation would be performed through the established tracts. Once the test revealed complete clearance, all nephrostomy tubes were removed. Peri- and postoperative clinical parameters and complications were observed. Clavien-Dindo classification [4] was used to grade the PCNL related complications.

To evaluate the impact from times of PCNL on surgical morbidity, we divided the patients into 3 groups according to the operation sessions. We compared the hospital stay and blood loss among the 3 groups. Statistics analyses were performed using the software IBM SPSS statistics 22. The results were considered significantly different when the p value was less than 0.05.

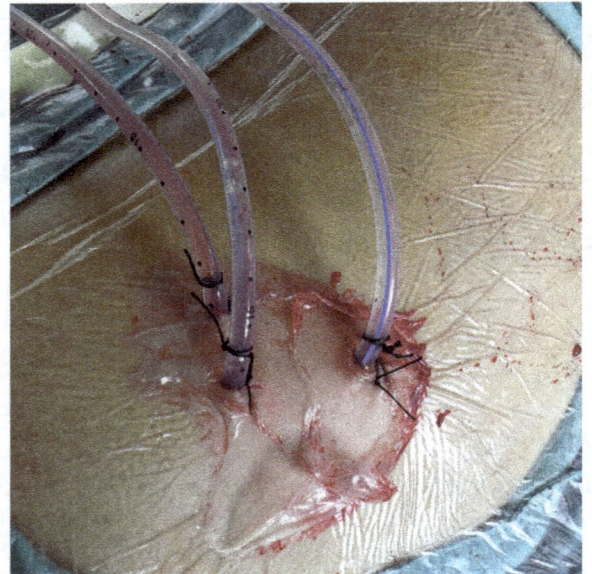

Fig. 1 The construction of multiple tracts

Results

All 54 kidney units in 27 patients were treated. Percutaneous punctures were performed under the guidance of ultrasonography. The serum creatinine ranged from 123.4 to 667.2 umol/L, and eight patients experienced renal insufficiency. Preoperative urine tests showed that leucocyturia existed in 13 cases, among which *Escherichia coli* was found in six patients. Patients with urinary tract infection were treated with culture-specific antibiotic therapy until the reexamine urine culture was negative. Meanwhile, those with negative urine cultures received empiric antibiotic therapy for 3 days before operation. The patient demographics are shown in Table 1.

Table 1 Patient demographics

Number of patients	27
Number of renal unit treated	54
Age, years, mean (range)	47.8 (41–63)
Gender, male/female	12/15
Preoperative body temperature, °C, mean (range)	37.0 (36.5–38.6)
Preoperative serum creatinine, umol/L, mean (range)	204.6 (123.4–667.2)
Mean stone size, cm	2.5–8.6
Urological anatomical abnormalities	Ureteropelvic Junction Obstruction (UPJO) 3
	Double renal pelvis 2
Other relevant conditions	Obesity 3
	Spine deformation 1
Previous stone surgeries	One side 5
	Both sides 3

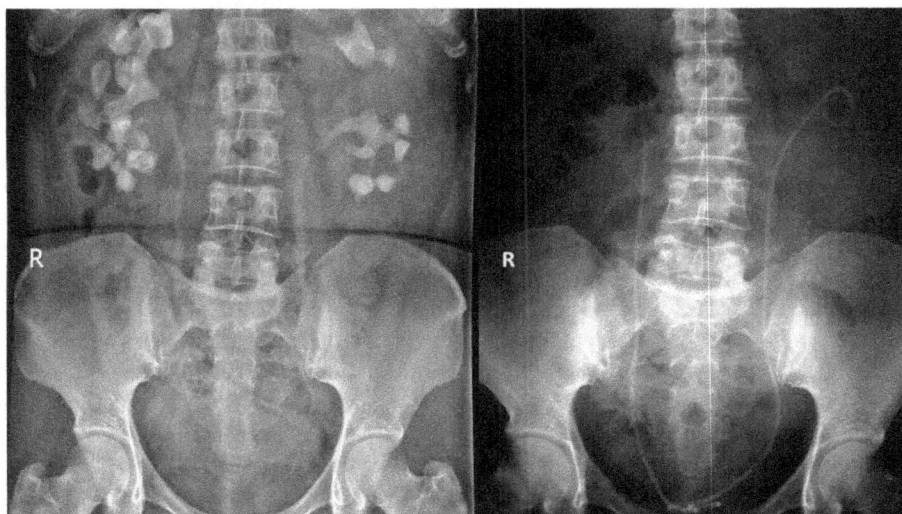

Fig. 2 The comparison of the KUBs before and after PCNL of one patient with bilateral complex renal stones

Complete clearance on both sides was achieved in 24 patients. The x-ray film of one example as complete clearance is shown in Fig. 2. Among them, four patients needed one single surgery session, 13 patients needed a secondary PCNL, and three sessions of PCNL were needed in seven patients. Three patients did not achieve complete clearance although one underwent two-stage and two underwent three-stage multi-tract PCNL. The total stone-free rate within three operations was 88.9%. The mean operation time was 78.7 (26–124) min. During surgeries the estimated blood loss was 97.3 (30–250) ml. Severe bleeding occurred in two patients due to mucous membrane injury and tearing of the calyx neck, although no patients required blood transfusion. Six patients had postoperative fever, and two were confirmed to have urinary infection. To prevent possible septic shock, patients with fever were treated with broad-spectrum antibiotics for 3 days, until body temperature and blood tests returned to normal. No patients suffered symptomatic hydrothorax or other visceral organ injury. The Clavien-Dindo classification was assessed as grade II in 6 patients because of the application of antibiotic, whereas the other 21 patients were assessed as grade I. The mean duration of hospital stay was 18 (10–31) days for total cases.

After leaving hospital, all patients accepted follow-up care for 20 (2–42) months. During the follow-up period, two treated kidney units progressed to nephrarctia. Serum creatinine increased by 13.4–132.6 umol/L in three patients compared with the level before surgery; however, for the other patients, serum creatinine decreased to or remained at a normal level. The mean serum creatinine was 116.8 (72.5–154.3) umol/L. Six patients experienced stone recurrence, which required further PCNL or extracorporeal shock wave lithotripsy (ESWL) combined with medical expulsion treatment. All surgical outcomes are shown in Table 2.

The statistical analyses revealed that, there was no significant difference in terms of estimated blood loss among the 3 groups ($p = 0.083$). However, more sessions of surgeries were associated with longer hospital stay ($p < 0.001$).

Table 2 Operative characteristics and results

Tracts in one renal unit, mean (range)	1.8 (1–4)
Number of patients who underwent different sessions of PCNL	One session 4
	Two sessions 14
	There sessions 9
Operation time, min, mean (range)	78.7 (26–124)
Estimated blood loss, ml, mean (range)	97.3 (30–250)
Hospital stay, days, mean (range)	18 (10–31)
1 session	11.8 (10–13)
2 sessions	14 (10–18)
3 sessions	27.7 (24–31)
Complete stone clearance rate within 3 sessions	24 (88.9%)
Postoperative serum creatinine, umol/L, mean (range)	116.8 (72.5–154.3)
Complications	Bleeding 2
	Fever 6
	Infection 2
Clavien-Dindo Classification, Grade (Number)	I (21); II (6)
Follow-up, months, median (range)	20 (2–42)
Recurrence	6
Nephrarctia	2

Discussion

Complex stones are extremely harmful to kidneys because they cause infection, atrophy, renal failure and cancerization. For treatment, multiple tracts are always required to achieve complete clearance and to avoid a second-look procedure such as ESWL or retrograde intrarenal surgery (RIRS). However, multiple tracts are often associated with a higher risk of bleeding [5]. In addition, multi-tract PCNL is very difficult to learn and requires much experience, despite the improvements in devices and techniques over past decades [6]. Some studies have suggested that open or laparoscopic stone surgery is an efficient method for the treatment of complex kidney stones, and is reported to be associated with higher one-session stone-free rate [7, 8]. However, PCNL can be repeated, whereas open or laparoscopic surgery would be increasingly difficult after the first procedure. Moreover, bilateral renal stones are difficult to be treated together in a single session by open or laparoscopic surgery. By contrast, in Cho's study, multi-tract PCNL had similar safety and effectiveness as conventional single-tract PCNL in patients with complex stones [9]. The AUA guideline also suggested that PCNL with multiple tracts was a safe and effective way for treating staghorn stones, with monotherapy stone-free rate of 79%, and acute complication rate of 15%[3].

A safe and efficient PCNL always begins with successful punctures, especially for complex stones. In our study, no severe complications occurred in any of the 27 patients, although we treated bilateral kidneys for each patient at a single time. We established the tracts under the guidance of ultrasonography. Compared with fluoroscopy, ultrasonography has advantages as it is more convenient without any radiation and it can present the three-dimensional structure of kidneys by turning the probe [10]. Based on our experience, ultrasonography could clearly show hydronephrosis calyces as well as anatomical abnormalities. All tracts could be accurately placed in the line collecting the calyx neck middle and the corresponding calyceal fornix middle. Thus, the tracts provided the least traumatic and most direct access for the fragment of calculi. At the same time, the injury to adjacent viscera was avoided. Moreover, the whole procedure was performed under ultrasonography until dilation was complete, and it was confirmed whether there was any sign of bleeding. It is possible to totally avoid severe bleeding as long as precise punctures are achieved.

Multi-tract PCNL is still controversial. The major area of criticism has been safety during the process, as more than one tract dilatation is considered to be associated with a higher complication rate. Except for a higher risk of bleeding, there might be a significant rise in serum creatinine and drop in creatinine clearance after multi-tract PCNL [11], which means that multiple tracts might cause damage to renal function. However, in our study, only three patients experienced increased postoperative serum creatinine, and based on other studies, there was no evidence to indicate that multiple tracts led to renal insufficiency [12–14]. Moreover, in a number of studies, when compared with single-tract PCNL, no significant difference was reported in terms of complications [9, 11]. In our study, no patients suffered severe perioperative and postoperative complications, and no patients required blood transfusion, showing that more than one tract in a single operation is not always accompanied by high risk. In Singla's study, the maximal number of tracts used in a single renal unit could be up to six with acceptable morbidity [15]. However, we have to admit, the safety should necessarily be the first principle when we treat complex stones, especially for bilateral stones. Although bilateral PCNL is more efficient and can be performed in both children and adults, it carries a higher rate of overall complications, such as fever, persistent pain, acute renal failure and vomiting, than unilateral PCNL [16]. In addition, once there is hematuria or leucocyturia after bilateral surgery, we cannot determine which is the disease-causing kidney. In consideration of these risks, we performed a careful assessment for every patient before operation to ensure that bilateral PCNL could proceed smoothly. We kept the operation time within 2 h and always started in the renal unit that seemed easier to treat, so that the risk of sepsis was controlled. For each patient, the first tract is the main one, through which we could clear most of the stone burden and relieve the obstruction. Once any severe bleeding or pyonephrosis was found, the operations were stopped immediately, and the tracts remained for the secondary procedure. On the other hand, we acknowledge that more sessions of surgery would inevitably prolong the mean hospital stay, which means more financial cost and higher risk of nosocomial infection, because of the necessary preparation before each session of PCNL, particularly for those with urinary infection. Given these factors, more experience is required to improve the efficiency without any decrease in safety.

For the fragmentation of complex stones, we used the fourth-generation EMS, applying pneumatic and ultrasonic energy together. The stone fragmenting and removal can be carried out at the same time through vacuum suction. The normal saline solution was hung approximately one metre higher than the renal location, which poured naturally as the washing flow, instead of using a pump. Combined with the suction system, a clear surgical field was provided with a low intrapelvis pressure. Using this device, the operation time was shortened and the safety together with efficacy was increased. In our study, only six patients developed postoperative fever, but recovered quickly. In Wang's study, EMS was even safe for the treatment of calculous pyonephrosis, which was considered as a contraindication of PCNL [17].

Even though most patients also needed more than one stage of operation, multi-tract PCNL significantly improved the clearance efficacy. The totally stone-free rate was 88.9% within three sessions of PCNL, while the recurrence rate was 6/23 within 42 months. Complex stones often result from inherent existing factors such as infection, metabolic disturbance or anatomical abnormality, which occurred in five patients in our series, indicating that prevention is a much more important and difficult task for urologists. Although multi-tract PCNL is an appropriate option to clear complex stones from kidneys with anatomical abnormality, it is of limited value to reduce the recurrence risk. Perhaps, the concomitant of laparoscopic and endoscopic treatment would be the further direction for the treatment of such cases [18, 19].

Conclusion

Ultrasonography together with pneumatic and ultrasonic endoscopic lithotripter is a widely used device in China for PCNL. With their help, multi-tract PCNL is an efficient and safe method for the treatment of bilateral complex renal stones. Given the limitation of the sample size and the retrospective nature of our study, more multi-center, randomized control studies with large sample size and high quality are required.

Abbreviations
PCNL: Percutaneous nephrolithotomy; EMS: Electro Medical Systems; CT: Computed Tomography; KUB: Kidney-ureter-bladder; ESWL: Extracorporeal Shock Wave Lithotripsy; RIRS: Retrograde intrarenal surgery

Acknowledgements
None.

Funding
None.

Authors' contribution
HY and TSL conceived and designed this study. TSL, GW, BTT, XDL, SGL and YD carried out surgeries on patients. XDL, YD, CMZ and HY contributed to the follow-up questionnaire. CMZ, HY, GW, BTT and SGL participated in data acquisition and interpretation. CMZ performed the statistics analyses and drafted the manuscript. HY, TSL and GW critically reviewed the manuscript. All the authors read and approved the final manuscript.

Competing interests
The authors declare that they have no competing interests.

Author details
[1]Department of Urology, Ruikang Hospital Affiliated to Guangxi University of Chinese Medicine, Nanning, China. [2]Department of Urology, Tongji Hospital, Tongji Medical College, Huazhong University of Science and Technology, Wuhan, China.

References
1. Patel SR, Nakada SY. The modern history and evolution of percutaneous nephrolithotomy. J Endourol. 2015;29(2):153–7.
2. Türk C, Knoll T, Petrik A, et al. Guidelines on urolithiasis. Eur Assoc Urol. 2015. https://uroweb.org/guideline/urolithiasis/?type=pocket-guidelines.
3. Assimos DG, Lingeman JE, et al. AUA guideline on management of staghorn calculi: diagnosis and treatment recommendations. J Urol. 2005; 173(6):1991–2000.
4. Clavien PA, Barkun J, de Oliveira ML, et al. The Clavien-Dindo classification of surgical complications: five-year experience. Ann Surg. 2009;250(2):187–96.
5. Akman T, Binbay M, Sari E, et al. Factors affecting bleeding during percutaneous nephrolithotomy: single surgeon experience. J Endourol. 2011;25(2):327–33.
6. Desai M, Jain P, Ganpule A, et al. Developments in technique and technology: the effect on the results of percutaneous nephrolithotomy for staghorn calculi. BJU Int. 2009;104(4):542–8.
7. Basiri A, Tabibi A, Nouralizadeh A, et al. Comparison of safety and efficacy of laparoscopic pyelolithotomy versus percutaneous nephrolithotomy in patients with renal pelvic stones: a randomized clinical trial. Urol J. 2014; 11(6):1932–7.
8. Haggag YM, Morsy G, Badr MM, et al. Comparative study of laparoscopic pyelolithotomy versus percutaneous nephrolithotomy in the management of large renal pelvic stones. Can Urol Assoc J. 2013;7(3–4):E171–175.
9. Cho HJ, Lee JY, Kim SW, et al. Percutaneous nephrolithotomy for complex renal calculi: is multi-tract approach ok? Can J Urol. 2012;19(4):6360–5.
10. Li J, Xiao B, Hu W, et al. Complication and safety of ultrasound guided percutaneous nephrolithotomy in 8,025 cases in China. Chin Med J (Engl). 2014;127(24):4184–9.
11. Hegarty NJ, Desai MM. Percutaneous nephrolithotomy requiring multiple tracts: comparison of morbidity with single-tract procedures. J Endourol. 2006;20(10):753–60.
12. Aron M, Yadav R, Goel R, et al. Multi-tract percutaneous nephrolithotomy for large complete staghorn calculi. Urol Int. 2005;75(4):327–32.
13. Fei X, Li J, Song Y, et al. Single-stage multiple-tract percutaneous nephrolithotomy in the treatment of staghorn stones under total ultrasonography guidance. Urol Int. 2014;93(4):411–6.
14. Chen J, Zhou X, Chen Z, et al. Multiple tracts percutaneous nephrolithotomy assisted by LithoClast master in one session for staghorn calculi: report of 117 cases. Urolithiasis. 2014;42(2):165–9.
15. Singla M, Srivastava A, Kapoor R, et al. Aggressive approach to staghorn calculi-safety and efficacy of multiple tracts percutaneous nephrolithotomy. Urology. 2008;71(6):1039–42.
16. Kadlec AO, Greco KA, Fridirici ZC, et al. Comparison of complication rates for unilateral and bilateral percutaneous nephrolithotomy (PCNL) using a modified Clavien grading system. BJU Int. 2013;111(4 Pt B):E243–248.
17. Wang J, Zhou DQ, He M, et al. One-phase treatment for calculous pyonephrosis by percutaneous nephrolithotomy assisted by EMS LithoClast master. Chin Med J (Engl). 2013;126(8):1584–6.
18. Yin Z, Wei YB, Liang BL, et al. Initial experiences with laparoscopy and flexible ureteroscopy combination pyeloplasty in management of ectopic pelvic kidney with stone and ureter-pelvic junction obstruction. Urolithiasis. 2015;43(3):255–60.
19. Zheng J, Yan J, Zhou Z, et al. Concomitant treatment of ureteropelvic junction obstruction and renal calculi with robotic laparoscopic surgery and rigid nephroscopy. Urology. 2014;83(1):237–42.

Application and analysis of retroperitoneal laparoscopic partial nephrectomy with sequential segmental renal artery clamping for patients with multiple renal tumor

Jundong Zhu[†], Fan Jiang[†], Pu Li[†], Pengfei Shao, Chao Liang, Aiming Xu, Chenkui Miao, Chao Qin[*], Zengjun Wang[*] and Changjun Yin

Abstract

Background: To explore the feasibility and safety of retroperitoneal laparoscopic partial nephrectomy with sequential segmental renal artery clamping for the patients with multiple renal tumor of who have solitary kidney or contralateral kidney insufficiency.

Methods: Nine patients who have undergone retroperitoneal laparoscopic partial nephrectomy with sequential segmental renal artery clamping between October 2010 and January 2017 were retrospectively analyzed. Clinical materials and parameters during and after the operation were summarized.

Results: Nineteen tumors were resected in nine patients and the operations were all successful. The operation time ranged from 100 to 180 min (125 min); clamping time of segmental renal artery was 10 ~ 30 min (23 min); the amount of blood loss during the operation was 120 ~ 330 ml (190 ml); hospital stay after the operation is 3 ~ 6d (5d). There was no complication during the perioperative period, and the pathology diagnosis after the surgery showed that there were 13 renal clear cell carcinomas, two papillary carcinoma and four perivascular epithelioid cell tumors with negative margins from the 19 tumors. All patients were followed up for 3 ~ 60 months, and no local recurrence or metastasis was detected. At 3-month post-operation follow-up, the mean serum creatinine was 148. 6 ± 28.1 μmol/L ($p = 0.107$), an increase of 3.0 μmol/L from preoperative baseline.

Conclusions: For the patients with multiple renal tumors and solitary kidney or contralateral kidney insufficiency, retroperitoneal laparoscopic partial nephrectomy with sequential segmental renal artery clamping was feasible and safe, which minimized the warm ischemia injury to the kidney and preserved the renal function effectively.

Keywords: Kidney neoplasms, Retroperitoneal laparoscopic operation, Partial nephrectomy, Segmental renal artery, Sequential clamping

* Correspondence: 13776678978@163.com; zengjunwang@njmu.edu.cn
[†]Equal contributors
Department of Urology, The First Affiliated Hospital of Nanjing Medical University, Nanjing, 300 Guangzhou Road, Nanjing 210029, China

Background

Current studies found that of retroperitoneal laparoscopic partial nephrectomy can be a nephron-sparing option which have no significant difference with radical nephrectomy in the aspect of oncologic efficacy to properly selected patients [1] and this novel technique has gained popularity widely in the world [2–4]. In regard to some patients with solitary kidney or contralateral kidney insufficiency, partial nephrectomy can effectively reduce the incidence of dialysis on account of postoperative kidney failure [5]. In traditional partial nephrectomy, surgeons conduct the tumor excision and wound suture in the state of complete renal ischemia with main renal artery clamped,which is usually complete within 20 ~ 30 min to avoid the kidney from irreversible injury [6]. It's extremely difficult to complete the surgery within a specified time when multiple renal carcinoma exist. In view of this, we retrospectively analyzed the clinical data of 9 patients from October 2010 to January 2017 who underwent retroperitoneal laparoscopic partial nephrectomy with sequential segmental renal artery clamping which avoided the complete renal ischemia during the whole surgical process. The curative effect is satisfied, report as follows.

Methods

Clinical data

From October 2010 to January 2017, a total of 756 partial nephrectomies were performed in our center and of these, a total of 9 patients including five male and four female underwent retroperitoneal laparoscopic partial nephrectomy with sequential segmental renal artery clamping, aging from 37 to 65 (mean of 51). Table 1 summarizes the demographic data for these patients. Six patients' tumors were located in the left renal and three

Table 1 Characteristics of the recruited patients

Age	
Mean (range), year	51 (37–65)
Gender	
Male (%)	5 (56)
Female (%)	4 (44)
Tumor side	
Right (%)	3 (33)
Left (%)	6 (67)
Number of tumor	
Two tumors (%)	8 (89)
Three tumors (%)	1 (11)
Tumor size	
Mean (range), cm	2.5 (1.8–3.5)
R.E.N.A.L score	
Mean (range)	4.4 (4–6)

were located in the right renal. There were three cases of contralateral renal atrophy and six of solitary kidney. All the nine patients were diagnosed by physical examination with no obvious symptom of lumbago and hematuria. Eight of them had two tumors and one had three tumors in unilateral renal. Tumors were exophytic with the R.E.N.A.L score ranged from 4 to 6 points (mean of 4.4 points) and the diameter of them ranged from 1.8 to 3.5 cm (mean of 2.5 cm). No lymph nodes, renal vein or inferior vena cava tumor thrombus and distant metastasis were found in any patients. CT arteriography (CTA) was used preoperatively to show the tumors' segmental arteries [7] (Figure 1). The first postoperative follow-up was performed at 1 month after operation with the examination of abdominal ultrasonography, chest radiography, hemogram, erythrocyte sedimentation rate (ESR) and blood biochemical tests. The follow-up of glomerular filtration rate (GFR), abdominal CT scan and hemogram were performed at 3th months postoperatively and reviewed every 3 months after that until 1 year. Afterwards, blood and imagine examinations were conducted annually.

Surgical methods

Patients were administered general anesthesia and placed in the lateral decubitus position. To establish the retroperitoneal space, the trocar was inserted according to the location of the tumors. Then, 2 cm incision was made via the median axillary line at the level of iliac crest. A self-made balloon was placed in the retroperitoneal space through the incision and infused 800 ml air to expand the retroperitoneal space. Under the guidance of fingers, a 12 mm trocar was inserted below the 12th rib at the posterior axillary line. Two 5 mm trocars were placed up and down at the anterior axillary line and observation mirror was inserted through the incision above the illac crest. Pneumoperitoneum pressure was maintained at 15 mmHg (1 mmHg = 0.133kpa). In the case of patients with ventral tumors needing to perform the segmental renal artery clamping in the front of renal hilar, all trocar would be moved toward anterior median line by 2 ~ 3 cm [8]. The fascia and adipose capsule of kidney were opened along the dorsal renal to make the kidney dissociative, revealing renal tumor and peripheral renal parenchyma. Instead of separating the renal artery trunk, we dissociated several segmental arteries of the tumor directly in the vicinity of the renal hilar under the guidance of the CTA (Fig. 2). Subsequently, the segmental artery was clamped and a scissor was used to resect the tumor in the renal parenchyma, 2 mm away from the tumor edge. After the wound was continuous sutured with absorbable suture, releasing the segmental arteries to check if any active bleeding existed. In the same manner, clamping the other segmental arteries sequentially to

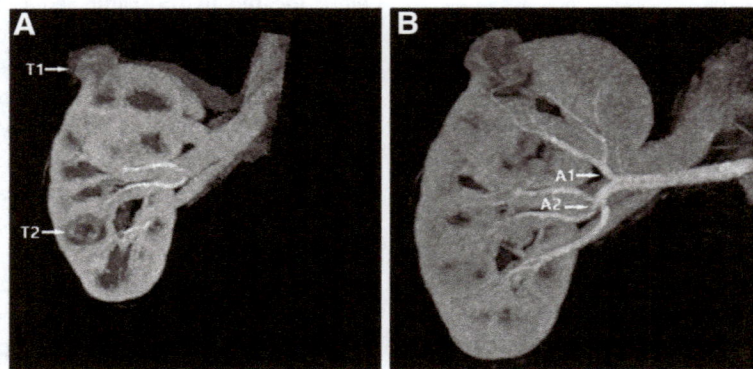

Fig. 1 CTA was used to position tumors and their corresponding segmental arteries. **a** CTA showed the tumors in the upper (T1) and lower pole (T2) of right renal; **b** Superior, anterior and posterior branch were separated from the right renal artery near the renal hilum. Superior branch supplied the lesions in the upper pole (A1) and anterior branch supplied the lesions in the lower pole (A2)

resect other tumors. After resecting all the renal tumors, renal blood flow was restored and no obvious hemorrhage should be confirmed again at the place of wound, renal hilar and every puncture hole. Finally, packing the resected tumors into the specimen bag to fetch them out, then indwelling the drainage tube and closing the incision.

Statistical analysis

Statistical analysis of pre- and postoperative serum creatinine (SCr) levels were performed using the student t test. All data are reported as mean and range, with $p < 0.05$ considered statistically significant.

Results

All operations were successfully completed and 19 tumors were cut off from nine patients. Operative characteristics are presented in Table 2. The operation time ranged from 100 to 180 min (125 min) and warm ischemia time of each 19 clamping was 10 ~ 30 min (23 min). The blood loss during operations was 120 ~ 330 ml (190 ml) and the postoperation hospital stays was 3 ~ 6 days (5 days). There was no complication

in perioperative period. After the surgery, we routinely conducted a clinicopathologic analysis and the results showed 13 renal clear cell carcinomas, two papillary carcinoma and four perivascular epithelioid cell tumors with negative margins from the 19 tumors. All patients had no local recurrence or metastasis with a 3 ~ 60 months follow-up visit (16.6 months).

Mean preoperative SCr was 145.6 ± 25.9 μmol/L respectively and the mean SCr increased to 182.1 ± 26.6 μmol/L ($p < 0.001$) at 1 day and 197.4 ± 34.2 μmol/L (p < 0.001) at 3 day after the operation. Mean SCr at 1-month follow-up showed dramatic recoveries and reached to 156.7 ± 28.4 μmol/L ($p = 0.002$). At 3-month post-operation follow-up, the mean SCr was 148.6 ± 28.1 μmol/L ($p = 0.107$), only an increase of 3.0 μmol/L from baseline (Table 3).

Discussion

Shortening the warm ischemia (WI) time and reducing the area of WI are the main methods to protect renal function in partial nephrectomy [9]. Nowadays, continuous main renal artery clamping is the main method to

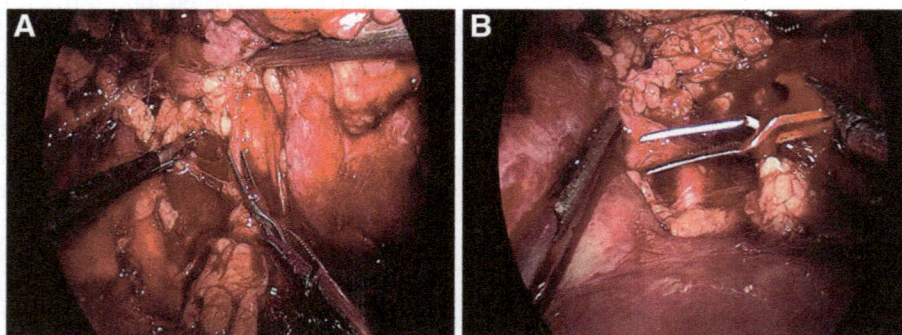

Fig. 2 Clamping the superior and anterior branch of the right renal artery during the operation. **a** clamping the superior branch before resecting the tumor in upper pole; **b** clamping the anterior branch before resecting the tumor in lower pole

Table 2 Operative characteristics of the operation

Operation time	
Mean (range), min	125 (100–180)
Warm ischemia time of each tumor	
Mean (range), min	23 (10–30)
Blood loss	
Mean (range), ml	190 (120–330)
Postoperation hospital stays	
Mean (range), day	5 (3–6)
Histology	
Clear cell carcinoma (%)	13 (68)
Papillary carcinoma (%)	2 (11)
Perivascular epithelioid cell tumors (%)	4 (21)
Postoperative follow-up time	
Mean (range), month	16.6 (3–60)

block the bloodstream in partial nephrectomy and studies show that the renal function will be damaged irreversibly if exceeding the renal tolerant time of WI for 30 min. Therefore, surgeons were supposed to complete the resection and suture within 30 min after clamping renal artery in partial nephrectomy. To reduce the area of WI, unblocking and segmental renal artery clamping technique was applied. Although the operation demand high equipment quality and operation technique, more and more departments carrying out these techniques in recent years [10–12]. What's more, our previous study has been demonstrated that patients underwent segmental artery clamping have better early recovery comparing by 3-month postoperative GFR levels [13].

In clinical practice, it is usually difficult to handle multiple renal tumors with solitary kidney and contralateral kidney insufficiency. Patients are supposed to receive postoperative dialysis treatment if underwent a radical nephrectomy. Because of multiple lesions, nephron-sparing operation is hardly to be completed within 30 min to protect renal away from irreversible damage. Therefore, some scholars have proposed a scheme to protect renal function by reducing renal temperature [14]. In addition, under the pressure of limited time for surgeons, the probability to rupture the tumor capsule, suture the wound and collection system imprecisely during the operation will increase and thus affect the prognosis and complications rates. For these special patients, we complete the partial nephrectomy by applying the technique of retroperitoneal laparoscopic partial nephrectomy with sequential segmental renal artery clamping and protecte the patient's renal function satisfyingly by reducing the area of WI during the operation. The advantages of this technique are as follows: ① Complete renal ischemia can be avoided during the operation and the blood supply of other parts of kidney is unaffected when segmental renal arteries are clamped, so that the renal function can be protected effectively. ②surgeons can complete each resection and wound suture carefully instead of dealing with several tumors in a hurry time, reducing surgical complications and ensuring the operation efficacy.

We believe that the key points of this technique are as follows:

① Before the operation, doctor should establish a three-dimensional renal artery reconstruction model by imagine techniques to determine the number and block position of target vessels, and design the path to separate the target vessels [7]. ② Position of the trocar should be adjusted according to the surgical approach which will make the the target vessels and tumors separated easily [8]. ③ After recognizing the anatomic spatial relationships according to the three-dimensional renal artery reconstruction model, surgeons can directly attempt to free the segmental artery in the renal hilum by a scissor instead of the equipment with heating effect such as coagulation hook and harmonic scalpel [13]. ④ Providing tumors are resected completely, interlobular vessels outside the tumor psuedocapsule should be reserved as much as possible in order to maximally save the blood supply of peripheral normal renal tissue.

Surgeons should adequately evaluate tumor location, size, exophytic or not and the complexity of feeding artery to each kidney segment if they decide to conduct sequential segmental renal artery clamping for patients with multiple renal tumor. If the tumor is too close to the hilum, it is hard to achieve clear exposure of segmental arteries and pelvis without compression of the tumor, so conventional method is more suitable for these cases. What's more, surgical method should also be considered cautiously for the patients with bigger or overmany tumors or already metastasize to peripheral renal tissue or lymph nodes. In our selected patients, the average diameter of these tumors is 2.5 cm and all of them were exophytic. Therefore, the surgical procedure was not difficult and the local WI time of each clamping can be controlled within 30 min during the operation.

Table 3 Pre-operative and post-operative comparisons of serum creatinine

	Pre-Operation	Post-Operation at 1 day	Post-Operation at 3 day	Post-Operation at 1 month	Post-Operation at 3 month
mean(μmol/L)	145.6 ± 25.9	182.1 ± 26.6	197.4 ± 34.2	156.7 ± 28.4	148.6 ± 28.1
P-value		<0.001	<0.001	0.002	0.107

Due to sufficient preoperative assessment, no cases converted to main renal artery clamping or open operation in our study. No lymph nodes, renal vein or inferior vena cava thrombus and distant metastasis were found among the nine patients, so that the renal function and oncological efficacy is better with no subsequent dialysis.

Nonetheless, limitations of this study exist regarding the sample size and retrospective nature of the study. Due to the case number constraints of multiple renal tumors with solitary kidney or contralateral kidney insufficiency, this study does not compare sequential selective clamping to main renal artery clamping for multiple tumor removal; rather, it presents a feasible technique for minimizing the warm ischemia injury to the kidney and preserving the renal function.

Conclusions

In conclusion, retroperitoneal laparoscopic partial nephrectomy with sequential segmental renal artery clamping can avoid complete renal WI injury and the operation is safe and feasible. This technique can be selectively applied according to the particular tumor situation for the patients with isolated kidney, contralateral renal insufficiency or bilateral multiple renal tumors.

Abbreviations
CT: Computed tomography; CTA: Computed tomography arteriography; ESR: Erythrocyte sedimentation rate; GFR: Glomerular filtration rate; SCr: Serum creatinine; WI: Warm ischemia

Acknowledgements
Not applicable.

Funding
The study was supported by the Priority Academic Program Development of Jiangsu Higher Education Institutions (PAPD), Program for Development of Innovative Research Team in the First Affiliated Hospital of Nanjing Medical University, Provincial Initiative Program for Excellency Disciplines of Jiangsu Province, National Natural Science Foundation of China (81,270,685, 81,372,757, 81,672,531).

Authors' contributions
ZW, CQ and CY: Protocol/project development; JZ, FJ, PL and CM: Data collection or management; PS, CL and AX: Data analysis; JZ and FJ: Manuscript writing/editing. All authors read and approved the final manuscript.

Competing interests
The authors declare that they have no competing interests.

References
1. Lane BR, Fergany AF, Weight CJ, et al. Renal functional outcomes after partial nephrectomy with extended ischemic intervals are better than after radical nephrectomy. J Urol. 2010;184(4):1286–90.
2. Porpiglia F, Fiori C, Bertolo R, et al. Long-term functional evaluation of the treated kidney in a prospective series of patients who underwent laparoscopic partial nephrectomy for small renal tumors. Eur Urol. 2012; 62(1):130–5.
3. Naghiyev R, Imamverdiyev S, Sanli O. The results of laparoscopic partial nephrectomy depending on the type of access and the tumour size. Georgian Med News. 2016;(259):10–7.
4. Guo J, Zhou X, Fu B, et al. Retroperitoneal laparoscopic partial nephrectomy for treatment of metanephric adenoma (report of 6 cases). Spring. 2016;5(1): 996.
5. Van Poppel H, Becker F, Cadeddu JA, et al. Treatment of localised renal cell carcinoma. Eur Urol. 2011;60(4):662–72.
6. Becker F, Van Poppel H, Hakenberg OW, et al. Assessing the impact of ischaemia time during partial nephrectomy. Eur Urol. 2009;56(4):625–34.
7. Shao P, Tang L, Li P, et al. Precise segmental renal artery clamping under the guidance of dual-source computed tomography angiography during laparoscopic partial nephrectomy. Eur Urol. 2012;62(6):1001–8.
8. Shao P, Tang L, Li P, et al. Application of a vasculature model and standardization of the renal hilar approach in laparoscopic partial nephrectomy for precise segmental artery clamping. Eur Urol. 2013;63(6): 1072–81.
9. Klatte T, Ficarra V, Gratzke C, et al. A literature review of renal surgical anatomy and surgical strategies for partial Nephrectomy. Eur Urol. 2015; 68(6):980–92.
10. Simone G, Gill IS, Mottrie A, et al. Indications, techniques, outcomes, and limitations for minimally ischemic and off-clamp partial nephrectomy: a systematic review of the literature. Eur Urol. 2015;68(4):632–40.
11. Desai MM, de Castro AA, Leslie S, et al. Robotic partial nephrectomy with superselective versus main artery clamping: a retrospective comparison. Eur Urol. 2014;66(4):713–9.
12. Zhang S, Zhao X, Ji C, et al. Radiofrequency ablation of synchronous bilateral renal cell carcinoma. Int J Urol. 2012;19(3):241–7.
13. Shao P, Qin C, Yin C, et al. Laparoscopic partial nephrectomy with segmental renal artery clamping: technique and clinical outcomes. Eur Urol. 2011;59(5):849–55.
14. Satkunasivam R, Tsai S, Syan S, et al. Robotic unclamped "minimal-margin" partial nephrectomy: ongoing refinement of the anatomic zero-ischemia concept. Eur Urol. 2015;68(4):705–12.

Single-stage laparoscopic surgery for bilateral organ tumors using a transumbilical approach with a zigzag incision

Yoichiro Kato[1*], Renpei Kato[1], Misato Takayama[1], Daiki Ikarashi[1], Mitsutaka Onoda[1], Tomohiko Matsuura[1], Mitsugu Kanehira[1], Ryo Takata[1], Shigeaki Baba[2], Toshimoto Kimura[2], Koki Otsuka[2], Jun Sugimura[1], So Omori[1], Akira Sasaki[2] and Wataru Obara[1]

Abstract

Background: Reduced port laparoscopic surgery (RPLS) is comparable to conventional multiport laparoscopic surgery and has the potential to provide improved cosmesis and decreased pain; as such, it satisfies a growing demand for less invasive surgical procedures. Moreover, a zigzag incision of the umbilicus results in a less visible scar in plastic surgery. Here we report a series of two cases with bilateral organ tumors treated by single-stage RPLS using a combination of a transumbilical approach and a zigzag incision.

Case presentation: Case 1: A 63-year-old man was diagnosed with right renal cell carcinoma (RCC) (clear cell carcinoma, pT1a, venous invasion (−)) and a splenic tumor (cavernous hemangioma). Case 2: An 84-year-old woman was diagnosed with concurrent left RCC (clear cell carcinoma, pT1b, 65 × 65 mm, venous invasion (+)) and ascending colon cancer (adenocarcinoma pT3 with no nodal involvement (0/48)). The perioperative course was uneventful in both cases. However, an additional incision was required in Case 2 for specimen excision. Therefore, the scars were more obvious in Case 2 than in Case 1.

Conclusions: Although more cases are required to evaluate the superiority of this technique, this novel procedure could be considered for patients with bilateral lesions.

Keywords: Reduced port laparoscopic surgery, Transumbilical approach, Zigzag incision

Background

Reduced port laparoscopic surgery (RPLS), especially single-port laparoscopic surgery for adrenalectomy, is recognized as a comparable approach to general laparoscopic surgery in terms of bleeding, complication rate, and operating time [1, 2]. Moreover, aesthetic outcomes and postoperative pain are favorable for RPLS [1, 2]. However, RPLS must be performed with great care and attention because of the difficulty of manipulating forceps in a small space, such as in nephrectomy [3]. A zigzag incision (ZI) has been reported as almost scar-less by plastic surgeons [4]. Hachisuka et al. applied this method with the transumbilical approach and reported being able to maintain the skin's cosmetic appearance [5]. Therefore, we aimed to perform single-site RPLS for multifocal lesions located at both ends of the body in two patients and followed the each scar.

Case presentation

The two patients provided informed consent for the publication of their case.

Case 1: A 63-year-old man who was diagnosed with a right renal tumor and a splenic tumor presented to our department. He was asymptomatic, but an ultrasonography scan performed during a routine medical examination revealed a right renal mass. Enhanced computed

---

* Correspondence: katoyooo@iwate-med.ac.jp
[1]Department of Urology, Iwate Medical University School of Medicine, 19-1 Uchimaru, Morioka 020-8505, Japan
Full list of author information is available at the end of the article

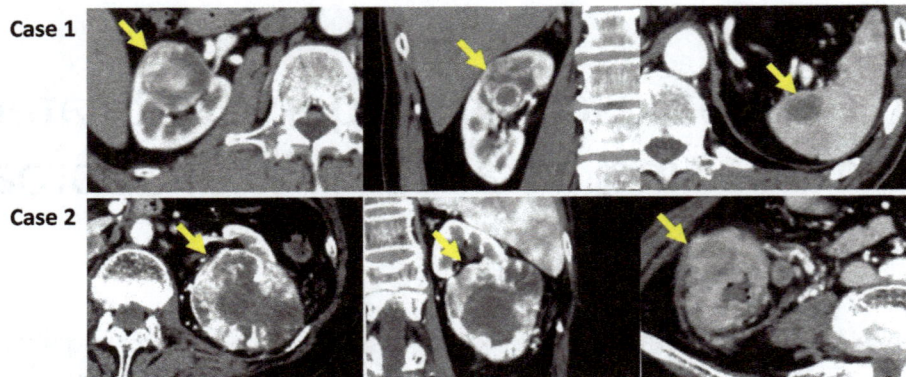

Fig. 1 Enhanced computed tomography (CT) showing renal tumor and suspected metastatic tumor or concurrent colon cancer. Above, well-enhanced right renal tumor and splenic tumor of Case 1.Below, large enhanced left renal tumor and ascending colon tumor with lymph node swelling of Case 2

tomography (CT) showed a 40-mm-diameter right renal mass with enhancement and a 21-mm diameter splenic mass with weak enhancement (Fig. 1). We diagnosed the asses as a right renal cell carcinoma (RCC) and a metastatic splenic tumor (cT1bN0M1) clinically. The patient's body mass index (BMI) was 22.8 kg/m^2 (Table 1).

Case 2: The next patient was an 84-year-old woman with concurrent left renal tumor and ascending colon cancer. She reported right flank pain and underwent

screening CT. Enhanced CT showed a 75-mm-diameter left renal tumor and invasive focal ascending colon cancer (Fig. 1). The renal tumor was cT2aN0M0 RCC and the ascending colon cancer was cT4aN2M0. The patient's BMI was 19.0 kg/m^2 (Table 1).

Surgical technique

Case 1: We performed a radical right nephrectomy and splenectomy using the transumbilical approach with a

Table 1 Patients characteristics and perioperative status

	Case 1	Case 2
Age (Y)	63	84
Gender	male	female
BMI (Kg/m^2)	22.8	19.0
Clinical diagnosis and stage	right renal tumor and spleen metastasis (cT1bN0M1)	concurrence of left renal tumor (cT2aN0M0) and ascending colon cancer (cT4aN2M0)
Operative procedure	right nephrectomy, splenectomy	left nephrectomy, right hemicolectomy
Incision of umbilicus	ZI	ZI
Total number of port	2	6
Placed the port status	GelPOINT® and single additional 12mm port	conventional
Conversion of the surgical position intraoperatively	left to right lateral decubitus position	lithotomy position to lateral decubitus position
Drain	none	2
Operation time Nephrectomy/the other (min)	284 123/161	505 177/328
Total blood loss (ml)	91	898
Perioperative transfusion (unit)	none	2
Resume oral intake (day)	3	3
Hospitalization period (day)	7	16
Additional postoperative analgesic[a]	drip of 50 mg of flubiprofen × 1	none
Renal tumor	clear cell carcinoma (pT1aN0), spleen: cavernous hemangioma (M0)	clear cell carcinoma (pT1bN0), colon cancer: adenocarcinoma (pT3N0)

BMI body mass index, *ZI* zigzag incision
[a]Except for epidural anesthesia

ZI in a single-stage laparoscopic surgery (Fig. 2). A Gel-POINT access platform (Applied Medical, CA, USA) was placed in the ZI, while a 12-mm assist port was placed at below the 12th rib costochondral margin on the left midclavicular line (Fig. 3a, c). We used ADACHI-TANKO Kanshi flexural forceps (ADACHI-INDUSTRY, Gifu, Japan) to reduce the interference between the laparoscope and the instruments (Fig. 3b, d). We first performed a right nephrectomy with the patient in the left lateral decubitus position and then converted from the left to the right position and performed a splenectomy. During the nephrectomy, beating of the renal artery was confirmed; thereafter, the inferior vena cava and renal vein were identified. One renal artery was blocked, but since the kidney did not shrink, another renal artery was identified and blocked. Soon thereafter, the kidney shrank and the renal vein was blocked and detached. Furthermore, at the time of the peritoneal incision and detachment of the upper pole of the kidney, the liver interfered and became difficult to maneuver around. Both specimens were extracted from the umbilical scar without extension of the wound (Fig. 2c). The surgery was completed without a blood transfusion or drain tube.

Case 2: We performed a right hemicolectomy followed by a left radical nephrectomy. The surgical position was converted from lithotomy for the hemicolectomy to lateral decubitus for the nephrectomy. The start of the midline incision included the umbilicus, and a port approximately 30 mm long accommodated the camera. Four other ports were used to perform the conventional laparoscopic hemicolectomy. An extra 12-mm port placed at below the 12th rib costochondral margin on the left anterior axillary line during the nephrectomy. First, an incision was made on a portion of the fused fascia, and then the space between the fascia and the Gerota fascia was carefully expanded during peeling to the renal pedicle. Upon reaching the renal pedicle, there was one renal artery and one vein and no obvious running abnormality. Moreover, the camera port was somewhat

caudal compared to a regular port, but the usual percutaneous approach was used and the vessels were processed in nearly the same way, although some bleeding from the renal vein occurred during the peeling process. A few pieces of tissue sealing sheet (Tachosil®) were used to manage this. Because the resected specimen was too large to extract from the umbilical scar, the total length of the skin incision of the six ports was extended to 99 mm. Two drains were placed, one in the pelvic cavity and one in the renal cavity.

Peri- and postoperative results

The perioperative results for both patients are shown in Table 1.

Case 1: The total operating time was 284 min: the right nephrectomy took 123 min, while the splenectomy took 161 min. Total blood loss was 91 mL. The pathological diagnosis of the renal tumor was clear cell carcinoma, pT1a, venous invasion (−). The splenic tumor was not diagnosed as metastatic RCC but rather as a cavernous hemangioma. The perioperative period was uneventful. Except for a general epidural, the only postoperative analgesic was a 50-mg flurbiprofen drip on postoperative day 2. He was discharged on postoperative day 7. Images of Case 1 show the condition of the umbilical region in the first postoperative month and the umbilical and whole abdominal regions in the sixth postoperative months, respectively (Fig. 4 above).

Case 2: The operating time totaled 505 min: the left nephrectomy took 177 min and the right hemicolectomy took 328 min. Total blood loss was 898 mL. The patient received 400 ml of red blood cell transfusion after surgery. The left RCC was diagnosed as clear cell carcinoma, pT1b, 65 × 65 mm, venous invasion (+). The pathological diagnosis of the ascending colon cancer was adenocarcinoma pT3 with no nodal involvement (0/48). The patient restarted oral intake on postoperative day 3. The only postoperative analgesic was the general epidural. The drain tubes were extracted on postoperative

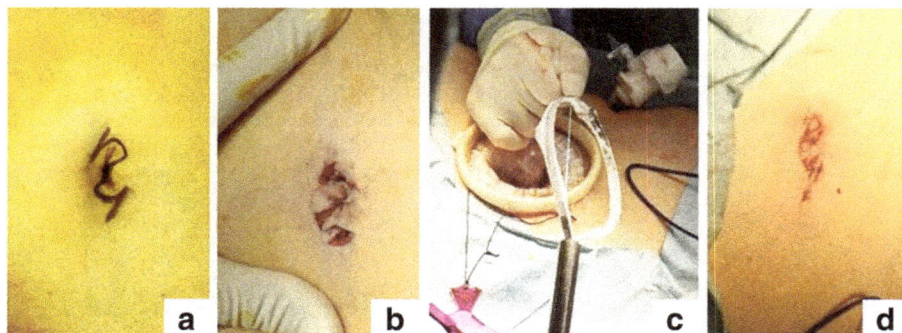

Fig. 2 Perioperative view of the zigzag incision (ZI) created in Case 1: (**a**) pre-incision, (**b**) post-incision, (**c**) extraction of the right kidney from the ZI, and (**d**) post-suture

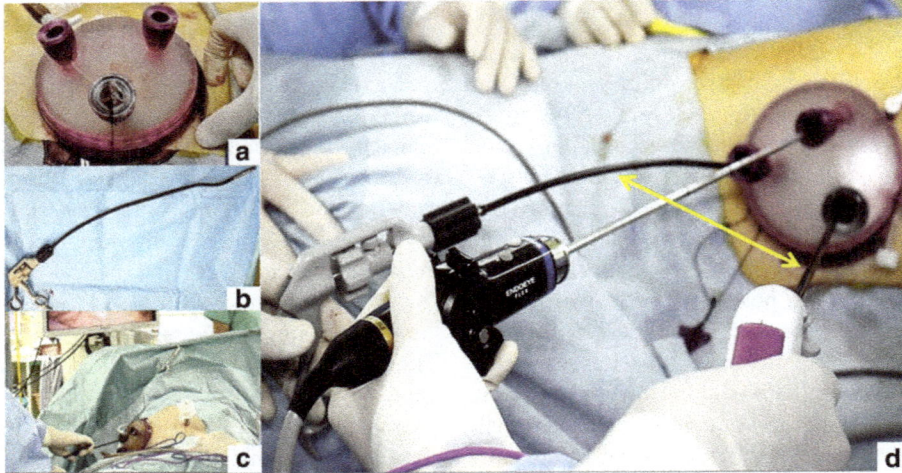

Fig. 3 Surgical equipment used in Case 1. **a** GelPOINT, the multiport system, can be placed in three ports at most. **b** The ADACHI-TANKO Kanshi forms the bending of the shaft. **c** Whole ports image at splenectomy, GelPOINT and only one 12 mm assist port are placed. **d** Intraoperative photo of Case 1 using an ADACHI-TANKO Kanshi placed at GelPOINT shows that the distance between instruments can be maintained because of its form (double-headed allowed)

day 12 and the patient was discharged on postoperative day 16. Images of Case 2, as same as Case 1, show the condition of the umbilical region and whole abdominal regions (Fig. 4 below). Currently, both cases show no evidenced recurrence sites.

Discussion

Here we performed single-stage laparoscopic surgery for several bilateral multifocal lesions. We approached the bilateral organ tumors by installing a GelPOINT in the navel at the center of the body's surface. Hachisuka et al. reported that the ZI method is indicated for use in the umbilical region [5]. RPLS with a ZI was especially useful in Case 1 because it allowed the use of a shorter incision with the flexural forceps that allowed extraction of the spleen or lumen organs, such as part of the resected colon. However, a large organ, such as one > 70 mm affected by RCC, is difficult to extract from the original incision and would require an additional incision. We completed the operations safely in both cases using single-stage surgery. Nephrectomy required 123 min in Case 1 and 177 min in Case 2, which seem not so long compared to other reports [6]. Furthermore, the common incision for the bilateral lesions was only a skin incision and other surgical procedures do not shorten the total operating time because they require separate delamination and incision. Considering that it was necessary to change the patients' positions for the bilateral tumors, the total operating time was acceptable. The perioperative courses in both case series were uneventful except for two units of blood transfused postoperatively in Case 2. When there is little perioperative bleeding, a drain tube may not be

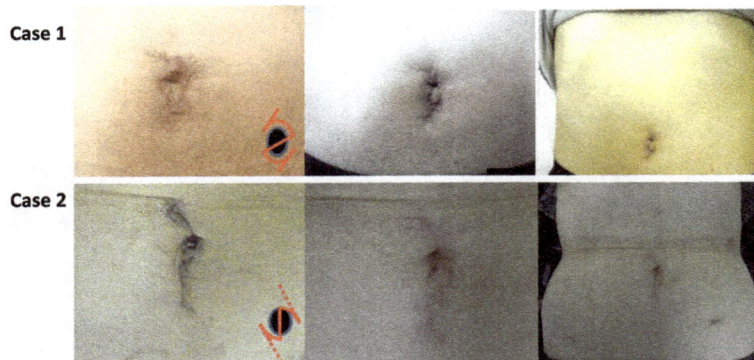

Fig. 4 First (left) and sixth (center) month postoperative clinical images of Case 1 (above) and Case 2 (below). Moreover, the right figures are the whole abdominal images of both cases at sixth month postoperatively. The left lower figures are the incision images (the dotted line represents additional incisions) from the first month images

necessary. Experience with more cases and improvements in laparoscopic skills are necessary, but our proposed procedure may be a reasonable approach for the management of bilateral organ tumors. The shorter the total incision length, the less prolonged the postoperative ileus [7]. Walz et al. reported that single foramen surgery was superior to conventional multi-port surgery for adrenalectomies in terms of postoperative analgesic frequency and hospitalization period [8]. Our cases involved the complexities of multiple bilateral lesions. Nonetheless, in Case 2, which had the most ports (six), the total incision length was 99 mm, the same as that in conventional laparoscopic nephrectomy.

The ZI method was originally developed to make surgical wounds less noticeable. Figure 4 shows the condition of the umbilical region in the first and sixth postoperative months for this case series. An additional incision was required in Case 2 to enable extraction of the specimens (Fig. 4, below). Therefore, the umbilical scar of Case 2 was more obvious than that in Case 1. However, it can be confirmed that the scar of the additional incision site in Case 2 at 6 months postoperative is becoming less noticeable. The limitation of a ZI is that some cases require additional incisions. We could not make incisions along the circumference of the umbilicus; rather, they were made to both ends of the linear incisions. We designed the upper or lower half of the incision at the beginning of the surgery and then created the additional incision based on the requirement for specimen extraction. From a cosmetic standpoint, it is necessary to use a more refined ZI method that considers specimen size and skin striae direction. Furthermore, in order to prove the superiority of these procedures, a larger clinical trial using a quantitative evaluation method such as Derriford Appearance Scale (DAS 59) should be necessary [9].

Conclusions

This is the first report describing single-stage surgery using a ZI and a transumbilical approach that can be accomplished safely and with a better aesthetic outcome than previous surgical methods for bilateral organ lesions. In conclusion, based on our experiences, this novel procedure could be considered for patients with bilateral lesions. However, in order to prove superiority of these procedures, this should be tested in a clinical trial setting.

Abbreviations

BMI: Body mass index; CT: Computed tomography; RCC: Renal cell carcinoma; RPLS: Reduced port laparoscopic surgery; US: Ultrasonography; ZI: Zigzag incision

Acknowledgments

We would like to thank the Department of Urology and Surgery, Iwate Medical University School of Medicine. In addition, we would like to thank the patients for giving us the permission to publish.

Authors' contributions

YK drafted the report. RK, MT, DI, MO, TM, MK, RT, SB, TK, KO, JS, and SO cared for the patients and collected the data. AS and WO performed the surgeries and revised the manuscript. All authors reviewed and approved the final version of the manuscript.

Competing interests

The authors declare no competing interests in this case series.

Author details

[1]Department of Urology, Iwate Medical University School of Medicine, 19-1 Uchimaru, Morioka 020-8505, Japan. [2]Department of Surgery, Iwate Medical University School of Medicine, 19-1 Uchimaru, Morioka 020-8505, Japan.

References

1. Jeong BC, Park YH, Han DH, et al. Laparoendoscopic single-site and conventional laparoscopic adrenalectomy:a matched case-control study. J Endourol. 2009;23:1957–60.
2. Tunca F, Senyurek YG, Terzioglu T, et al. Single-incision laparoscopic adrenalectomy. Surg Endosc. 2012;26:36–40.
3. Desai MM, Rao PP, Aron M, et al. Scarless single-port transumbilical nephrectomy and pyeloplasty: first clinical report. BJU Int. 2008;101:83–8.
4. Borges AF. Timing of scar revision techniques. Clin Plast Surg. 1990;17(1):71–6.
5. Hachisuka T, Kinoshita T, Yamakawa T, et al. Transumbilical laparoscopic surgery using GelPort through an umbilical zigzag skin incision. Asian J Endosc Surg. 2012;5(1):50–2.
6. Antonelli JA, Bagrodia A, Odom C, et al. Laparoendoscopic single-site nephrectomy compared with conventional laparoscopic nephrectomy: a 5-year, single-surgeon experience. Eur Urol. 2013;64(3):412–8.
7. Vather R, Josephson R, Jaung R, et al. Development of a risk stratification system for the occurrence of prolonged postoperative ileus after colorectal surgery: a prospective risk factor analysis. Surgery. 2015;157(4):764–73.
8. Walz MK, Petersenn S, Koch JA, et al. Endoscopic treatment of large primary adrenal tumours. Br J Surg. 2005;92:719–23.
9. Harris DL, Carr AT. The Derriford appearance scale (DAS59): a new psychometric scale for the evaluation of patients with disfigurements and aesthetic problems of appearance. Br J Plast Surg. 2001;54(3):216–22.

Circumcision-related tragedies seen in children at the Komfo Anokye Teaching Hospital, Kumasi, Ghana

Kwaku Addai Arhin Appiah[1]*⦿, Christian Kofi Gyasi-Sarpong[2], Roland Azorliade[1], Ken Aboah[2], Dennis Odai Laryea[3], Kwaku Otu-Boateng[1], Kofi Baah-Nyamekye[1], Patrick Opoku Manu Maison[1], Douglas Arthur[1], Isaac Opoku Antwi[1], Benjamin Frimpong-Twumasi[1], Edwin Mwintiereh Yenli[4], Samuel Kodzo Togbe[1] and George Amoah[1]

Abstract

Background: Circumcision is a common minor surgical procedure and it is performed to a varying extent across countries and religions. Despite being a minor surgical procedure, major complications may result from it. In Ghana, although commonly practiced, circumcision-related injuries have not been well documented. This study is to describe the scope of circumcision-related injuries seen at the Komfo Anokye Teaching Hospital in Kumasi, Ghana.

Methods: The study was conducted at the Urology Unit of the Komfo Anokye Teaching Hospital in Kumasi. Consecutive cases of circumcision-related injuries seen at the unit over an 18 month period were identified and included in the study. Data was collected using a structured questionnaire. Data was entered and analysed using SPSS version 16. Charts and tables were generated using Microsoft Excel.

Results: A total of 72 cases of circumcision-related injuries were recorded during the 18 month period. Urethrocutaneous fistula was the commonest injury recorded, accounting for 77.8 % of cases. Other injuries recorded were glans amputations (6.9 %); iatrogenic hypospadias (5.6 %), and epidermal inclusion cysts (2.8 %). The majority of children were circumcised in health facilities (75 %) and nurses were the leading providers (77.8 %). The majority of circumcisions were conducted in the neonatal period (94.7 %).

Conclusion: Circumcision-related injuries commonly occurred in the neonatal period. Most of the injuries happened in health facilities. The most common injury recorded was urethrocutaneous fistula but the most tragic was penile amputation. There is the need for education and training of providers to minimise circumcision-related injuries in Ghana.

Keywords: Circumcision, Penile amputation, Circumcision injury, Urethrocutaneous fistula, Ghana

Background

Circumcision is routinely performed in most parts of Ghana as a tradition. While generally regarded as a minor surgical procedure, major complications may result from it [1–4]. Although circumcision injuries are unintended, the prominence of circumcision as a cause of major injury in children is not recognised, as the world report on injury in children did not identify circumcision-related injuries as significant causes of injury-related morbidity and mortality in children [5]. This notwithstanding, some circumcision injuries may be associated with long term social and psychological challenges including the inability to have a fulfilling sexual life as the case may be in penile amputations [6] and even death in some cases of severe haemorrhage [6, 7]. In Nigeria, circumcision-related injuries have been on the ascendancy with an estimated 20 % circumcisions resulting in one form of complication or the other [3]. Various degrees of circumcision-related injuries occur. However, severe ones seldom occur in developed countries [2] where circumcision is practised by well-

* Correspondence: addaiarhin@yahoo.com
[1]Department of Surgery, Komfo Anokye Teaching Hospital, Kumasi, Ghana
Full list of author information is available at the end of the article

trained personnel [8]. Circumcision injuries have been associated with all the methods of circumcisions [1, 4] especially in untrained hands [3, 6–8]. In Ghana, data on circumcision-related injuries is scanty. This cross-sectional observational study was designed to describe the scope of circumcision-related injuries seen at the Komfo Anokye Teaching Hospital in Kumasi, Ghana.

Methods

The study was conducted at the Urology Unit of the Directorate of Surgery, Komfo Anokye Teaching Hospital (KATH). KATH is a major referral centre for the middle and northern zones of Ghana.

All male children below 18 years of age referred to the Komfo Anokye Teaching Hospital's Urology Unit for treatment of early and late complications of circumcision as determined by our eligibility criteria were included in the study. Urologists at the unit conducted penile examinations and assigned eligible patients specific injury categories as haemorrhage, urethrocutaneous fistula, penile amputation, iatrogenic hypospadias, skin bridges, excess foreskins, epidermal inclusion cysts, buried penis or any other injury that was deemed to be as a result of circumcision. Guardians/parents of eligible children were approached for inclusion in the study. The aim of the study was explained to them and informed consent obtained. Ethical approval was obtained from the Committee on Human Research, Publications and Ethics of the Kwame Nkrumah University of Science and Technology and the Komfo Anokye Teaching Hospital. Data collection involved a structured questionnaire administered by a trained research assistant. Data collected included demographic information, place of circumcision, person circumcising, age at circumcision and clinical examination findings. Data was collected over an 18 month period from September 2012 to February 2014.

Data was entered into SPSS version 16 and the same was utilized for statistical analysis. Microsoft Excel was used to generate the tables and charts.

Results

A total of 72 cases of children with circumcision-related complications were seen during the 18 month period. The youngest case was recorded in a 2-day old neonate and the oldest case recorded was in an 11-year-old boy. The majority of the children were resident in urban communities (54.0 %).

Over 87 % of children in this study were circumcised before they were 2 weeks old. Only 5.6 % were circumcised after 4 weeks of age (Table 1).

The majority of children were circumcised in a hospital (65.3 %). The place of circumcision is as shown in Fig. 1. Nurses accounted for the majority of circumcision-related injuries recorded in this study, 77.8 %. Doctors and

Table 1 Age at circumcision for circumcision-related injuries recorded in Kumasi

Age at Circumcision	Frequency	%
≤1 week	34	47.2
>1–2 weeks	29	40.2
>2–3 weeks	3	4.2
>3–4 weeks	2	2.8
>4 weeks	4	5.6
Total	72	100.0

traditional circumcisers (Wanzams) accounted for 8.3 and 20.8 % of circumcision-related injuries respectively. None of the children seen during the period under review reported within 24 h of injury. The majority of injuries (80.5 %) were seen within 2 weeks of circumcision. Twelve (16.7 %) cases presented within 3 months of circumcision and the remaining 2.8 % presented more than a year after circumcision.

In 37 (51.4 %) of the cases studied, the exact method of circumcision could not be ascertained from the parents of affected children. Figure 2 details the methods of circumcision as recorded among cases seen during this study.

Complications

The commonest complication recorded in this study was urethrocutaneous fistula (77.8 %). The various categories of complications recorded in this study are as shown in Table 2. There were five cases of glans penis amputations accounting for 6.9 % of complications recorded.

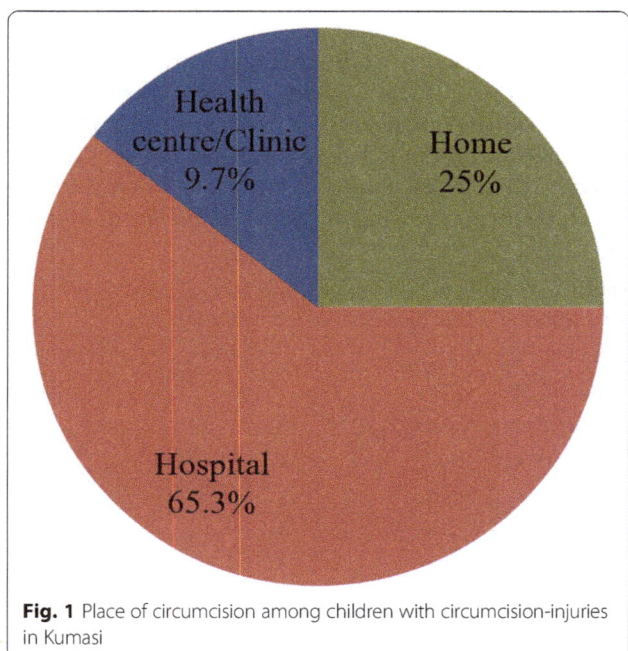

Fig. 1 Place of circumcision among children with circumcision-injuries in Kumasi

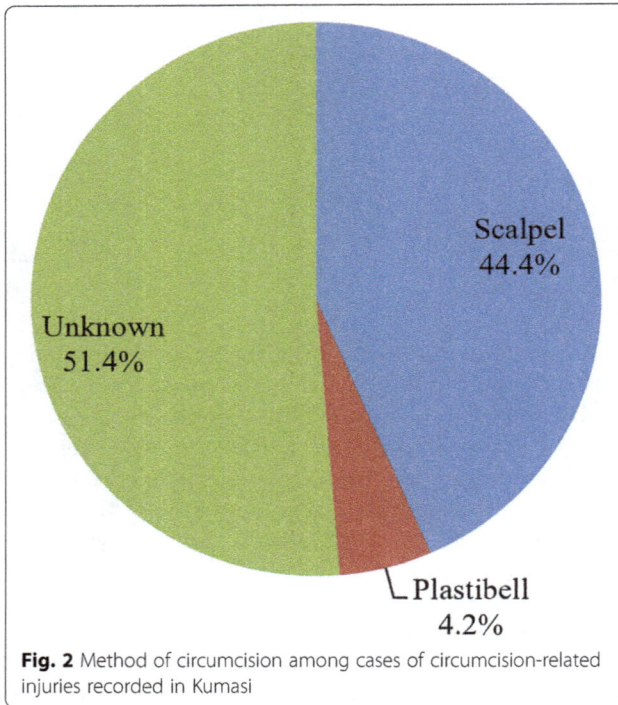

Fig. 2 Method of circumcision among cases of circumcision-related injuries recorded in Kumasi

Three (60 %) were complete amputations of the glans penis, with the remaining 40 % being partial amputations.

Discussion

Circumcision remains one of the oldest and commonest surgical procedures performed on young boys worldwide [9, 10]. It is widely practiced in the United States [2] and especially in Israel where virtually every male child is circumcised [11]. However in Europe it is rarely performed [12]. The notable advantages of circumcision include: reduction in early childhood urinary tract infections, which is also noted in adult men [13–17], reduction of HIV transmission by almost 60 % [18–21], and reduction in the incidence of penile cancer [22–24]. Ghana's circumcision rate is estimated to be on the high side as the majority of ethnic groups and religions identify

Table 2 Categories of complications among children with circumcision-related injuries recorded in Kumasi

Type of Complication	Frequency	Percentage
Urethrocutaneous fistula	56	77.8
Complete Penile Amputation	3	4.1
Iatrogenic Hypospadias	4	5.6
Epidermal Inclusion cyst	3	4.1
Partial Penile Amputation	2	2.8
Skin Bridges	2	2.8
Excess Foreskin	2	2.8
Total	72	100.0

circumcision as an appropriate religious or cultural practice for males to undergo [7].

The timing of circumcision among children in this study suggests an early age of circumcision in Ghana as over 87 % of cases had circumcision done in the neonatal period (Table 1). This is similar to findings by Osifo and Oraifo [7] and Chaim et al. [11]. However, in Eastern and Southern Africa and some parts of the pacific, circumcision is performed far beyond the neonatal period [6, 25, 26]. For some, it is a rite of passage into adulthood [6, 25]. Only 5.6 % of our cases were circumcised beyond the neonatal period. While our study population may not be representative of the population of Ghana, it provides an indication that most circumcisions are being performed during the neonatal period. This may have implications for interventions in the areas of circumcision such as persons to target for training, timing of educational messages on circumcision and the location of circumcision services.

In this study, over 65 % of children with the complications recorded had their circumcisions done in a hospital. The proportion is even higher (75 %) when lower level health facilities (health centres and clinics) are included. Similarly in Nigeria, more circumcisions were done in orthodox medical centres (66.9 %) than traditional settings (33.1 %) [27]. Our findings however, contrast sharply with studies from Southern and Eastern Africa where virtually all circumcisions are performed outside hospitals as part of traditional rites of passage into manhood with high complication rates [6, 25]. In Israel, however, although a significant proportion of circumcisions are undertaken outside health facilities by the ritual circumciser, a lower proportion of complications have been recorded because they are well trained and the practice is regulated [11].

In this study, nurses accounted for the majority of circumcision-related injuries - 77.8 % of cases. Doctors and traditional circumcisers (locally referred to as Wanzams) accounted for 8.3 and 20.8 % of the circumcision-related complications respectively. Likewise in Nigeria, nurses were found to account for the majority of complications (55.9 %) with doctors and traditional circumcisers accounting for 35.1 and 9 % respectively [3]. In a comparative study by Atikeler et al., it was found that circumcisions done by unlicensed circumcisers resulted in more early phase complications as well as late lifelong complications compared with licensed surgeons [8]. Even among physicians performing circumcisions, there is evidence that there a is lack of formal training amongst them as to how to perform circumcision correctly and providers also lack the requisite skills to manage the complications of circumcisions [4, 7]. Our findings indicate gaps either in knowledge and/or practice among persons providing circumcision services in health facilities in Ghana and it is therefore imperative that training workshops are organised for all providers especially nurses to reduce the incidence of circumcision-related injuries in the future.

The method of circumcision was unknown in 37 (51.4 %) of the cases. A significant proportion (91.4 %) of the cases for which the method of circumcision was known underwent surgical circumcision with a scalpel and this is still consistent with other studies that have examined circumcision-related injuries and complications in the West African sub-region [3, 7]. Due to the high proportion (51.4 %) of cases for which the method of circumcision was unknown in this study, we are unable to associate the method of circumcision with the complications observed. However, there is evidence that the Plastibel device poses a higher risk of complication compared with conventional dissection [1].

The majority of our cases (77.8 %) had urethrocutaneous fistulae. Urethrocutaneous fistulae have largely been associated with hypospadias repair in developed countries [28, 29] and not circumcision. The proportion of urethrocutaneous fistulae recorded in this study contrasts sharply with findings in Nigeria by Osifo and Oraifo et al. in which urethrocutaneous fistula accounted for only 21 % of complications recorded [7] and that of Okeke et al., where no fistula was recorded [3]. The urethrocutaneous fistulae in the present study ranged in sizes from pinhole defects (<5 mm) to very big defects (>10 mm) on the ventral aspect of the glans penis (Fig. 3a-c). We think the management of haemorrhage/bleeding during circumcision may be accounting for the high numbers of urethrocutaneous fistulae observed. The ligation of bleeding sites with larger-sized sutures and

direct laceration into the urethra during circumcision may be responsible for the high numbers of urethrocutaneous fistulae observed in this study [30]. The occurrence of urethrocutaneous fistula has also been associated with the Plastibel device [28].

There were four cases (5.6 %) of iatrogenic hypospadias (Fig. 4a-b). This is one of the worse forms of circumcision-related injuries. Complete ligation of the artery to the frenulum may cause extensive tissue necrosis on the ventrum of the glans penis leading to the iatrogenic hypospadias [30]. Isolated cases of iatrogenic hypospadias have been reported after the circumciser performed a ventral rather than a dorsal slit prior to the start of circumcision. It is imperative that the proper plane is entered into for the initial separation of adhesions so that the meatus is not inadvertently entered into, and then damaged [2].

The iatrogenic hypospadias seen in this study may not necessarily be as a result of complications of circumcision but may have been missed mega meatus with intact prepuce variants before circumcision and only found thereafter. This study is unable to determine whether the iatrogenic hypospadias observed had megameatus with intact prepuce before circumcision. Clinically, these are difficult to distinguish after circumcision [2].

The most tragic form of circumcision-related injury is penile amputation and it was the second leading complication recorded in this study, accounting for 6.9 % overall. Complete penile amputation accounted for 4.1 % of all complications. This is higher compared with the 3.1 % recorded in Nigeria by Okeke et al. [3] but lower than the 8 % recorded in a study in Turkey by Ceylan et al. [31]. One case of partial penile amputation recorded

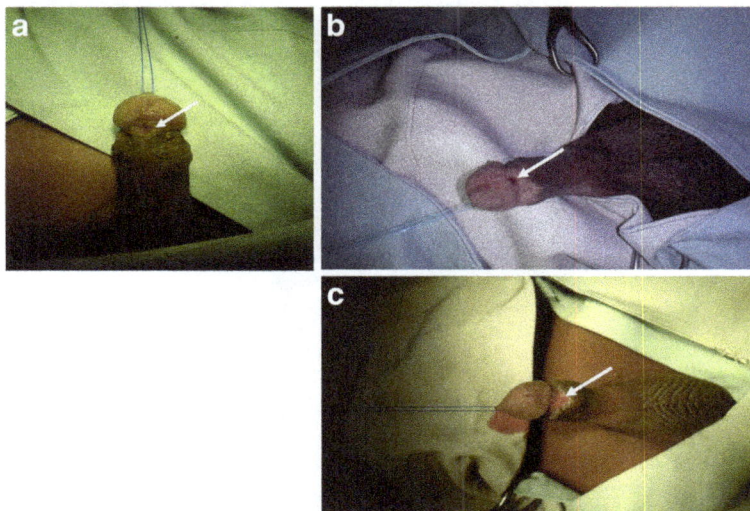

Fig. 3 a A small (<5 mm) sized urethrocutaneous fistula (*arrowed*). **b** Medium sized (5–10 mm) urethrocutaneous fistula (*arrowed*). **c** Large sized (>10 mm) urethrocutaneous fistula (*arrowed*)

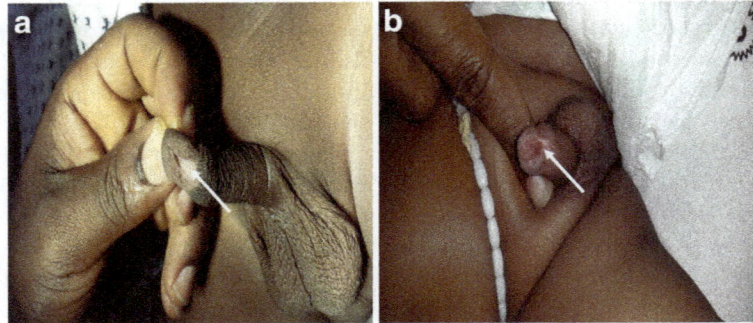

Fig. 4 a Iatrogenic hypospadias (*arrowed*). **b** Iatrogenic hypospadias (*arrowed*)

in this study was reported within 48 h and this was repaired successfully (Fig. 5a-c). However, the other case reported after six months and presented with a healed wound with a constriction band and urethrocutaneous fistula (Fig. 6). In all the cases of complete penile amputations, the parents of the babies were falsely reassured that all was well by the circumcisers either because of ignorance on their part or for fears of litigation against them. As a result they all presented late with difficulty passing urine as wound healing with scarring at the stump ends caused meatal stenosis (Fig. 7a-c). Penile glans amputation like many others is a preventable complication of circumcision if proper attention is paid to detail and the circumcision is carried out by properly trained personnel [32–34]. Again if the practitioners were trained to recognise these complications, they would have

referred such patients immediately with the severed penile tissue properly preserved on ice so that penile reattachment could be attempted. This may have resulted in better cosmetic outcomes for such patients [32, 35, 36].

There were four cases of epidermal inclusion cysts (Fig. 8) with the youngest aged 7 months presenting with a painless swelling on the dorsum of the penis. Epidermal inclusions cysts are known to result from the implantation of skin in the subcutaneous tissue during circumcision [37]. They are considered rare in some countries [36, 37]. Our findings may suggest that these may not be rare. They are known to be usually asymptomatic and may not be reported unless issues bordering on aesthetics or pain from infection emerge [37]. Skin bridges (Fig. 9) are also recognised minor complications of circumcision and are easily treated

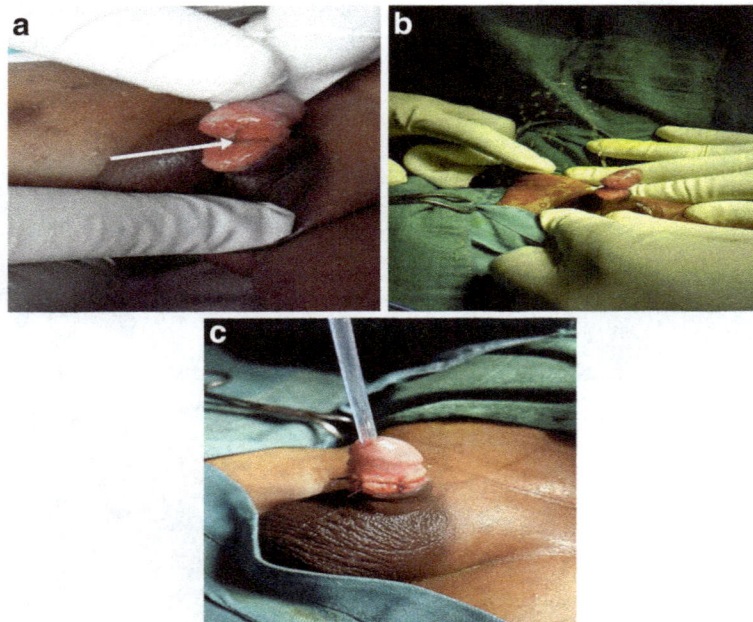

Fig. 5 a Partial penile amputation from tourniquet effect of a suture material (*arrowed*) seen within 48 h. **b** Patient urinating immediately after release of tourniquet. **c** Immediate post-repair

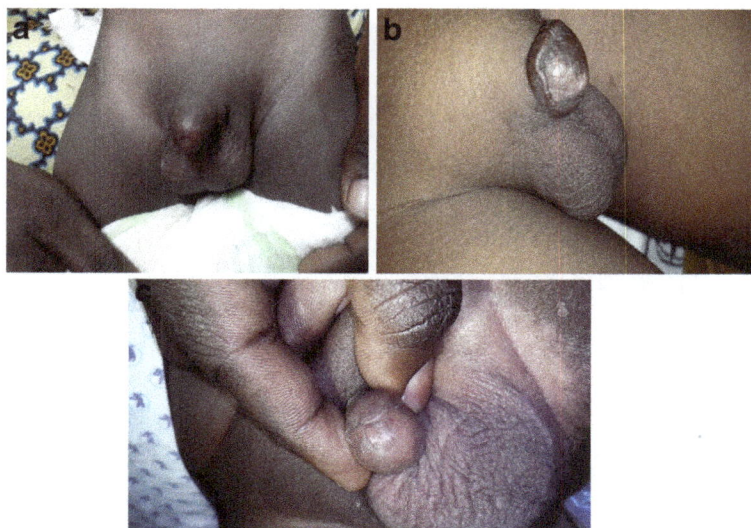

Fig. 6 a Complete glans penis amputation seen 3 years post circumcision with scarred stump end. **b** near total penile amputation seen 2 years post circumcision. **c** Complete glans penis amputation from plastibel circumcision seen 3 months post circumcision with meatal occlusion

[38]. They may go unnoticed unless cosmetic issues or pain and infection occur. In our study, these two categories of complications each accounted for 2.8 % of all complications. There were two cases of excess foreskin. This results from inadequate excision of the foreskin. The parents brought them because they were dissatisfied with the cosmetic appearance of the penis. In other studies, excess foreskin constituted the predominant late complication of circumcision [11].

Our study did not record any case of haemorrhage which was among the leading complications recorded by Gee and Ansell [39]. Haemorrhage, most likely, will occur in the first few hours of circumcision. We surmise that late reporting may account for the non-recording of haemorrhage as a complication in our study. It may also be due to clients accessing acute care in lower level health facilities and only reporting severe complications to the Urology Unit. This may also imply that the complete spectrum of circumcision-related injuries may not have been fully covered in our study, thus a bigger burden may exist.

Circumcision has social, cultural and religious implications and this may account for the high uptake of the procedure despite the associated complications [1, 6, 8]. It is imperative that the procedure is made safe in order to ensure that children undergoing the procedure in the future do not develop complications. Persons who have not been circumcised have been ostracised in some parts of Africa; this can take the form of denial of marriage since uncircumcised men were frowned upon [6, 35, 36] in the past and such stereotypes may still exist.

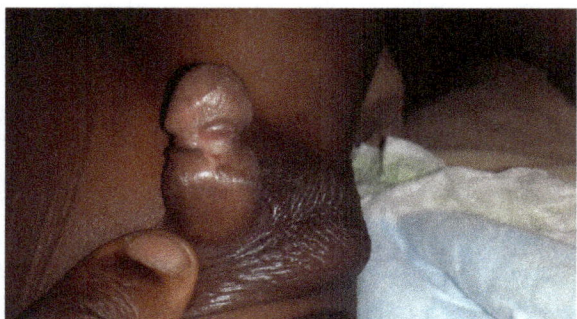

Fig. 7 Healed partial penile amputation from tourniquet effect with a constriction ring and urethrocutaneous fistula

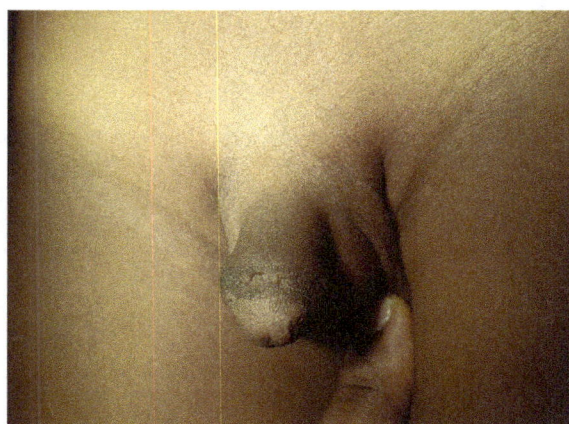

Fig. 8 Skin bridges in an 8year old boy

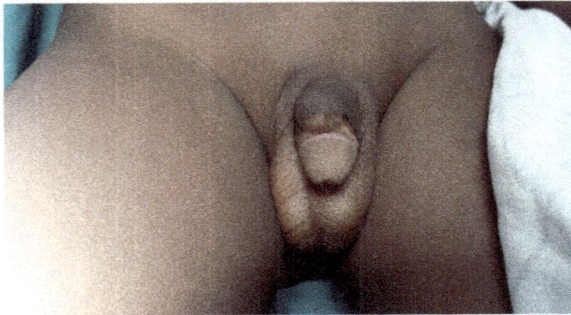

Fig. 9 Epidermal inclusion cyst seen 7 months post circumcision

Conclusion

Neonatal circumcision, a common practice in Ghana is associated with several and sometimes tragic complications such as penile amputations. The high proportion of urethrocutaneous fistulae recorded in this study requires further investigation to determine the underlying causes and allow for the institution of appropriate preventive measures. There is the need for further studies focusing on the immediate or early complications following circumcision including injuries related to specific methods of circumcision. The training of providers in order to reduce the incidence of injuries is also recommended.

Abbreviations

HIV: Human Immunodeficiency virus; KATH: Komfo Anokye Teaching Hospital; SPSS: Statistical Software Package for Social Sciences

Acknowledgements

We would like to acknowledge the immense contributions of Prof Francis Abantanga and Prof Peter Donkor both of KATH for critically reviewing this manuscript before final submission. We are grateful to them for their words of wisdom and encouragement. We will also like to thank Ms Portia Adutwumwaa, our research assistant who typed and administered the questionnaires and helped enter them into SPSS. Location of Work: Komfo Anokye Teaching Hospital.

Funding

The study received no funding.

Authors contributions

KAAA: Conceived and designed the study and was involved in all stages of the manuscript writing. RA: drafting of manuscript, literature search and critical revision of manuscript for important intellectual content. CKG-S: Literature search, drafting of manuscript and helped in the analysis and interpretation of data. KA: Literature search, manuscript drafting and final approval for submission of manuscript. PM: Helped in data acquisition and was involved in drafting the manuscript at all stages. DOL: Helped in designing the manuscript, was involved in the drafting as well as the critical revision for important intellectual content and approved the final submission of the manuscript. KNB: Was involved in data collection and helped with data analysis and interpretation and approved the final submission of manuscript. KO-B: Data acquisition and interpretation of data. Approved the final submission of manuscript. BF-T: Data acquisition and interpretation, drawing of figures and approval of final submission of manuscript. DA: Data acquisition and analysis, drafting of manuscript and approval for final submission of manuscript. IOA: Data acquisition and analysis, drafting of manuscript and approval for final submission of manuscript. EMY: Data acquisition and interpretation, helped generate the tables and figures. He approved the final submission of manuscript. GA: Was involved in designing the study, helped with data acquisition and interpretation, was involved in drafting of the manuscript and revised it critically for important intellectual content. He also gave approval for the final submission of manuscript. SKT: Data acquisition and interpretation, helped generate the tables and figures. He approved the final submission of manuscript. All authors read and approved the final manuscript.

Competing interests

The authors declare that they have no competing interests.

Author details

[1]Department of Surgery, Komfo Anokye Teaching Hospital, Kumasi, Ghana.
[2]Department of Surgery, School of Medical Sciences-KNUST, Kumasi, Ghana.
[3]Public Health Unit, Komfo Anokye Teaching Hospital, Kumasi, Ghana.
[4]Department of Surgery, Tamale Teaching Hospital, Tamale, Ghana.

References

1. Mousavi SA, Salehifar E. Circumcision complications associated with the Plastibell device and conventional dissection surgery: a trial of 586 infants of ages up to 12 months. Adv Urol [Internet]. 2008 [cited 2014 Nov 9]; 2008. Available from: http://www.ncbi.nlm.nih.gov/pmc/articles/PMC2581731/
2. Krill AJ, Palmer LS, Palmer JS. Complications of circumcision. Sci World J. 2011;11:2458–68.
3. Okeke LI, Asinobi AA, Ikuerowo OS. Epidemiology of complications of male circumcision in Ibadan, Nigeria. BMC Urol. 2006;6(1):21.
4. Moslemi MK, Abedinzadeh M, Aghaali M. Evaluation of epidemiology, safety, and complications of male circumcision using conventional dissection surgery: experience at one center. Open Access J Urol. 2011;3:83–7.
5. Peden M, Ozanne-Smith J, Branche C, Fazlur Rahman AKM, Rivara F, Kidist Bartolomeos. World report on child injury prevention [Internet]. Geneva, Switzerland; 2008 [cited 2014 Nov 9]. Available from: http://www.preventionweb.net/files/8438_9789241563574eng1.pdf
6. Mogotlane SM, Ntlangulela JT, Ogunbanjo BGA. Mortality and morbidity among traditionally circumcised Xhosa boys in the Eastern Cape Province, South Africa. Curationis [Internet]. 2004 Sep 28 [cited 2014 Nov 9];27(2). Available from: http://www.curationis.org.za/index.php/curationis/article/view/980
7. Osifo OD, Oriaifo IA. Circumcision mishaps in Nigerian children. Ann Afr Med. 2009;8(4):266–70.
8. Atikeler MK, Geçit I, Yüzgeç V, Yalçin O. Complications of circumcision performed within and outside the hospital. Int Urol Nephrol. 2005;37(1):97–9.
9. Hutcheson JC. Male neonatal circumcision: indications, controversies and complications. Urol Clin North Am. 2004;31(3):461–7. viii.
10. Nelson CP, Dunn R, Wan J, Wei JT. The increasing incidence of newborn circumcision: data from the nationwide inpatient sample. J Urol. 2005;173(3):978–81.
11. Ben Chaim J, Livne PM, Binyamini J, Hardak B, Ben-Meir D, Mor Y. Complications of circumcision in Israel: a one year multicenter survey. Isr Med Assoc J IMAJ. 2005;7(6):368–70.
12. Schoen EJ. Benefits of newborn circumcision: is Europe ignoring medical evidence? Arch Dis Child. 1997;77(3):258–60.
13. Craig JC, Knight JF, Sureshkumar P, Mantz E, Roy LP. Effect of circumcision on incidence of urinary tract infection in preschool boys. J Pediatr. 1996;128(1):23–7.
14. Crain EF, Gershel JC. Urinary tract infections in febrile infants younger than 8 weeks of age. Pediatrics. 1990;86(3):363–7.
15. Spach DH, Stapleton AE, Stamm WE. Lack of circumcision increases the risk of urinary tract infection in young men. JAMA. 1992;267(5):679–81.
16. Wiswell TE, Geschke DW. Risks from circumcision during the first month of life compared with those for uncircumcised boys. Pediatrics. 1989; 83(6):1011–5.

17. Wiswell TE, Miller GM, Gelston HM, Jones SK, Clemmings AF. Effect of circumcision status on periurethral bacterial flora during the first year of life. J Pediatr. 1988;113(3):442–6.

18. Bailey RC, Egesah O, Rosenberg S. Male circumcision for HIV prevention: a prospective study of complications in clinical and traditional settings in Bungoma, Kenya. Bull World Health Organ. 2008;86(9):669–77.

19. Gray RH, Kigozi G, Serwadda D, Makumbi F, Watya S, Nalugoda F, et al. Male circumcision for HIV prevention in men in Rakai, Uganda: a randomised trial. Lancet. 2007;369(9562):657–66.

20. Millett GA, Flores SA, Marks G, Reed J, Herbst JH. Circumcision status and risk of hiv and sexually transmitted infections among men who have sex with men: a meta-analysis. JAMA. 2008;300(14):1674–84.

21. Young MR, Odoyo-June E, Nordstrom SK, Irwin TE, Ongong'a DO, Ochomo B, et al. Factors associated with uptake of infant male circumcision for HIV prevention in western Kenya. Pediatrics. 2012;130(1):e175–82.

22. Kochen M, McCurdy S. Circumcision and the risk of cancer of the penis. A life-table analysis. Am J Dis Child 1960. 1980;134(5):484–6.

23. Morris BJ, Gray RH, Castellsague X, Bosch FX, Halperin DT, Waskett JH, et al. The strong protective effect of circumcision against cancer of the penis. Adv Urol. 2011;2011, e812368.

24. Schoen EJ. The relationship between circumcision and cancer of the penis. CA Cancer J Clin. 1991;41(5):306–9.

25. Wilcken A, Keil T, Dick B. Traditional male circumcision in eastern and southern Africa: a systematic review of prevalence and complications. Bull World Health Organ. 2010;88(12):907–14.

26. Afsari M, Beasley SW, Maoate K, Heckert K. Attitudes of pacific parents to circumcision of boys. Pac Health Dialog. 2002;9(1):29–33.

27. Osarumwense DO, Ovueni EM. Current views, levels of acceptance, and practice of male circumcision in Africa subregion. Ann Pediatr Surg. 2009;5(4):254–60.

28. Elbakry A. Management of urethrocutaneous fistula after hypospadias repair: 10 years' experience. BJU Int. 2001;88(6):590–5.

29. Richter F, Pinto PA, Stock JA, Hanna MK. Management of recurrent urethral fistulas after hypospadias repair. Urology. 2003;61(2):448–51.

30. Ikuerowo SO, Bioku MJ, Omisanjo OA, Esho JO. Urethrocutaneous fistula complicating circumcision in children. Niger J Clin Pract. 2014;17(2):145–8.

31. Ceylan K, Burhan K, Yilmaz Y, Can S, Kuş A, Mustafa G. Severe complications of circumcision: an analysis of 48 cases. J Pediatr Urol. 2007;3(1):32–5.

32. Kaplan GW. Complications of circumcision. Urol Clin North Am. 1983; 10(3):543–9.

33. Mazza ON, Cheliz GM. Glanuloplasty with scrotal flap for partial penectomy. J Urol. 2001;166(3):887–9.

34. Shaeer O, El-Sebaie A. Construction of neoglans penis: a new sculpturing technique from rectus abdominis myofascial flap. J Sex Med. 2005;2(2):259–65.

35. Gluckman GR, Stoller ML, Jacobs MM, Kogan BA. Newborn penile glans amputation during circumcision and successful reattachment. J Urol. 1995;153(3 Pt 1):778–9.

36. Essid A, Hamzaoui M, Sahli S, Houissa T. Glans reimplantation after circumcision accident. Prog En Urol J Assoc Fr Urol Société Fr Urol. 2005;15(4):745–7.

37. Hamoudi A, Shier M. Late complications of childhood female genital mutilation. J Obstet Gynaecol Can JOGC J Obstétrique Gynécologie Can JOGC. 2010;32(6):587–9.

38. Naimer SA, Peleg R, Meidvidovski Y, Zvulunov A, Cohen AD, Vardy D. Office management of penile skin bridges with electrocautery. J Am Board Fam Pract Am Board Fam Pract. 2002;15(6):485–8.

39. Gee WF, Ansell JS. Neonatal circumcision: a ten-year overview: with comparison of the Gomco clamp and the Plastibell device. Pediatrics. 1976;58(6):824–7.

Continuous saline bladder irrigation for two hours following transurethral resection of bladder tumors in patients with non-muscle invasive bladder cancer does not prevent recurrence or progression compared with intravesical Mitomycin-C

Andrew T. Lenis[1,2,3] (iD), Kian Asanad[1], Maher Blaibel[4], Nicholas M. Donin[1,2,3] and Karim Chamie[1,2,3*]

Abstract

Background: Intravesical Mitomycin-C (MMC) following transurethral resection of bladder tumor (TURBT), while efficacious, is associated with side effects and poor utilization. Continuous saline bladder irrigation (CSBI) has been examined as an alternative. In this study we sought to compare the rates of recurrence and/or progression in patients with NMIBC who were treated with either MMC or CSBI after TURBT.

Methods: We retrospectively reviewed records of patients with NMIBC at our institution in 2012–2015. Perioperative use of MMC (40 mg in 20 mL), CSBI (two hours), or neither were recorded. Primary outcome was time to recurrence or progression. Descriptive statistics, chi-squared analysis, Kaplan-Meier survival analysis, and Cox multivariable regression analyses were performed.

Results: 205 patients met inclusion criteria. Forty-five (22.0%) patients received CSBI, 71 (34.6%) received MMC, and 89 (43.4%) received no perioperative therapy. On survival analysis, MMC was associated with improved DFS compared with CSBI ($p = 0.001$) and no treatment ($p = 0.0009$). On multivariable analysis, high risk disease was associated with increased risk of recurrence or progression (HR 2.77, 95% CI: 1.28–6.01), whereas adjuvant therapy (HR 0.35, 95% CI: 0.20–0.59) and MMC (HR 0.43, 95% CI: 0.25–0.75) were associated with decreased risk.

Conclusions: Postoperative MMC was associated with improved DFS compared with CSBI and no treatment. The DFS benefit seen with CSBI in other studies may be limited to patients receiving prolonged irrigation. New intravesical agents being evaluated may consider saline as a control given our data demonstrating that short-term CSBI is not superior to TURBT alone.

Keywords: Bladder cancer, Therapeutic irrigation, Mitomycin-C, Recurrence, Outcome assessment

* Correspondence: kchamie@mednet.ucla.edu
[1]David Geffen School of Medicine at the University of California Los Angeles, 300 Stein Plaza, Suite 348, Los Angeles, California 90095, USA
[2]Department of Urology, Health Services Research Group, David Geffen School of Medicine at UCLA, Los Angeles, California, USA
Full list of author information is available at the end of the article

Background

Non-muscle invasive bladder cancer (NMIBC) accounts for approximately 70% of new cases of urothelial carcinoma of the bladder. [1] NMIBC has been considered a chronic disease due to its high risk of future complications, including recurrence, which necessitates frequent monitoring and surveillance. The lifelong risk of recurrence and repeated interventions contributes to poor physician and patient compliance with published guidelines, and it significantly burdens the healthcare system from a financial standpoint. [2, 3] Therefore, strategies to prevent recurrence and future complications are paramount to reducing long-term morbidity and mortality.

The standard adjuvant therapy following transurethral resection of bladder tumor (TURBT) for NMIBC is intravesical instillation of Mitomycin-C (MMC), which has been shown to decrease rates of recurrence by approximately 11%, although this is variable depending on the number of and time from prior recurrences. [4, 5] The posited mechanism of action is to prevent free-floating tumor cells in the urine following TURBT from re-implanting onto the bladder wall. Although rare, MMC can potentially cause several significant side effects, including severe lower urinary tract symptoms, persistent chronic bladder pain, and even bladder necrosis in case reports. [6] Furthermore, MMC is contraindicated when there is a concern for bladder perforation and when there is significant post-operative gross hematuria. Considering these limitations, there is an urgent need for alternative strategies to prevent the re-implantation of tumor cells following TURBT, to reduce recurrence and minimize the morbidity of the disease. A 2012 Cochrane review of intravesical gemcitabine yielded conflicting results. [7] Apaziquone is a novel intravesical alkylating agent that has demonstrated safety and tolerability in patients as a post-TURBT instillation and is being evaluated in Phase 3 clinical trials (NCT02563561). [8] Alternatively, several groups have utilized sterile water and saline irrigation over 18–24 h as a strategy to lyse floating tumors cells and prevent the re-implantation of cells into the bladder wall. [9, 10] In our current study, we sought to evaluate continuous bladder irrigation with isotonic (0.9% NaCl) normal saline (CBSI) for two hours following TURBT as a strategy to reduce recurrence or progression in patients with NMIBC.

Methods

Patient cohort

Patients undergoing endoscopic resection of bladder tumors at our institution between March 2012 and July 2015 were identified from the medical record by Current Procedure Terminology (CPT)-4 codes for transurethral biopsy and resection (52204, 52214, 52224, 52234, 52235, 52240). Pathologic and clinical reports were reviewed, and patients with NMIBC were selected for inclusion in the cohort. We excluded all patients with variant histology, including small cell, squamous cell, adenocarcinoma, lymphepithelioid, sarcomatoid, and micropapillary disease. We also excluded patients with a diagnosis of upper tract urothelial carcinoma within one year, unresectable volume of tumor, known metastatic disease, less than three months of follow-up, or patients who underwent cystectomy within three months of diagnosis. Patients were categorized based on a modified AUA Risk Stratification for NMIBC. [11] Low risk was defined as a solitary LG lesion < 2 cm. Intermediate risk was defined as any LG T1, solitary LG Ta > 2 cm, multiple LG Ta, solitary HG Ta < 2 cm, or a history of LG NMIBC. High risk was defined as any CIS, HG T1, HG Ta > 2 cm, multiple HG Ta, or any history of HG Ta lesions or BCG recurrence. Modification of the AUA risk groups was made in order to conform to the size criteria used in the current procedural terminology codes for TURBT. Follow-up was calculated based on the time of the last cystoscopy. All study conduct was approved by the Institutional Review Board at our institution.

Independent variables

All patients received adjuvant CSBI, adjuvant MMC, or no adjuvant treatment at the discretion of the operating surgeon. Typically, patients for whom there was a concern for bladder perforation were not given CSBI or MMC. MMC was given as an instillation of 40 mg in 20 mL of saline. Following a dwell time of 60–90 min, the MMC was drained from the bladder and the catheter was left in place if deemed necessary by the surgeon. CSBI was performed by placement of a three-way Foley catheter at the conclusion of the case and was left running for approximately two hours post-operatively. The rate was kept at maximum flow without titration for this time. Patients did not require an overnight stay specifically for CSBI.

Dependent variables

Our dependent variable of interest was time to recurrence or progression. Recurrence was defined as the presence of pathologically confirmed urothelial carcinoma on biopsy or repeat resection. Patients who were found to have a lesion visible on cystoscopy that warranted intervention in the office (e.g. fulguration) were also classified as having disease recurrence. Cytology results obtained at the time of office fulguration were recorded. Progression was defined as any increase in grade or stage of disease.

Statistical analysis

Comparisons between categorical variables were tested using Chi-squared analysis and Fisher's exact test when appropriate. The two-sample Student's t-test was used to test for differences between continuous variables. Differences in disease-free survival (DFS) were analyzed using the Kaplan-Meier method. Cox proportional hazards models were used to estimate hazards ratios for covariates of interest. All statistical analyses were performed with Stata statistical software version 14 (StataCorp, College Station, TX).

Results

A total of 205 patients underwent TURBT for NMIBC during the study period and met all inclusion criteria. Mean age was 71.9 (SD = 11.4) years and 81.5% were male. Low grade (LG) and high grade (HG) were the primary grades in 105 (51.2%) and 100 (48.8%) patients, respectively. Stage was Ta without CIS, Ta with CIS, T1 without CIS, T1 with CIS, and CIS alone in 126 (61.5%), 12 (5.9%), 36 (17.6%), 13 (6.3%), and 18 (8.8%) patients, respectively. Tumor size was < 0.5 cm, 0.5–2 cm, 2–5 cm, and > 5 cm in 20 (9.8%), 90 (43.9%), 45 (21.9%), and 50 (24.4%) patients, respectively. Multiple tumors were present in 105 (51.2%) patients and 75 (36.6%) had a history of NMIBC. A modified AUA risk stratification as discussed in the methods resulted in 23 (11.2%) low risk patients, 80 (39%) intermediate risk patients, and 102 (49.8%) high risk patients. As immediate perioperative therapy, a total of 45 (22.0%) patients had CSBI, 71 (34.6%) had MMC, and 89 (43.4%) had no perioperative therapy. Only 36 (19.8%) of patients with intermediate or high risk disease underwent a restaging TURBT. Eighty-six (42.0%) patients received adjuvant intravesical therapy, most commonly with bacillus Calmette-Guérin (BCG $n = 76$), BCG + interferon ($n = 6$), Gemcitabine ($n = 2$), or MMC (n = 2). Table 1 and Table 2 summarize the cohort characteristics stratified by perioperative treatment and recurrence and progression, respectively.

Median follow-up time for the entire cohort was 16 [Interquartile range (IQR): 8–28] months. A total of 74 (36.1%) patients recurred at a median of 9.5 [IQR: 4–14] months and 16 (7.8%) progressed at a median of 16 [IQR: 6–31.5] months. The median DFS was 25 months for those who received no perioperative treatment, 55 months for those receiving MMC, and 16 months for those receiving CSBI. The Kaplan-Meier survival curve is presented in Fig. 1 and demonstrates a significant DFS advantage of MMC compared with either CSBI or no perioperative treatment (log rank test: $p < 0.01$). Kaplan-Meier curves for patients with a combination of low and intermediate risk NMIBC (log rank test: $p = 0.02$) and high risk NMIBC (log rank test: $p = 0.04$), and are presented in Figs. 2 and 3, respectively.

Lastly, we created a multivariable model incorporating age, AUA risk stratification, use of additional adjuvant therapy, and type of perioperative therapy (None, MMC, or CSBI). On Cox multivariable modeling, high risk was

associated with increased risk of recurrence or progression (HR 2.77, 95% CI: 1.28–6.01), whereas adjuvant therapy (HR 0.35, 95% CI: 0.20–0.59) and MMC (HR 0.43, 95% CI: 0.25–0.75) were associated with decreased risk of recurrence or progression (Table 3).

Discussion

The burden of NMIBC includes high financial costs to the healthcare system, significant risk of recurrence that necessitates life-long invasive surveillance, and uncertainty of possible progression that would prompt future radical operative intervention, especially in the highest-risk patients. Strategies to reduce the risk of recurrence and progression, including intravesical chemotherapy and immunotherapy, have been shown to be effective. [4, 12] However, none of these are without risk of potential significant side effects. In our current study we sought to utilize postoperative CSBI in a fashion similar to MMC, as an immediate, one-time postoperative treatment following surgery. This strategy avoids the toxicity of intravesical chemotherapy, as well as the inconvenience of an overnight hospital stay for prolonged CSBI.

In our cohort, however, post-operative CSBI for two hours was not equivalent to a single dose of perioperative MMC. Given the small numbers of patients in the low risk subgroup, we combined patients from low risk and intermediate risk groups for analysis. In the low and intermediate risk patients, there was a significant improvement in DFS with MMC compared with CSBI. In fact, CSBI performed no better than no perioperative treatment. In the high risk subgroup, a similar trend was observed. In our study the absolute risk reduction of postoperative MMC compared with no treatment at one year was 12.3%, which is similar to what is reported in the literature (11.7%). [4, 13] This benefit of MMC holds true even in our Cox multivariable model.

With respect to the efficacy of CSBI, our data stands in contrast to results published by others, albeit with some important differences in study design. Onishi et al. performed a non-randomized study comparing 18–22 h of post-operative CSBI to a full year of induction and maintenance MMC in patients with European Organization for Research and Treatment of Cancer (EORTC) intermediate risk NMIBC and showed no difference in several outcomes, including recurrence-free rates, time to first recurrence, and frequency of recurrences. [10] In this manuscript, the authors alluded to a planned prospective study that was recently published. [14] In their follow-up study, 227 patients with primary EORTC low- to intermediate-risk (all LG) NMIBC were randomized 1:1 to receive CSBI for 18 h or a single dose of 30 mg of MMC in 30 mL of saline. After a median follow-up of 37 months, 29% of patients experienced a recurrence. Recurrence-free rates at 1, 3, and 5 years were similar between the CSBI

Table 1 Cohort characteristics stratified by perioperative treatment

Variable	No treatment	MMC	CSBI	p-value
Total no. of patients	89	71	45	–
Age, mean (SD)	73.2 (11.2)	68.2 (12.3)	75.3 (8.9)	< 0.002+
Gender, n (%)				0.54
Male	75 (84.3)	55 (77.5)	37 (83.2)	
Female	14 (15.7)	16 (22.5)	8 (17.8)	
Grade, n (%)				0.9
High	45 (50.6)	34 (47.9)	21 (46.7)	
Low	44 (49.4)	37 (52.1)	24 (53.3)	
Stage, n (%)				0.03*
Ta without CIS	55 (61.8)	41 (57.8)	30 (66.7)	
Ta with CIS	3 (3.4)	4 (5.6)	5 (11.1)	
T1 without CIS	13 (14.6)	18 (25.4)	5 (11.1)	
T1 with CIS	4 (4.5)	6 (8.5)	3 (6.7)	
CIS only	14 (15.7)	2 (2.8)	2 (4.4)	
Tumor size, n (%)				0.12*
< 0.5 cm	11 (12.36)	3 (4.2)	6 (13.3)	
0.5–2.0 cm	33 (37.1)	41 (57.8)	16 (35.6)	
2.0–5.0 cm	22 (24.7)	13 (18.3)	10 (22.2)	
> 5.0 cm	23 (25.8)	14 (19.7)	13 (28.9)	
Multiple tumors, n (%)	47 (52.8)	36 (50.7)	22 (48.9)	0.91
Recurrent disease, n (%)	40 (45.0)	23 (32.4)	12 (26.7)	0.08
AUA Risk Stratification				0.72
Low risk	10 (11.2)	6 (8.5)	7 (15.6)	
Intermediate risk	34 (38.2)	31 (43.7)	15 (33.3)	
High risk	45 (50.6)	34 (47.9)	23 (51.1)	
Restaging resection, n (%)	8 (9.0)	18 (25.4)	10 (22.2)	0.02
Adjuvant therapy, n (%)	35 (39.3)	35 (49.3)	16 (35.6)	0.28
Follow-up in months, median [IQR]	14 [6–28]	23 [11–32]	13 [9–19]	< 0.01§

MMC Mitomycin-C, *CSBI* continuous saline bladder irrigation, *SD* standard deviation, *CIS* carcinoma in situ. +One-way ANOVA. *Fisher's exact test. §non-parametric equality of medians test

and MMC groups on Kaplan-Meier analysis. Subgroup analysis showed no difference when stratified between the low- and intermediate-risk tumors. Adverse events were also compared and the MMC group was found to have significantly higher rates of gross hematuria, irritative bladder symptoms, and dysuria (including retention). While the equivalence of CSBI and MMC demonstrated by Onishi et al. could be explained in part by patient selection (all LG patients), we did not replicate this result even in the low and intermediate risk subgroups of our cohort. One important difference in our protocols is the dose of MMC, which was the standard 40 mg in our study and 30 mg in the study by Onishi et al. The most striking difference between our studies, however, is in the duration of CSBI. We intentionally restricted CSBI to two hours to limit the need for overnight hospital stays. While similarly

efficacious to one instillation of MMC, CSBI used by Onishi et al. was titrated over 18 h, and it was not reported how many of these patients required an overnight stay. While the authors debate the cost advantages of saline compared with MMC, we question whether this may be offset by even a small fraction of patients requiring overnight admissions for CSBI. Nevertheless, this data demonstrates that in addition to a standard dose of 40 mg of MMC, duration may be an important component of the efficacy of CSBI in preventing tumor cell reimplantation.

Our results also appear to conflict with the results of a recent meta-analysis utilizing individual patient data from randomized trials comparing immediate intravesical instillation of various chemotherapy agents to TURBT alone or instillation of control solution (saline

Table 2 Cohort characteristics stratified by Recurrence or Progression

Variable	Recurrence or Progression	No Recurrence or Progression	p-value
Total no. of patients	90	115	–
Age, mean (SD)	73.6 (10.8)	70.6 (11.8)	0.07+
Gender, n (%)			0.81
Male	74 (82.2)	93 (80.9)	
Female	16 (17.8)	22 (19.1)	
Grade, n (%)			0.38
High	47 (52.2)	53 (46.1)	
Low	43 (47.8)	62 (53.9)	
Stage, n (%)			0.09*
Ta without CIS	55 (61.1)	71 (61.7)	
Ta with CIS	3 (3.3)	9 (7.8)	
T1 without CIS	14 (15.6)	22 (19.1)	
T1 with CIS	5 (5.6)	8 (7.0)	
CIS	13 (14.4)	5 (4.4)	
Tumor size, n (%)			0.09
< 0.5 cm	14 (15.6)	6 (5.2)	
0.5–2.0 cm	37 (41.1)	53 (46.1)	
2.0–5.0 cm	17 (18.9)	28 (24.4)	
> 5.0 cm	22 (24.4)	28 (24.3)	
Multiplicity of tumor, n (%)	56 (62.2)	49 (42.6)	< 0.01
Recurrent disease, n (%)	42 (46.7)	33 (28.7)	< 0.01
AUA Risk Stratification			0.07
Low risk	9 (10.0)	14 (12.2)	
Intermediate risk	28 (31.1)	52 (45.2)	
High risk	53 (58.9)	49 (42.6)	
Restaging resection, n (%)	12 (13.3)	24 (20.9)	0.16
Adjuvant therapy, n (%)	32 (35.6)	54 (47.0)	0.10
Perioperative treatment, n (%)			0.004
None	47 (52.2)	42 (36.5)	
MMC	20 (22.2)	51 (44.4)	
CSBI	23 (25.6)	22 (19.1)	

MMC Mitomycin-C, *CSBI* continuous saline bladder irrigation, *SD* standard deviation, *CIS* carcinoma in situ. +One-way ANOVA. *Fisher's exact test

or water). [5] Upon closer examination, however, we are unable to compare the protocols included as published in the meta-analysis or in the original manuscripts to our brief post-operative irrigation protocol. Of the 13 included studies, the use of post-operative irrigation was only documented as consistently used in four of these studies. Irrigation protocols were not detailed in the meta-analysis and review of the original data could not identify specific protocols. Furthermore, at least one study utilized distilled water for irrigation, which has the theoretical advantage of an osmotic cytotoxic effect but the disadvantages of being hypotonic. Therefore, despite a 21% relative reduction in recurrences found in this meta-analysis with use of post-operative irrigation alone, we can only cautiously compare this result with our data without more detailed information about the irrigation protocols used.

The concept of utilizing irrigation for eradication of residual tumor cells following surgery for cancer is not a new concept, nor is it limited to urology or even endoscopic surgery. Surgeons have traditionally irrigated surgical sites to mechanically wash away debris, dilution of bacterial loads, and as a method of tumor cell lysis, depending on the tonicity of the fluid. A survey in England found that 74% of general surgeons perform intraoperative peritoneal lavage during cancer operations (36%

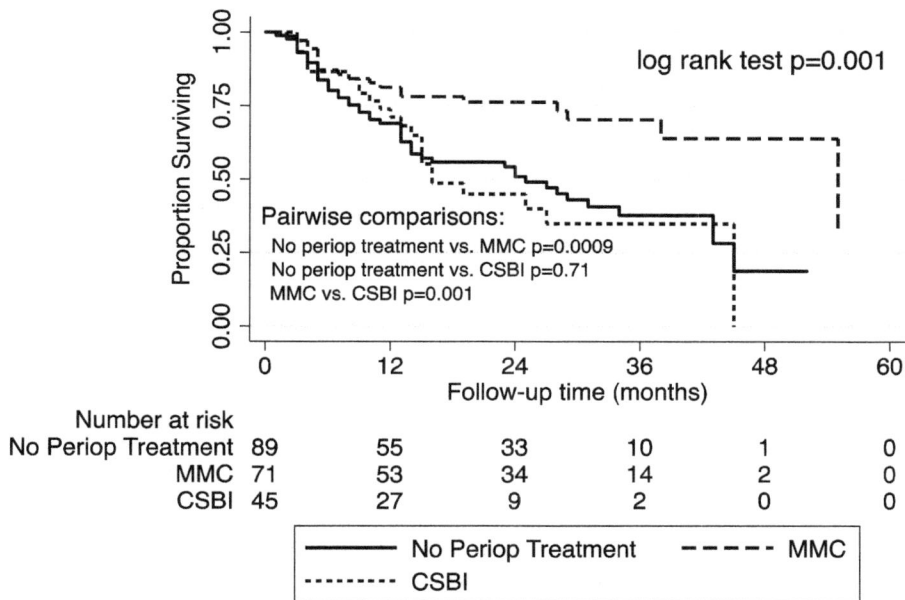

Fig. 1 "DFS in Patients with NMIBC". Kaplan-Meier survival curve for all patients with NMIBC stratified by perioperative treatment. MMC, Mitomycin-C. CSBI, continuous saline bladder irrigation

with water, 21% with saline, and 17% with betadine). [15] However, efficacy data on irrigation type is conflicting. Sweitzer et al. designed an experiment in mice to evaluate whether distilled water or sterile saline irrigation could reduce the burden of orthotopically implanted melanoma tumor cells. [16] Unfortunately, they found that neither the mechanical process of irrigation nor the hypotonicity of water reduced the tumor burden. In contrast, Fumito et al. demonstrated the superiority of water irrigation to saline irrigation following laparotomy in a mouse model of colorectal cancer tumor spillage. [17] In head and neck cancer models, both the type of irrigation and type of cancer cell line contributed to efficacy. [18, 19] These and other conflicting data suggest that multiple

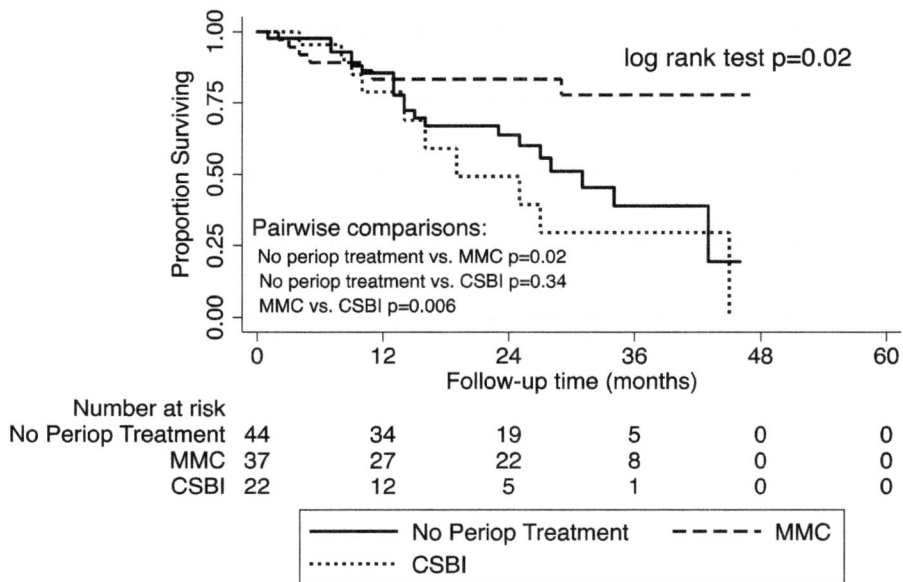

Fig. 2 "DFS in Patients with Low and Intermediate Risk". Kaplan-Meier survival curve for patients with low and intermediate risk disease stratified by perioperative treatment. MMC, Mitomycin-C. CSBI, continuous saline bladder irrigation

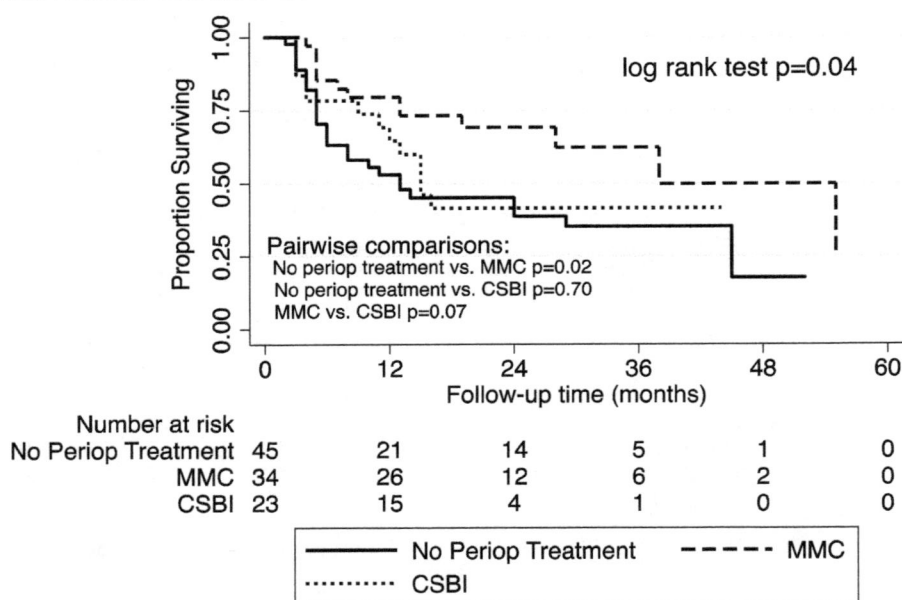

Fig. 3 "DFS in Patients with High Risk". Kaplan-Meier survival curve for patients with high risk disease stratified by perioperative treatment. MMC, Mitomycin-C. CSBI, continuous saline bladder irrigation

factors play a role with respect to the eradication of residual tumor burden, potentially related to the microenvironment and tumor cell-specific factors, such as cell adhesion properties and degree of de-differentiation.

The literature does strongly support irrigation following intra-luminal surgery in other surgical fields. For example, Zhou et al. performed a meta-analysis of studies evaluating intra-luminal washout following anterior resection for rectal cancer and concluded that washout leads to reduced rates of local recurrence. [20] In the urologic literature, Moskovitz et al. first postulated in

1987 that intravesical irrigation with distilled water during and after TURBT would lead to fewer recurrences. [21] While several small studies have demonstrated conflicting results regarding the use of water irrigation compared with no perioperative treatment, no studies have compared CSBI to MMC until the aforementioned studies by Onishi et al. [10, 14, 22, 23] Our study is the first to compare a shorter, perioperative duration of CSBI to both MMC and no perioperative treatment, and to evaluate this strategy in a heterogeneous patient population with low, intermediate, and high risk disease.

Table 3 Cox multivariable model for Recurrence or Progression

Variable	Hazard Ratio	95% Confidence Interval	p-value
Age (per year of age)	1.00	0.98–1.02	0.92
AUA Risk Stratification			
Low Risk	Reference	Reference	
Intermediate Risk	0.84	0.39–1.80	0.66
High Risk	2.77	1.28–6.01	0.01
Adjuvant therapy			
No	Reference	Reference	
Yes	0.35	0.20–0.59	< 0.001
Perioperative treatment			
No perioperative treatment	Reference	Reference	
MMC	0.43	0.25–0.75	0.003
CSBI	0.96	0.58–1.60	0.89

LG low grade, *HG* high grade, *CIS* carcinoma in situ, *MMC* Mitomycin-C, *CSBI* continuous saline bladder irrigation

Our results, however, should be considered within the context of several limitations. Although this was a hypothesis-based study driven by pre-clinical and clinical data, it was not a randomized controlled study, and was limited to the data available in medical records. Furthermore, the study is underpowered and longer term follow-up is required to fully realize the potential differences between treatment groups. It is possible that a larger cohort with longer term follow up could confirm the null hypothesis, suggesting that no difference exists between treatment groups. However, at our institution we are mainly utilizing intravesical gemcitabine based on recently published data that suggests efficacy at a fraction of the cost and with reduced side effects compared with MMC. [24] Consequently, in combination with the current data that suggests inefficacy of 2 h of CSBI, we are unlikely to treat more patients with adjuvant CSBI. Primarily one surgeon (KC) performed CSBI during the study period while most other surgeons in the department utilized either MMC or no additional perioperative therapy. Therefore, referral patterns may have contributed to patient heterogeneity between groups. Despite some baseline differences between treatment groups described in our results, the data remains consistent when controlling for factors such as tumor grade, stage, and recurrence disease, among others, in a multivariable model. A consistent surveillance cystoscopy protocol was not used for all patients and could have helped standardize follow-up and limit detection bias. Finally, we utilized a clinical definition of recurrence that included any suspicious lesion during office cystoscopy that warranted an intervention (usually fulguration), which may have artificially increased our recurrence rates.

Nevertheless, our study comparing perioperative CSBI, perioperative MMC, and no perioperative treatment answers important questions regarding CSBI as prophylaxis following endoscopic resection for NMIBC. While CSBI for two hours postoperatively should not replace current guideline-recommended perioperative MMC, it does appear that longer duration of CSBI may increase its efficacy. [10, 14] Research is needed to determine whether the duration can be reduced to limit the number of additional hospital stays and whether other, novel perioperative instillations may reduce recurrences and limit side effects.

Conclusions

Our data demonstrates that perioperative CSBI for two hours following TURBT is not equivalent to postoperative MMC in terms of rates of recurrence or progression. CSBI for two hours appears to be equivalent to no perioperative treatment, regardless of tumor grade. It is possible that CSBI may be required for a longer duration to reduce tumor cell re-implantation and, in turn, decrease rates of recurrence or progression.

Acknowledgements
This work was supported by the National Institutes of Health Loan Repayment Program (L30 CA154326 (Principal Investigator: KC)), the STOP Cancer Foundation (Principal Investigator: KC), the H & H Lee Surgical Resident Research Award (Recipient: ATL), and the Short Term Training Program (STTP) at the David Geffen School of Medicine at UCLA (Recipient: KA).

Authors' contributions
ATL was primarily involved in protocol/project development, data collection/ management, data analysis, manuscript writing/editing. KA was involved in data collection/management and manuscript writing. MB was involved in data collection/management and manuscript writing. NMD was involved in protocol/project development, data collection/management, data analysis, manuscript writing/editing. KC supervised and was responsible for all study oversight. All authors read and approved the final manuscript.

Competing interests
The authors declare that they have no competing interests.

Author details
[1]David Geffen School of Medicine at the University of California Los Angeles, 300 Stein Plaza, Suite 348, Los Angeles, California 90095, USA. [2]Department of Urology, Health Services Research Group, David Geffen School of Medicine at UCLA, Los Angeles, California, USA. [3]Jonsson Comprehensive Cancer Center, David Geffen School of Medicine at UCLA, Los Angeles, California, USA. [4]Riverside School of Medicine, University of California, Riverside, California, USA.

References
1. Clark PE, Agarwal N, Biagioli MC, Eisenberger MA, Greenberg RE, Herr HW, et al. Bladder cancer J Natl Compr Canc Netw. 2013:446–75.
2. James AC, Gore JL. The costs of non-muscle invasive bladder cancer. Urol. Clin. North Am. 2013;40:261–9 Available from: http://www.ncbi.nlm.nih.gov/ pubmed/23540783.
3. Chamie K, Saigal CS, Lai J, Hanley JM, Setodji CM, Konety BR, et al. Compliance with guidelines for patients with bladder cancer: variation in the delivery of care. Cancer. 2011;117:5392–401 Available from: http://www. pubmedcentral.nih.gov/articlerender.fcgi?artid=3206145&tool= pmcentrez&rendertype=abstract.
4. Sylvester RJ, Oosterlinck W, van der Meijden APM. A single immediate postoperative instillation of chemotherapy decreases the risk of recurrence in patients with stage ta T1 bladder cancer: a meta-analysis of published results of randomized clinical trials. J Urol. 2004;171:2186–90 quiz2435.
5. Sylvester RJ, Oosterlinck W, Holmäng S, Sydes MR, Birtle A, Gudjonsson S, et al. Systematic review and individual patient data meta-analysis of randomized trials comparing a single immediate instillation of chemotherapy after transurethral resection with transurethral resection alone in patients with stage pTa-pT1 urothelial carcinoma of the bladder: which patients benefit from the instillation? Eur Urol. 2016;69:231–44.
6. Doherty AP, Trendell-Smith N, Stirling R, Rogers H, Bellringer J. Perivesical fat necrosis after adjuvant intravesical chemotherapy. BJU Int. 1999;83:420–3.
7. Jones G, Cleves A, Wilt TJ, Mason M, Kynaston HG, Shelley M. Intravesical gemcitabine for non-muscle invasive bladder cancer. Cochrane Database Syst Rev John Wiley & Sons, Ltd. 2012;1:CD009294.
8. Hendricksen K, Cornel EB, de Reijke TM, Arentsen HC, Chawla S, Witjes JA. Phase 2 study of adjuvant intravesical instillations of apaziquone for high risk nonmuscle invasive bladder cancer. J Urol. 2012;187:1195–1199.
9. Taoka R, Williams SB, Ho PL, Kamat AM. In-vitro cytocidal effect of water on bladder cancer cells: the potential role for intraperitoneal lavage during radical cystectomy. CUAJ. 2015;9:E109–13.
10. Onishi T, Sasaki T, Hoshina A, Yabana T. Continuous saline bladder irrigation after transurethral resection is a prophylactic treatment choice for non-muscle invasive bladder tumor. Anticancer Res. 2011;31:1471–4.

11. Chang SS, Boorjian SA, Chou R, Clark PE, Daneshmand S, Konety BR, et al. Diagnosis and treatment of non-muscle invasive bladder Cancer: AUA/SUO guideline. J Urol. 2016;196:1021–9.

12. Sylvester RJ, van der Meijden APM, Lamm DL. Intravesical bacillus Calmette-Guerin reduces the risk of progression in patients with superficial bladder cancer: a meta-analysis of the published results of randomized clinical trials. J Urol. 2002;168:1964–70 Available from: http://www.ncbi.nlm.nih.gov/pubmed/12394686.

13. Abern MR, Owusu RA, Anderson MR, Rampersaud EN, Inman BA. Perioperative intravesical chemotherapy in non-muscle-invasive bladder cancer: a systematic review and meta-analysis. J Natl Compr Cancer Netw. 2013;11:477–84.

14. Onishi T, Sugino Y, Shibahara T, Masui S, Yabana T, Sasaki T Randomized controlled study of the efficacy and safety of continuous saline bladder irrigation after transurethral resection for the treatment of n... - PubMed - NCBI. BJU international. 2016.

15. Whiteside OJH, Tytherleigh MG, Thrush S, Farouk R, Galland RB. Intra-operative peritoneal lavage--who does it and why? Ann R Coll Surg Engl. 2005;87:255–8.

16. Sweitzer KL, Nathanson SD, Nelson LT, Zachary C. Irrigation does not dislodge or destroy tumor cells adherent to the tumor bed. J Surg Oncol. 1993;53:184–90.

17. Ito F, Camoriano M, Seshadri M, Evans SS, Kane JM, Skitzki JJ. Water: a simple solution for tumor spillage. Ann Surg Oncol Springer-Verlag. 2011;18:2357–63.

18. Lodhia KA, Dale OT, Winter SC. Irrigation solutions in head and neck cancer surgery: a preclinical efficacy study. Ann Otol Rhinol Laryngol SAGE Publications. 2015;124:68–71.

19. Hah JH, Roh DH, Jung YH, Kim KH, Sung M-W. Selection of irrigation fluid to eradicate free cancer cells during head and neck cancer surgery. Head neck. Wiley subscription services, Inc. A Wiley Company. 2012;34:546–50.

20. Zhou C, Ren Y, Li J, Li X, He J, Liu P. Systematic review and meta-analysis of rectal washout on risk of local recurrence for cancer. - PubMed - NCBI. J Surg Res. 2014;189:7–16.

21. Moskovitz B, Levin DR. Intravesical irrigation with distilled water during and immediately after transurethral resection and later for superficial bladder cancer. Eur Urol. 1987;13:7–9.

22. Sakai Y, Fujii Y, Hyochi N, Masuda H, Kawakami S, Kobayashi T, et al. A large amount of distilled water ineffective for prevention of bladder cancer cell implantation at the time of transurethral resection. Hinyokika Kiyo. 2006;52:173–5.

23. Amos S, Gofrit ON. Prevention of bladder tumor recurrence. Evolving trends in urology. In: Sashi S Kommu, editor. 1st ed. Rijeka, Croatia: InTech; 2012. pp. 69–76. https://doi.org/10.5772/38495.

24. Messing EM, Tangen CM, Lerner SP, Sahasrabudhe DM, Koppie TM, Wood DP, et al. Effect of Intravesical instillation of gemcitabine vs saline immediately following resection of suspected low-grade non-muscle-invasive bladder Cancer on tumor recurrence: SWOG S0337 randomized clinical trial. JAMA. 2018;319:1880–8.

Acceptability of dietary and physical activity lifestyle modification for men following radiotherapy or radical prostatectomy for localised prostate cancer

Lucy E. Hackshaw-McGeagh[1,2]*, Eileen Sutton[2], Raj Persad[3], Jonathan Aning[4], Amit Bahl[5], Anthony Koupparis[3], Chris Millett[6], Richard M. Martin[1,2] and J. Athene Lane[1,2]

Abstract

Background: The experience and acceptability of lifestyle interventions for men with localised prostate cancer are not well understood, yet lifestyle interventions are increasingly promoted for cancer survivors. We explored the opinions, experiences and perceived acceptability of taking part in nutritional and physical activity interventions amongst men with prostate cancer and their partners; with the ultimate plan to use such information to inform the development of nutritional and physical activity interventions for men with prostate cancer.

Methods: Semi-structured interviews with 16 men, and seven partners, undergoing curative surgery or radiotherapy for prostate cancer. Interviews explored experiences of lifestyle interventions, acceptable changes participants would make and perceived barriers and facilitators to change. Interviews were thematically analysed using the framework approach.

Results: Men were frequently open to lifestyle modification and family support was considered vital to facilitate change. Health beneficial, clinician endorsed, understandable, enjoyable interventions were perceived as attractive. Barriers included 'modern' digital technology, poor weather, competing commitments or physical limitations, most notably incontinence following radical prostatectomy. Men were keen to participate in research, with few negative aspects identified.

Conclusions: Men are willing to change behaviour but this needs to be supported by clinicians and health professionals facilitating lifestyle change. An 'intention-behaviour gap', when an intended behaviour does not materialise, may exist. Digital technology for data collection and lifestyle measurement may not be suitable for all, and post-surgery urinary incontinence is a barrier to physical activity. These novel findings should be incorporated into lifestyle intervention development, and implemented clinically.

Keywords: Clinical implications, Intervention, Interview, Lifestyle, Nutrition, Physical activity, Prostate cancer, Qualitative, Radical prostatectomy, Radiotherapy

* Correspondence: lucy.hackshaw@bristol.ac.uk
[1]University of Bristol, NIHR Biomedical Research Centre - Nutrition, Diet and Lifestyle Theme, Level 3, University Hospitals Bristol Education Centre, Upper Maudlin Street, Bristol BS2 8AE, England, UK
[2]University of Bristol, Bristol Medical School: Population Health Sciences, Canynge Hall, 39 Whatley Road, Bristol BS8 2PS, England, UK
Full list of author information is available at the end of the article

Background

Approximately one in eight men will be diagnosed with prostate cancer in the UK, and it is the most common male cancer in the Western world [1]. Cancer risk and disease progression have been linked to a variety of lifestyle factors and it has been estimated that up to one third of all cancers may be attributed to poor diet, lack of physical activity and obesity [2].

Physical activity and nutrition are thought to benefit physical and psychological health in cancer survivors [3]. Accumulating observational evidence suggests that physical activity and a healthy diet improve overall survival in men with prostate cancer [4, 5], yet most men with prostate cancer do not spontaneously alter their diet or physical activity following a diagnosis [6, 7].

Due to this lack of spontaneous change, much research, including randomised controlled trials, have attempted to influence lifestyle changes in men with prostate cancer; however, these are often underpowered, at high risk of bias, inadequately reported or of short duration, prohibiting reliable conclusions from being drawn [8]. For example, in a systematic review of dietary, nutritional and physical activity interventions in men with prostate cancer half of the 44 trials identified had high risk of bias for sequence generation and blinding of participants, and 21 of the 44 failed to report whether the trial was sufficiently powered [8].

Previous qualitative research to evaluate the experiences of men with prostate cancer, and their attitudes towards participating in lifestyle behaviour change interventions, concluded that men were often positive about making such changes, were optimistic about participation in an intervention and expressed a desire to 'give something back' by participating in research [9]. Group interventions were favoured over individual activities [10], but the shock, distress and anxiety of a diagnosis led to sometimes strained relationships with partners [9] and it was (perhaps surprisingly) often not desired that partners took part in an intervention alongside the men [10]. This is in contrast to studies supporting the efficacy of couple based interventions [11]. Previous research exploring lifestyle interventions have often included men undergoing watchful waiting [9] and androgen deprivation therapy [10]. Our focus was on men who had previously undergone, or were currently undergoing, radical prostatectomy or radiotherapy for localised prostate cancer. This is a population of men who are expected to survive after their prostate cancer treatment for a long period of time, but who nevertheless have a risk of either prostate cancer recurrence or a second primary cancer [12]. These survivors will be at risk of competing medical comorbidities such as cardio-respiratory mortality [13] and in addition to the cardio-metabolic effects of androgen deprivation therapy or later salvage treatments and so might benefit from making long-term dietary and physical activity changes [3].

We explored the opinions, experiences and perceived acceptability of taking part in nutritional and physical activity interventions amongst men with localised prostate cancer, who had previously undergone, or were currently undergoing, radical prostatectomy or radiotherapy, and their partners; with the ultimate plan to use such information to inform the development of nutritional and physical activity interventions for men with prostate cancer [14].

Methods

Participants and recruitment

Men were recruited from one hospital urology outpatient clinic in England between July and December 2013. Using a convenience sampling approach [15], consecutively eligible men with clinically localised prostate cancer, who had recently undergone robotic radical prostatectomy or were undergoing radiotherapy, and with sufficient understanding of the English language, were introduced to the researcher by the clinicians. Men thought not to be suitable for interview by their Urology health care team were excluded. Those who agreed to participate were invited to invite their partner, where applicable, to take part in the interview process. This was optional and reasons for partners being included, or not, were not explored further.

Procedures and data collection

Interviews were conducted by either LHM (n = 13) or ES (n = 10). Participants were interviewed individually, except where men and their partners chose to be interviewed together (n = 5). The majority (n = 16) were conducted at the participant's home, or within a private location at the urology clinic. However, some (n = 7) took place via telephone at the participant's request. Interviews lasted from between 26 and 95 min (mean 49 min).

Following a general introduction, an example 6 month lifestyle intervention was described by the researcher, where men would be asked to walk briskly for an additional 30 min, 5 days a week, alongside either taking a daily lycopene supplement or increasing fruit and vegetable intake and reducing dairy milk intake. The semi-structured interviews included the following topics: previous experience of nutritional and physical activity interventions, lifestyle behaviours that the men would and would not be happy to change, expected gains and costs of participating in an intervention, and perceived barriers and facilitators to change. An interview schedule, developed through reviewing previously discussed existing literature, acted as a guide, but allowed the researcher flexibility to examine the participants' perspectives and gain an insight in to their thoughts and feelings. Additionally, all participants provided a range of demographic data.

Analysis

Interviews were digitally audio-recorded and transcribed verbatim. Thematic analysis was conducted using the framework approach by LHM [16]. Transcripts of five participants (22%) were analysed by both LHM and ES to ensure validation triangulation of themes. NVivo (NVivo10, QSR International, 2012) was used to assist with the analysis. Here we present only the analysis relating to behaviour change and intervention development; other topics will be reported elsewhere, for example patient's views and experiences of advice provision by health care professionals [17]. The COREQ (COnsolidated criteria for REporting Qualitative research) Checklist was used to guide the design, implementation and analysis of this research.

The NHS North West - Lancaster NRES Committee approved the study (13/NW/0228). All participants provided fully informed consent.

Results

In total 16 men with prostate cancer (mean age 67 years; range 53 – 79) and seven partners (mean age 65 years; range 47 – 77), were interviewed. Aggregated demographic information is shown in Table 1 and individual level characteristics are illustrated in Table 2. Twelve men had surgery (on average 6 months prior to the interview, range 2 – 15 months) and 4 were undergoing radiotherapy as treatment for their prostate cancer. Seven men declined the invitation to participate, equating to a recruitment rate of 70% (16/23). The following reasons were given for not wanting to participate; unable to be contacted (n = 2), too overwhelmed by cancer experience or incontinence (n = 2), felt too unwell (n = 1),

Table 1 Demographic characteristics of the men with prostate cancer and their partners

	Men with prostate cancer: 12 surgery; 4 radiotherapy	Partners: 3 surgery; 4 radiotherapy
Mean age in years (range)	67 (53–79)	66 (47–77)
Ethnicity	White British (100%)	White British (100%)
Gender	Male (100%)	Female (86%)
Highest level of education	Attended school to 16 years or less (60%)	Attended school to 16 years or less (57%)
Completed university	2 (13%)	1 (14%)
Marital status	Married (81%)	Married (86%)
Occupation	Retired (50%)	In work (75%)
Drinking alcohol	Drink on 1 or 2 days per week (31%)	Drink almost every day (33%)
Smoking	Non-smoker (88%)	Non-smoker (86%)

simply did not want to (n = 1) and finally 'concerned about computer hacking' (n = 1).

All participants were generally very positive about the proposed 6 month lifestyle intervention. Five main themes emerged: three related to motivations, facilitators and barriers to change; one related to research participation; and one related to lifestyle intervention characteristics.

Motivations for change

Motivations for change were discussed and were often supported by a partner. Shock at the time of diagnosis were frequently discussed, and on many occasions, this had resulted in participants taking stock of their current lifestyle behaviour, identifying that change may be necessary.

If it meant that I could prolong my life to a certain extent, without having to suffer, I would most probably consider it....If it meant I had to cut out certain food, because they're the ones that do the problem to my body, then I would. I wouldn't hesitate. Because if it's doing damage to me, that's it (Patient14-RAD)

If somebody said to me, "You've got to walk from here to the ring road" which is probably five minutes, ten minutes' walk, a fast walk, "And back every day, otherwise you'll be dead in six months" I would do it without hesitation (Patient6-RAD)

It should be noted that both men quoted here suggested that they were motivated by reducing mortality and suffering, not specifically by improving health and wellbeing.

Facilitators of change
Family support

Almost all men discussed the benefits of family or social support and as the majority (81%) of the men were married; subsequently, many suggested that their wife would either join in with an activity or assist with preparation of food.

I think [wife's name] would be very encouraging because you know, she thinks I don't eat healthily enough, so I think she would, there wouldn't be a problem in that sense, if I suddenly went vegetarian or I had to [eat] fish....if I was doing this I would do the same and eat the same as [wife's name], because I think that would probably help if we were both eating the same....she'd love it, if you know what I mean. She'd have a right grin on her face I think as she's cooking it for me (Patient6-RAD)

Table 2 Participant ID and key individual characteristics of the men with prostate cancer and their partners

Participant ID	Age group	Relationship	Treatment	Duration since end of treatment at time of interview
Patient1	71–76	Married	Surgery	4–6 months
Patient2 & Partner1	65–70 & 59–64	Married	Surgery	1–3 months
Patient3	65–70	Not married	Surgery	10–12 months
Patient4 & Partner2	NK & 71–76	Married	Surgery	> 12 months
Patient5	71–76	NK	Surgery	> 12 months
Patient6 & Partner3	65–70 & 65–70	Married	Radiotherapy	< 1 month
Patient7	53–58	Not married	Surgery	1–3 months
Patient8	71–76	Married	Surgery	1–3 months
Patient9	59–64	Married	Surgery	1–3 months
Patient10 & Partner4	59–64 & 65–70	Married	Surgery	1–3 months
Patient11	65–70	Married	Surgery	7–9 months
Patient12	65–70	Married	Surgery	4–6 months
Patient13 & Partner5	77–82 & 77–82	Married	Radiotherapy	< 1 month
Patient14 & Partner6	65–70 & NK	Married	Radiotherapy	< 1 month
Patient15 & Partner7	59–64 & 47–52	Not married	Radiotherapy	< 1 month
Patient16	65–70	Married	Surgery	1–3 months

The importance of involving a partner in an intervention to change behaviour was discussed by many, independent of whether a partner was present in the interview. It was generally felt that the support of a partner would be a facilitator to successful implementation.

Interviewer: So what about your typical diet, what would you say you eat ....?

Patient: Well [Laughter]

Partner: Do you want to answer that?

Patient: I eat whatever I'm given (Patient4 & Partner2-SUR)

This highlights the need to ensure that partners, where applicable, are involved in all elements of an intervention. For example, by inviting the partner along to a recruitment appointment, and ensuring that they are aware of the specific nature of the intervention, particularly for dietary elements. This may not be the case for all; however, in this specific population, the partners, often a wife, were key to the purchase and preparation of food.

Others discussed their partner, children, or friends providing emotional, informational, tangible support (eg. providing financial assistance or material goods) [18]. Such support may involve making healthy snacks for work or no longer buying unhealthy food for the home and it was believed that this social support

would help promote success. One participant discussed the impact of his recent divorce, and subsequently being less physically active, as this was something that he and his former partner had previously done together.

It's extremely difficult for an isolated individual to make that [behaviour] change (Partner7-RAD)

Health gains and clinical advice

Personal motivators to change varied and included weight loss or expectancy to improve general health. Weight gain was often discussed as a stimulus for carrying out physical activity or dietary interventions, especially if a health care professional had raised the issue.

A couple of years ago, I don't know how long it is, two, maybe three years, he went to have a health check at the surgery. He came back horrified because he said, "The nurse told me I'm obese." And that really upset him....that affected him. He then watched what he ate....he stopped having breakfasts and he wasn't eating anything....I think he was frightened of being fat (Partner3-RAD)

If a current behaviour was seen as potentially life threatening, this was also reported to be a personal motivator for change, with enhanced impact if recommendations for behaviour change were delivered by a health care professional.

"Well, I mean, you're... You tend to be in the hands of, of your consultants and, and the team, so if they, if they tell you something should be done for your benefit, then you probably do it" (Patient3-SUR)

If you take alcohol, if [health care professional] said ..."You will not survive another five years if you continuing drinking one unit a day" or something. I'd have to make a change (Patient4-SUR)

Rationale for change

Many men explained that knowing the reasons for lifestyle changes or understanding the underlying science, or how the specific change would benefit them, would help facilitate change.

I suppose if you've got a, a definite link between; "If you eat that, then..." You know, in 10 years' time, such and such might happen, then obviously it makes you think (Patient3-SUR)

If someone had turned round and said, "Look, these are the benefits of changing your diet," I would have done. But you know ... I'd have to be shown and say, "Right, this is the situation, this is - if you change and have these, this would be an improvement," that's fine I would do that (Patient12-SUR)

Anticipated enjoyment of lifestyle changes

Increased enjoyment of a behaviour was thought to encourage perseverance; likewise, it may prevent uptake if the activity is perceived to be boring or unenjoyable. For example, some suggested that they would be more likely to participate if they were walking for a purpose, such as to buy a newspaper.

My physical activity has always been doing things, going with dogs walking, diving, doing things in that way, rather than just going and work on a treadmill, that would bore... I wouldn't... If you asked me to do that I'd say, "No." (Patient12-SUR)

Others discussed that liking the taste of what they had been asked to consume would make them more likely to continue with it in the longer term.

Barriers to lifestyle change

Although men were generally positive about changing their behaviour and specifically in relation to the proposed intervention, there were several potential barriers to change.

Poor weather

Weather was discussed by many of the men and their partners. It was often implied that despite enjoying an activity, poor weather conditions could prevent the activity taking place, for example:

If it was raining, I'd sit on my backside [laughter] (Patient2-SUR)

I cycle when it's dry (Patient8-SUR)

It's a cold time of year, obviously, which limits you a little bit (Patient16-SUR)

During shorter winter days, some of the men suggested that they may be less inclined to go out walking; however, others talked about working outside, and this not being a problem for them; it was explained that in poor conditions they would carry out household chores or another task, and then do additional walking when the weather improved.

If it's pouring with rain, I would say no, but the thing is....you do other things....other weeks may compensate for your bad weeks....if I went out Monday, and the weather's bad on Tuesday, we may go somewhere Thursday, or Wednesday (Patent14-RAD)

This barrier could be seasonal; however, in countries where weather is often unpredictable it should be considered.

Urinary incontinence

Incontinence is a well-established potential side effect of radical prostatectomy and almost all men who had undergone surgery identified incontinence as an important barrier to physical activity. This was not discussed by those who had undergone radiotherapy.

The thing is, when you've had the operation walking is a problem, initially. Until....you can control yourself a bit better. Then walking is a, it acts like a pump, you know what I mean? So you'd have to wait....before you were quite confident walking a long way anyway (Patient5-SUR)

I think perhaps I could do a bit more, bit more walking, but at the moment I'm still got problems with this, the incontinence so I don't like to go too far (Patient9-SUR)

Men described fear of leakage whilst participating in physical activity as often debilitating and causing embarrassment.

I'm still incontinent ... I wear pads and I do find that if I'm walking around I obviously leak a bit and I can feel myself getting, you know, the pads getting full, if you like. And I have to then go and then sort it out (Patient10-SUR)

Ways to overcome issues surrounding incontinence were discussed with the participants, for example finding well-fitting and comfortable pads, exercising when it was darker, so leaks were less noticeable, or mastering pelvic floor exercises, which can help to control urinary incontinence.

Time pressures and overall health
A further barrier to making changes to behaviour could be competing time interests, as illustrated below.

That's a problem, you know with all the activity wot I do now....some days, some days I probably would [be able to do additional walking], but won't be every day I shouldn't think, because it's a time factor, it's a time factor, to put in with my schedule wot I do on a week (Patient1-SUR)

Although others suggested that they would be prepared to incorporate activities like walking into their routine.

The only cost would be would you'd have to organise your day, your time to fit it in. You could either do it first thing in the morning or when you get home from work. Go for a walk, you know, before lunch- before dinner or probably try and fit in a bit more exercise at work, a bit more walking in at work. I could probably rearrange a few things so that I could do a bit more, bit more walking at work (Patient9-SUR)

Other unrelated health conditions such as knee replacements, arthritis, bowel problems, stroke and heart attacks were discussed as individual physical barriers to making changes.

It's alright if you're in, in reasonable physic... Good physical health, but if you're not then these things become more difficult (Patient3-SUR)

Partner: The only thing I'm thinking is, is your leg going to let you do that? Not because he wouldn't want to do it, but I'm not sure if your leg would let you do that.

Patient: No, not going too fast, that's the problem. I've had a new knee in there (Patient13 & Partner5-RAD)

Research participation
The overall opinion portrayed by the men was that once they had committed to participating in the research, then they would do whatever was asked of them. Some referred to this as being stubborn, others as being determined to support research, but it was implied that once they agreed to be involved, they would not change their mind.

Interviewer: So if you were in our trial and we said to you, "Please drink three cups of green tea a day"?

Patient: I'd do it. 'cause you've asked. I always do what I'm told, almost....Well just to say that I'm doing it for this particular purpose. It's a good enough reason for me to do it (Patient10-SUR)

This may be due to an altruistic wish to help provide research data, an intention to improve one's own or other people's health, having a specific interest in the study or simply a desire to see a 'project' through once committed to it.

Interviewer: If we had asked you to walk an additional 30 minutes at a brisk pace every day, how would you feel about that?

Patient: Yes... Well I suppose if it was part of a trial, I'd, I'd do it for the, sort of, esoteric act of being part of a trial (Patient3-SUR)

I'm quite open to try anything, because....this is really an experiment that may benefit people in the future....to really benefit the people for the future as a younger generation....I thought if it could help someone in future years, it's well worth it (Patient14-RAD)

We also explored any anticipated negative aspects of participation in an intervention trial. Some men mentioned specific foods that they would find challenging to eat (one example given was curry) or would find hard to give up (such as cheese).

If I tried it and I liked it, I'd eat it, if I didn't like it, I wouldn't eat it (Patient1-SUR)

One participant explained that despite being committed, if asked to do something he did not wish to, it would be unlikely to happen.

Interviewer: If it's something you didn't like, is there any way to get you to do it?

Patient: You'd have to work hard [laughter]....

Interviewer: Are there any techniques we could use to get you to do something that you weren't keen on?

Partner: No, because I think, he would sort of, "Do you want to..?" "No". "Right, okay, I'm off, then." you've always been like that.

Patient: Always been like it, I think (Patient2 & Partner1-SUR)

The majority of men, and their partners, described busy lifestyles, including carrying out odd jobs, sitting and reading or 'pottering', and some were still in full time work. Generally, however, participants illustrated that it would not be a sacrifice, implied that they would be happy to make changes, and would try to find time to do so.

If you want to do something you always fit it in somewhere....you should hopefully lose a bit of weight, feel better, you know, so there's no real losses except a bit of time (Patient12-SUR)

Lifestyle intervention characteristics
Research data collection methods: Internet, phone and paper
There was a general mistrust regarding e-technology and online data collection.

Interviewer: So what about having records like that, on that kind of technology? Would that be okay?

Patient: I don't really know how these things work, but I am worried. I had a [company] phone and [the company] are beginning to worry me a bit 'cause they, they might well intercept and take all that information as well. [They] do take a lot of information in your transmission of data....

Partner: I don't use the computer at all. I think it's intrusive and dangerous (Patient4 & Partner2-SUR)

This sentiment was further illustrated by lack of use of social media, which was recommended for younger people, and was seen to be too intrusive.

I think it would appeal to ... the younger people. I mean, and I'm personally not on Twitter or Facebook (Patient3-SUR)

I don't take part in Twitter or, or any of those. They're for children aren't they, really? (Patient4-SUR)

That's a bit personal if you ask me. I'm not a Facebook person; I don't understand it, I don't understand it at all. I know how it works, but for me it just baffles me. I can't understand why somebody would write on Facebook, "Had a hard day at work, now I'm sat down drinking a cup of tea." I'm thinking, "Okay, fair enough. Why do you want to say that?" But people do, so it's just me being old fashioned I suppose (Patient7-SUR)

Some participants regularly used their mobile phone for sending text messages, kept it turned on and would be comfortable to use it for research purposes. However the majority of men said that they either did not own a mobile phone, they rarely turned it on, or they would not know how to respond to a text message.

Interviewer: Do you use electronic devices, at all? Do you have a mobile phone?

Patient: Yes, with difficulty. I've got a mobile phone....For emergencies only

Partner: He never uses it....

Patient: My phone's from the Ark. I dial, and I can text

Partner: It might take him several days to text [laughter]

Patient: It's not something that I am partial to doing. It's easier to go, "Hello?"....I've never got the phone on....I don't very often pick my phone up, you wouldn't get an answer. That's basically the bottom line (Patient2 & Partner1-SUR)

Participants were more positive about computers and email, appearing comfortable to open and reply to an email, download attachments and use a printer. Further to this, many mentioned that neighbours, or children, would be on hand to help out if necessary.

Oh, I use a computer, no problems at all with a computer, and you know, save paper, do it on the computer. I think that would be a good idea (Patient6-RAD)

Some participants did not have, or express a desire for, access to a computer or the internet. It was noted, that for the majority of the men, their preferred method of contact was via the post.

I think I'd rather have a booklet that you fill in. Like, you know, weekly, daily or... something you can actually write in (Patient5-SUR)

It should be noted that there did not appear to be any demographic or other differences between those who responded positively or negatively to e-technology.

Group versus individual interventions

Those men in favour of individual physical activity interventions enjoyed the peace and quiet of being alone, or believed that others could slow them down.

> *I think I probably would be able to motivate myself. But probably my wife would probably join in with me. She used to do a little bit of running, a little bit of running before with me, not as much, but she would probably be receptive to the idea. She'd probably say, "Yeah, I'll come along with you" (Patient9-SUR)*

Alternatively, those who preferred a group intervention felt that other members could motivate them, as well as providing social support.

> *If you did it as a, as a group activity. You could join a walking club or... Or, I think the medical practice here runs a sort of, a weekly, healthy walking morning or something....you get the, sort of, support of others. It's a, it's a mutual support organisation, isn't it, when you join something like that? (Patient3-SUR)*

In this particular population, participants tended to favour individual interventions, yet with added spousal or other social support.

Dietary modification through supplements

Some men were positive about a daily supplement; feeling that it was an easy, efficient way to provide additional nutritional content to their daily diet.

> *Interviewer: Do you take any supplements currently, either of you?*
>
> *Partner: You take cod liver oil...*
>
> *Interviewer: So you're quite comfortable taking supplements?*
>
> *Patient: Yeah.*
>
> *Partner: Oh yeah (Patient13 & Partner5-RAD)*

In contrast, others disagreed with taking supplements, and would not choose to do so in their general diet. There often appeared to be a sense of disbelief at their efficacy.

> *Eating a more of a natural food like tomatoes, I'd be more inclined to do than taking supplements. I try and avoid pills when I can (Patient3-SUR)*

> *As for supplements, I think they're a total waste of time personally....it's all about intake again. You know, like a lot of people I know take garlic, but if you eat three or four garlic cloves a week, and that's a lot more than what a tablet a day would do or a capsule a day would do, you know? It's all about intake and volume. And I'd rather eat the food what gives you those vitamins rather than take supplements (Patient11-SUR)*

However, all men reported that if they were randomised to a supplement in a research study, they would try to incorporate it into their daily routine.

Discussion

Men with localised prostate cancer, who were undergoing or had completed radical treatment, were generally open to lifestyle modification and were motivated to engage in positive health behaviours. This willingness may result from disbelief, shock or fear at diagnosis and the findings support previous literature, whereby a cancer diagnosis can result in positive behaviour change [3, 9, 10]. Receiving a diagnosis of prostate cancer is considered to be a potential 'teachable moment': a naturally occurring health event thought to motivate individuals to spontaneously adopt risk-reducing behaviours [19]. Our findings further substantiate the concept that the period following a cancer diagnosis may be an ideal opportunity to engage with patients to implement diet and physical activity interventions [20].

The men in this study identified the importance of family and friends in motivating them to embrace change, in line with previous findings [21]. As such, when planning behaviour change interventions it is imperative that men taking part are made aware of what additional support is available and where to seek it. Additionally, behaviour change interventions should be tailored, and enjoyable, so that an individual has personal motivation to change; although this may not always be possible for all individuals. Supplements can be an efficient way to enhance the positive nutritional elements that are consumed, where an individual may not like or be able to access a food type [22]. Our findings suggested that knowing that there is an evidence based reason to change, may help assist behaviour change maintenance, particularly if the proposed change is already acceptable to the individual.

Increasingly, research data are being collected using electronic methods, such as web based surveys, text message or social media [23–25]. This is especially true with nutritional data [26]. Engaging the target population with suitable data collection methods is essential, as is avoiding social media if it does not appear to be acceptable to the target population. This is of importance, as many new intervention programmes have a strong technological slant and not considering the accessibility or acceptability to the particular target population may compromise their effectiveness. As technology develops, it could be easy to assume that all research should be collected in such a manner and that research populations would prefer the most high-tech methodologies. However, this may not always be true, as illustrated by many of the current sample preferring to respond to paper based questionnaires. One must always be mindful of an individual's level of understanding, acceptance and ability to use the technology in question.

Identifying and finding solutions to potential barriers, such as poor weather, competing time commitments or physical limitations such as incontinence, prior to them arising, will make these barriers easier to overcome and less likely to reduce compliance. For example, poor weather could lead to reduced physical activity; however, suggesting participation in indoor physical activities, or swapping the day that the activity is completed on, to avoid poor weather, yet still reaching the week's intended activity levels, could prove successful. To alleviate incontinence related barriers, well-fitting and comfortable pads could be sourced or men could be supported in the practice of pelvic floor exercises; this could reduce the likelihood of incontinence being a barrier to change.

Elements of the current findings are in line with previous literature derived from men undergoing androgen deprivation therapy [10] and watchful waiting [9], such as the level of shock or disbelief experienced at diagnosis, being motivated to make changes to lifestyle behaviours and having a desire to engage in research. However differing and novel findings emerged from our target group of men undergoing radical prostatectomy or radiotherapy. Men were encouraging of partner support and welcomed input from friends and family, with a preferred emphasis for tailored individual interventions. The use of electronic methods to collect data was suggested to be a potential barrier to participation or change in some men, but not all, as were physical limitations, such as incontinence or underlying unrelated health complaints. Endorsement for change by clinicians was seen to be a motivator for change, along with understanding the rationale behind the suggested change.

Men with prostate cancer demonstrated great intention to commit to research, with few sacrifices identified. It should be considered that social desirability response bias may have been evident, where participants seek the approval of the researcher by trying to give the 'correct' answer [27]. Men often stated that they would intend to

change their behaviours if requested. However, an 'intention-behaviour gap' may exist; this is a social construct that attempts to understand the psychological processes underlying whether or not intentions are translated into action, where what one says he or she plans to do, is not always translated into behaviour [28].

Analysis must be interpreted with caution, as those who had agreed to be interviewed for the current qualitative research may not be representative of the general prostate cancer population. Additionally, this research involved an exclusively White British population and the convenience sampling technique may have resulted in a non-representative sample. However, the men had undergone a range of treatments and varied in age, education level and occupation status. Thus, the data reported are believed to be representative of Caucasian men with prostate cancer and their partners, across the UK. Future research should aim to explore more diverse populations, particularly with regards to ethnicity. It should be noted that there are differences between the experience of surgery and radiotherapy, and that men were at different stages of their treatment pathway, and this could have resulted in differing responses based on treatment mode, for example when referring to incontinence. Despite this however, differences in responses were not always split depending upon treatment type, suggesting relevant similarities were evident across the two treatment types. Future research should consider approaching patients either prior to treatment or at a fixed time after treatment. Additionally, we did not systematically record the dietary or physical activity habits of the participants, or record their current BMI. This may have influenced their responses to the discussion; however it was felt that this level of quantitative data collection was not appropriate for a qualitative study. Finally, we note that two interviewers conducted the interviews, across different locations. This may have influenced the data collection process, however, both interviewers were experienced qualitative researchers, the interview schedule was used during data collection and data triangulation was carried out throughout the data processing and analysis period.

Clinical implications

Lessons learnt can be implemented in clinical practice. The finding that men could be more likely to make changes if encouraged to do so by their clinician, is an ideal opportunity to engage with patients about such changes. Clinicians should be aware of potential barriers to behaviour change, possible solutions to such barriers should be discussed. The current sample were highly willing to participate in research, and clinicians should feel confident discussing research participation with their patients. These implications for practice are in line with the Living With and Beyond Cancer Programme [29], which resulted from the National Cancer Survivorship Initiative [29], and state that all cancer patients should have access to a holistic needs assessment, patient education and support, which should include post treatment management and the promotion of health and wellbeing, such as physical activity. With this support, new behaviours that are made may have a greater chance of lasting, and short-lived changes avoided [30].

Conclusion

Generally, men facing a prostate cancer diagnosis are willing to make changes to their diet and physical activity, and this potential teachable moment should be embraced. Social support, tailored enjoyable interventions and background knowledge should be incorporated into an intervention package. Potential barriers should be pre-empted, and addressed in advance. Data illustrated that the proposed intervention would be well received in this population, with support for an individual physical activity intervention, provision of supplements and involvement of a partner throughout. Of note was the novel finding that modern technology and use of social media may not be suitable to all research populations, and thus the individual characteristics of the target population need to be considered. This research will be used to inform the development of a diet and physical activity intervention which is acceptable to prostate cancer patients who have undergone treatment. The research has additionally provided further information about the attitudes of Caucasian British men with prostate cancer, and their experiences of and preferences for different aspects of behaviour change, which can be implemented into clinical practice.

Acknowledgements
We thank the men with prostate cancer, and their partners, for dedicating their time to the research and welcoming us into their homes; the urology and oncology consultants who provided access to their patients and support with recruitment; and the urology CNS nurses and those working at the urology clinic, for the specialist knowledge and support with recruitment. We additionally thank members of the Bristol National Institute for Health Research Biomedical Research Unit in Nutrition, Diet and Lifestyle Prostate Cancer Patient and Public Involvement group for their input during the developmental stages of this research.

Funding
The current research was funded by the National Institute for Health Research (NIHR) Bristol Nutrition Biomedical Research Unit based at University Hospitals Bristol NHS Foundation Trust and the University of Bristol. The views expressed are those of the authors and not necessarily those of the NHS, the NIHR or the Department of Health.
RMM and JAL are supported by a Cancer Research UK (C18281/A19169) programme grant (the Integrative Cancer Epidemiology Programme). The funding bodies had no role in design, collection, analysis or interpretation of data, writing of the manuscript or decision to submit the manuscript.

Authors' contributions
LHM contributed to conception and design, collected data, led the analysis and interpretation of data, drafted the manuscript and revised it critically for important intellectual content, ES contributed to collection of data, contributed to the analysis and interpretation of data, helped draft the manuscript and helped revise it critically for important intellectual content, RP contributed to collection of data and helped revise the manuscript critically for important intellectual content, JA contributed to collection of data and helped revise the manuscript critically for important intellectual content, AB contributed to collection of data and helped revise the manuscript critically for important intellectual content, AK contributed to collection of data and helped revise the manuscript critically for important intellectual content, CM contributed to analysis and interpretation of data, RMM contributed to conception and design, analysis and interpretation of data and helped revise the manuscript critically for important intellectual content, JAL contributed to conception and design, analysis and interpretation of data and helped revise the manuscript critically for important intellectual content. All authors read, approved and agree to be accountable for the final manuscript.

Competing interests
The authors declare that they have no competing interests.

Author details
[1]University of Bristol, NIHR Biomedical Research Centre - Nutrition, Diet and Lifestyle Theme, Level 3, University Hospitals Bristol Education Centre, Upper Maudlin Street, Bristol BS2 8AE, England, UK. [2]University of Bristol, Bristol Medical School: Population Health Sciences, Canynge Hall, 39 Whatley Road, Bristol BS8 2PS, England, UK. [3]Bristol Urological Institute, Southmead Hospital Bristol, Southmead Road, Westbury-on-Trym, Bristol BS10 5NB, England, UK. [4]Freeman Hospital, Freeman Road, Newcastle upon Tyne, Tyne and Wear NE7 7DN, England, UK. [5]Bristol Haematology & Oncology Centre, Horfield Road, Bristol BS2 8ED, England, UK. [6]Member of the NIHR Biomedical Research Centre - Nutrition, Diet and Lifestyle Theme Prostate Cancer Patient and Public Involvement Group, Bristol, England, UK.

References
1. Cancer Research UK. Cancer incidence for common cancers. 2014. http://www.cancerresearchuk.org/health-professional/cancer-statistics/incidence/common-cancers-compared. Accessed 1 June 2015.
2. American Cancer Society. In: American Cancer Society, editor. Cancer facts and figures. Atlanta; 2008.
3. Demark-Wahnefried W, Aziz NM, Rowland JH, Pinto BM. Riding the crest of the teachable moment: promoting long-term health after the diagnosis of cancer. J Clin Oncol. 2005;23(24):5814–30.
4. Kenfield SA, Stampfer MJ, Giovannucci E, Chan JM. Physical activity and survival after prostate cancer diagnosis in the health professionals follow-up study. J Clin Oncol. 2011;29(6):726–32.
5. WCRF. Diet, nutrition, physical activity and prostate cancer. London: World Cancer Research Fund International; 2014.
6. Avery KN, Donovan JL, Gilbert R, Davis M, Emmett P, Down L, et al. Men with prostate cancer make positive dietary changes following diagnosis and treatment. Cancer Causes Control. 2013;24(6):1119–28.
7. Hackshaw-McGeagh L, Penfold CM, Walsh E, Donovan JL, Hamdy FC, Neal DE, et al. Physical activity, alcohol consumption, BMI and smoking status before and after prostate cancer diagnosis in the ProtecT trial: opportunities for lifestyle modification. Int J Cancer. 2015;137(6):1509–15.
8. Hackshaw-McGeagh L, Perry R, Leach V, Qandil S, Jeffreys M, Martin R, et al. A systematic review of dietary, nutritional and physical activity interventions for the prevention of prostate cancer progression and mortality. Cancer Causes Control. 2015; doi:10.1007/s10552-015-0659-4.
9. Kronenwetter C, Weidner G, Pettengill E, Marlin R, Crutchfield L, McCormac P, et al. A qualitative analysis of interviews of men with early stage prostate cancer: the prostate cancer lifestyle trial. Cancer Nurs. 2005;28(2):99–107.

10. Bourke L, Sohanpal R, Nanton V, Crank H, Rosario DJ, Saxton JMA. Qualitative study evaluating experiences of a lifestyle intervention in men with prostate cancer undergoing androgen suppression therapy. Trials. 2012;13:208.

11. Regan T, Lambert S, Girgis A, Kelly B, Turner J, Kayser K. Do couple-based interventions make a difference for couples affected by cancer? A systematic review. BMC Cancer. 2012;12(279) doi:10.1186/1471-2407-12-279.

12. Freedland SJ, Humphreys EB, Mangold LA, Eisenberger M, Dorey FJ, Walsh PC, et al. Risk of prostate cancer-specific mortality following biochemical recurrence after radical prostatectomy. JAMA. 2005;294(4):433–9.

13. Aziz NM, Rowland JH. Trends and advances in cancer survivorship research: challenge and opportunity. Semin Radiat Oncol. 2003;13(3):248–66.

14. Craig P, Dieppe P, Macintyre S, Michie S, Nazareth I, Petticrew M. Developing and evaluating complex interventions: the new Medical Research Council guidance. Int J Nurs Stud. 2013;50(5):587–92.

15. Bowling A, Ebrahim S. Handbook of health research methods. Investigation, measurement and analysis. Berkshire: Open University Press; 2006.

16. Ritchie J, Spencer L. Qualitative data analysis for applied policy research. London: Sage Publications; 2002.

17. Sutton E, Hackshaw-McGeagh LE, Aning J, et al. The provision of dietary and physical activity advice for men diagnosed with prostate cancer: a qualitative study of the experiences and views of health care professionals, patients and partners. Cancer Causes Control. 2017;28:319. https://doi.org/10.1007/s10552-017-0861-7.

18. Burleson BR. The experience and effects of emotional support: what the study of cultural and gender differences can tell us about close relationships, emotion, and interpersonal communication. Pers Relat. 2003;10(1):1–23.

19. McBride CM, Emmons KM, Lipkus IM. Understanding the potential of teachable moments: the case of smoking cessation. Health Educ Res. 2003;18(2):156–70.

20. Demark-Wahnefried W, Peterson B, McBride C, Lipkus I, Clipp E. Current health behaviors and readiness to pursue life-style changes among men and women diagnosed with early stage prostate and breast carcinomas. Cancer. 2000;88(3):674–84.

21. Stacey FG, James EL, Chapman K, Courneya KS, Lubans DRA. Systematic review and meta-analysis of social cognitive theory-based physical activity and/or nutrition behavior change interventions for cancer survivors. J Cancer Surviv. 2014;9:305–38.

22. Ward E. Addressing nutritional gaps with multivitamin and mineral supplements. Nutr J. 2014;13:72.

23. Coons SJ, Eremenco S, Lundy JJ, O'Donohoe P, O'Gorman H, Malizia W. Capturing patient-reported outcome (PRO) data electronically: the past, present, and promise of ePRO measurement in clinical trials. Patient. 2014;8(4):301–9.

24. Brabyn S, Adamson J, MacPherson H, Tilbrook H, Torgerson DJ. Short message service text messaging was feasible as a tool for data collection in a trial of treatment for irritable bowel syndrome. J Clin Epidemiol. 2014;67(9):993–1000.

25. Cavallo DN, Chou WY, McQueen A, Ramirez A, Riley WT. Cancer prevention and control interventions using social media: user-generated approaches. Cancer Epidemiol Biomark Prev. 2014;23(9):1953–6.

26. Carter MC, Burley VJ, Nykjaer C, Cade JE. Adherence to a smartphone application for weight loss compared to website and paper diary: pilot randomized controlled trial. J Med Internet Res. 2013;15(4):e32.

27. Krumpal I. Determinants of social desirability bias in sensitive surveys: a literature review. Qual Quant. 2013;47:2025–47.

28. Sheeran P. Intention—behavior relations: a conceptual and empirical review. Eur Rev Soc Psychol. 2002;12(1):1–36.

29. Department of Health, Macmillan Cancer Support and NHS Improvement. Living with and beyond cancer: Taking action to improve outcomes (an update to the 2010 The National Cancer Survivorship Initiative Vision). London: Department of Health; 2013.

30. Galvão DA, Newton RU, Gardiner RA, Girgis A, Lepore SJ, Stiller A, Occhipinti S, Chambers SK. Compliance to exercise-oncology guidelines in prostate cancer survivors and associations with psychological distress, unmet supportive care needs, and quality of life. Psychooncology. 2015;24:1241–9. doi:10.1002/pon.3882.

Pattern of varicocele vein blood gases in patients undergoing microsurgical Varicocelectomy

Khaleeq ur Rehman[1*], Hafsa Zaneb[2], Abdul Basit Qureshi[3], Ahsan Numan[4], Muhammad Shahbaz Yousaf[5], Imtiaz Rabbani[5] and Habib Rehman[5]

Abstract

Background: Varicocele is known to be associated with infertility and sperm disorders. The exact cause of this ailment is not fully understood. There are limited numbers of studies where venous blood gases (VBGs) of varicocele veins were determined with conflicting results. Therefore, we have investigated the pattern of VBGs in both internal spermatic and external spermatic varicocele veins and correlation with semen quality parameters in infertile individuals who underwent left microsurgical varicocelectomy.

Methods: Patients ($n = 27$) undergoing left microsurgical varicocelectomy at a tertiary care hospital, were included in the study. Before surgery, semen parameters and scrotal color Doppler ultrasonography was performed. During surgery, blood sample was drawn from varicocele veins (internal spermatic and external spermatic veins) and a peripheral arm vein of the same patient as a control. The VBGs of all veins under study were estimated and compared with each other. The VBGs were also correlated with various semen quality parameters. Data, expressed as Mean ± SD, regarding VBGs in three veins were analyzed using one-way ANOVA. The correlation between VBGs and semen quality parameters was determined using Pearson's correlation. Differences were considered significant at $p < 0.05$.

Results: The pH was found to be higher ($p < 0.01$) in the internal spermatic vein compared with the external spermatic and the peripheral veins. Partial pressure of oxygen (pO_2) and oxygen saturation (sO_2) were higher ($p < 0.01$) in the internal spermatic vein compared with the peripheral vein. However, concentration of bicarbonate ($HCO_{3)}$) was lower ($p < 0.01$) in both veins compared with the peripheral vein. Partial pressure of carbon dioxide (pCO_2) was also lower ($p < 0.01$) in the varicocele veins compared with the control vein.

Conclusion: The internal spermatic veins had higher pH and oxygen tension, but lower HCO_3 and pCO_2 levels compared with the control peripheral veins. External spermatic veins had lower pCO_2 and HCO_3 but other VBGs were similar to the peripheral veins. The shift of VBGs of internal spermatic vein toward arterial blood pattern may be a missing link to understand the pathophysiology of varicocele.

Keywords: Venous blood gases, Varicocele, Scrotal Doppler ultrasonography, Infertility, Testicular blood flow

* Correspondence: khaleeqr@hotmail.com
[1]Department of Urology & Andrology, FMH College of Medicine & Dentistry, Shadman, Lahore, Pakistan
Full list of author information is available at the end of the article

Background

Varicocele is known to be associated with infertility and sperm disorders. Most researchers believe that renospermatic reflux is the main mechanism behind all mal-effects of varicocele [1–6]. There is a possibility that varicocele has various types that exert influence through different mechanisms. We have already reported an interesting example of varicocele that appeared in 23% hypogonadotropic hypogonadism patients after treatment with gonadotropins [7]. The variable behaviour of varicocele on spermatogenesis is intriguing and far from being understood. Why some individuals with varicocele develop sperm disorders but others don't is not clear. It appears that some other mechanisms coexist. A previous experimental study described the presence of an arteriovenous communications between testicular artery and adjacent veins [8]. In spermatic cord of bull, when gas was pushed into the testicular venous system, it could be recovered from the arterial side [9]. Arteriovenous anastomosis has been reported in human spermatic cord as well [10]. It was reported that a periarterial capillary network exists that connects the human testicular artery with adjacent pampiniform plexus [11–13]. These findings have not been given due importance. Based on the animal experimental studies mentioned, we presumed that these types of communications might be present in the human varicocele veins and subsequently may change VBG patterns of varicocele veins. There are only a limited numbers of studies where VBGs of the varicocele veins of testes were determined. These studies had unfortunately conflicting results [14–16]. To the best of our knowledge, there is no study that describes the VBGs profile of both internal and external spermatic varicocele veins in a single subject and its relation with semen quality. Therefore, the present study aimed at investigating the profile of VBGs in the varicocele veins (internal spermatic and external spermatic veins) of infertile individuals and to compare these variables with peripheral vein blood from the same individual undergoing left microsurgical varicocelectomy. Attempts were also carried out to explore a possible correlation between various variables of VBGs and semen quality parameters like semen volume, appearance, sperm count, progressive and non-progressive sperm motility and sperm morphology.

Methods

Subjects

Twenty-seven consecutive patients diagnosed with infertility and varicocele, undergoing microsurgical varicocelectomy under spinal anaesthesia, were included in the study after informed written consent. The calculated sample size was 23 using the following equation:

$N = [(Z_\alpha + Z_\beta)/C]^2 + 3$. The values for α (two tailed), β and r were 0.050, 0.300 and 0.500 respectively.

The study was approved by the Institutional Review Board of Fatima Memorial Hospital, College of Medicine & Dentistry Lahore-Pakistan.

Study design

Twenty to 45 years-old individuals with Grade 2 or 3 varicocele [17] having varicocele vein diameter of > 2.5 mm on scrotal color Doppler ultrasonography (CDUS) [18] with at least 1-year of infertility were included in the study. Semen analysis was carried out at least twice to confirm semen disorders. Patients with any chronic illness (hepatitis C or B, cardiac or pulmonary disorders), on prolonged drugs having side effects for spermatogenesis (e.g., antiviral drugs, chemotherapeutic agents), hormonal disorders (hypogonadism, hypothyroidism etc.), on prolonged antidepressants or drugs addicts were excluded from study. Patients with male or female sexual dysfunction leading to decreased frequency of intercourse (less than twice per week) and patients with significant female factor infertility were also excluded from the study.

Semen collection and analysis

Semen samples were collected at 3–4 days of abstinence and were processed for determination of semen quality parameters (semen volume, appearance, sperm count, progressive and non-progressive motility, morphology and other microscopic details) as suggested by the World Health Organization [19].

Scrotal ultrasonography for varicocele and scrotal contents

Scrotal CDUS was performed (Voluson General Electronics 30) using 10 mHz linear probe [20]. Briefly, grey scale ultrasonography was done to detect any other associated abnormality. Testicular and epididymal diameters were noted. Using CDUS, peak systolic velocities (PSVs) and resistive indices (RIs) of the subcapsular and intraparenchymal branches of testicular artery were determined. Diameter and backflow status of varicocele veins was recorded in lying and standing position. Subinguinal microsurgical varicocelectomy was performed as per standard practice [20, 21] under spinal anaesthesia.

Acquisition of blood gases

During surgery just before ligation of varicocele veins, 2.0 mL blood was drawn with a 27G needle inserted towards the direction of testes, in a heparinized syringe, from 1 to 2 internal spermatic veins and from external spermatic vein if found dilated (> 2.5 mm diameter). Peripheral blood sample from same individual was also drawn simultaneously from the wrist vein as a control. The patients did not receive oxygen inhalation at the time of blood sampling as well as for the previous 15 min at minimum. All patients maintained 97% or more oxygen saturation at room air. The blood samples were taken free of air, sealed, and blood gas analysis was performed immediately with a blood-gas analyser (Cobas b 121–Hoffmann La Roche, Inc., Germany). The pH, partial pressure of oxygen (pO_2), partial pressure of carbon dioxide (pCO_2), oxygen saturation (sO_2), and bicarbonate (HCO_3) values were determined.

Statistical methods

Data are represented as mean ± standard deviation. Means values of VBGs in all 3 veins were compared with one-way analysis of variance using SPSS software (SPSS Inc., USA). Tukey's post hoc test was carried out to identify individual differences. The Pearson correlation test was employed to determine correlations between different variables. Level of significance was set at $p < 0.05$.

Results

Out of twenty-seven patients, twenty-three (85.18%) had G2 varicocele and 4 (14.8%) had G3 varicocele. Age of

the patients ranged from 20 to 43 (29.38 ± 7.94) years. Ten (37.04%) patients were 20–30 years old, 13 (48.15%) were between 31 to 40 years and 4 (14.81%) patients were 41–43 years old. Most of them (81.48%) were non-smokers.

Baseline semen and scrotal CDUS findings

The mean diameters of the varicocele veins of the patients were 3.40 ± 0.86 mm and 3.74 ± 0.86 mm at lying and standing positions, respectively. The PSV and RI of subcapsular and intraparenchymal artery along with testicular volume are summarized in Table 1. The semen quality parameters in terms of sperm count, progressive motility, non-progressive motility, immotililty, and morphology of spermatozoa of the studied individuals were 33.45 ± 27.78 × 10^6 per mL, 16.89 ± 14.4%, 17.59 ± 13.49%, 58.11 ± 27.43%, and 7.11 ± 7.00% respectively (Table 1). Among semen parameters, sperm morphology had significant correlation ($r = 0.463$; $p < 0.05$) with PSV of subcapsular artery of left testes, testicular volume ($p < 0.05$, $r = 0.407$) and transverse diameter of testes. ($p < 0.05$; $r = 0.439$). Sperm count had significant negative correlation ($r = -0.76$; $p < 0.05$) with RI of left

Table 1 Baseline characteristics of various parameters of varicocele patients ($n = 27$)

Variables	Mean	±SD	Minimum	Maximum
Sperm count (million/mL)	33.45	27.78	0.01	110.00
Progressive motility (%)	16.89	14.47	0.00	60.00
Non progressive motility (%)	17.59	13.49	0.00	48.00
Immotile (%)	58.11	27.43	0.01	100.00
Morphology (%)	7.11	7.01	1.00	25.00
Right transverse epididymal diameter (mm)	7.54	1.99	4.40	11.70
Left transverse epididymal diameter (mm)	7.51	1.67	5.30	11.50
Left Varicocele Lying (mm)	3.40	0.86	2.40	4.60
Left Varicocele Standing (mm)	3.74	0.95	2.50	5.80
Follicle Stimulating Hormone (mIU/ml)	6.44	4.23	2.5	21
Right longitudinal diameter of testes (mm)	41.15	3.90	32.00	48.00
Right transverse diameter of testes (mm)	21.00	2.66	17.00	28.00
Left longitudinal diameter of testes (mm)	40.11	3.89	32.00	48.00
Left transverse diameter of testes (mm)	20.33	2.80	16.00	27.00
Left testicular volume (mL)	8.9	2.96	4.93	14.41
Right PSV of sub capsular artery (cm/sec)	6.35	1.95	3.43	11.39
Left PSV of sub capsular artery (cm/sec)	6.36	1.28	4.22	9.50
Right PSV of intra parenchymal artery (cm/sec)	4.95	1.03	3.43	8.20
Left PSV of intra parenchymal artery (cm/sec)	5.46	1.67	3.37	11.71
Right RI of sub capsular artery	0.75	1.07	.35	6.10
Left I RI of sub capsular artery	0.54	0.08	.32	.70
Right RI of intra parenchymal artery	0.52	0.07	.40	.67
Left RI of intra parenchymal artery	0.49	0.14	.26	1.00

PSV peak systolic velocity; *RI* resistive index

intraparenchymal artery, whereas progressive motility of sperms had negative correlation ($r = -0.498$; $p < 0.01$) with RI of left intraparenchymal artery as well as RI of left subcapsular artery ($r = -0.505$; $p < 0.01$) (Table 2). On comparison between varicocele diameter and semen parameters, no correlations were appreciated.

VBGs analysis

Table 3 summarizes the comparison of various parameters of VBGs analysis of varicocele veins (internal and external spermatic) with the peripheral vein. Generally, the changes in VBG determinants were more pronounced in the internal spermatic vein than in the peripheral vein. The pH was higher ($p < 0.01$) in the internal spermatic vein compared with the external spermatic and the peripheral veins. The pO_2 and sO_2 were elevated ($p < 0.01$) in the internal spermatic vein compared with the peripheral vein. Serum HCO_3 concentration was lower ($p < 0.01$) in both internal and external spermatic veins compared with the peripheral vein. The pCO_2 was also lower ($p < 0.01$) in both varicocele veins compared with the peripheral veins (Table 3). There was no significant correlation between various parameters of VBGs of both internal and external spermatic varicocele veins with their respective testicular blood flow, semen quality parameters and the diameter of varicocele veins and testicular volume (data not shown).

Discussion

The current study demonstrates unique characteristics of the VBGs of internal spermatic varicocele veins, which are different from the peripheral veins. The internal spermatic veins have higher pH, sO_2, and pO_2 levels but lower HCO_3 and pCO_2 levels in comparison to the peripheral vein. On the other hand, the external spermatic varicocele veins revealed different VBGs profile that was similar to the peripheral veins, except lower HCO_3 and pCO_2 levels. Previously, between 1968 and 1989, there were only three studies that addressed the composition of venous blood in varicocele veins [14–16]. However, there were conflicting results. Today,

we have better methods of measuring blood gas levels and a better opportunity of measuring VBGs during the microsurgical varicocelectomy. This procedure is performed under microsurgical magnification and allows isolation of individual groups of veins thus providing better opportunity of precise blood sampling from different groups of varicocele veins before their ligation. In current study, the VBGs analysis was determined from venous blood, drawn individually from the internal spermatic varicocele veins, the external spermatic varicocele veins, and the peripheral vein. A single surgeon, who is also the principal investigator, performed all the procedures and was blinded to the results until the end of study.

Our results have shown a clear shift of VBGs profile of the internal spermatic veins toward an arterial pattern. The exact mechanism is not clear, but renospermatic backflow, low oxygen consumption due to lower testicular function, or the presence of arterio-venous communications may be a possible clue to this change. There are a few human and multiple animal studies that demonstrate the presence of an arterio-venous shunt in the spermatic cord and testes [8–12]. Based on the available anatomical findings reported in literature [8–12], we suspected that varicocele veins might have different venous composition of blood gases than the classical VBG levels. At the completion of study, it was confirmed that sO_2 and pO_2 levels were significantly higher in the internal spermatic varicocele vein compared with the peripheral vein. Nevertheless, further anatomical documentation of an arterial venous shunt mechanism is still required. Donhue and Brown reported in 1969 that the internal spermatic veins of varicocele patients had higher oxygen tension when the blood was drawn from the vein by inserting cannula in the direction of kidney. Anyhow this was not seen when the cannula was directed towards the testes. The authors proposed that the reflux of renal blood might be responsible for this mechanism [15]. In our experience, although we have drawn blood by inserting cannula towards the direction of testes, still we have observed higher oxygen tension in venous blood of internal spermatic veins. In contrast to our

Table 2 Correlation coefficient (r) between semen quality parameters and testicular blood flow in varicocele patients (n = 27)

Variable	Sub capsular artery				Intra parenchymal artery			
	Peak systolic velocity		Resistive index		Peak systolic velocity		Resistive index	
	r	p-value	r	p-value	R	p-value	r	p-value
Sperm count (million/mL)	0.329	0.094	−0.194	0.332	0.001	0.998	−0.76	0.012
Progressive motility (%)	0.094	0.640	−0.505	0.007	−0.160	0.424	−0.498	0.008
Non-progressive motility (%)	0.209	0.296	−0.194	0.333	−0.098	0.626	−0.325	0.098
Immotile (%)	0.220	0.270	0.291	0.141	0.226	0.258	0.206	0.304
Morphology (%)	0.463	−0.015	−0.157	0.43	0.14	0.48	−0.152	0.45

Table 3 Comparison of venous blood gas analysis of varicocele veins with peripheral vein

Items	Veins			p-value
	Internal spermatic n = 27	External spermatic n = 9	Peripheral n = 22	
pH	7.38 ± 0.04[a]	7.34 ± 0.05[b]	7.34 ± 0.04[b]	0.004
pO$_2$ (mm of Hg)	86.36 ± 40.47[a]	49.98 ± 7.45[b]	52.64 ± 34.01[b]	0.002
sO$_2$ (%)	91.02 ± 7.18[a]	81.24 ± 7.30[ab]	71.06 ± 18.60[b]	< 0.001
pCO$_2$ (mm of Hg)	36.87 ± 7.02[b]	40.03 ± 6.58[b]	46.47 ± 7.55[a]	< 0.001
HCO$_3$ (mEq/L)	21.4 ± 3.53[b]	21.23 ± 2.91[b]	24.60 ± 3.19[a]	0.003

Values (mean ± SD) with different superscripts in a same row differ significantly. p and s stand for partial pressure and saturation respectively. n shows the number of blood samples analyzed

findings, Yan reported in 1989 that oxygen saturation was lower in varicocele veins, and suggested that hypoxemia and metabolic acidosis affected spermatogenic function [16]. There is a possibility that the authors might have taken samples from the most accessible external spermatic veins. These veins exhibit lesser increase in intravenous pressure on valsalva compared to internal spermatic veins [22] and have oxygen tension similar to the peripheral veins.

In order to understand the significance of these findings, we determined the correlation of VBGs with testicular blood flow and semen parameters but no significant correlation was found.

Conclusion
Internal spermatic varicocele veins have significantly higher oxygen content and pH but lower HCO$_3$ and pCO$_2$ compared with the peripheral veins. The clinical importance of VBGs is difficult to ignore and the above-mentioned variation in blood gases may be a missing link or this may be another possible cause of higher intravenous pressure in these veins, to understand the pathophysiology of varicocele [22]. Further investigations are required to determine the significance of these findings.

Abbreviations
CDUS: Scrotal Color Doppler ultrasonography; HCO$_3$: Bicarbonate; pCO$_2$: Partial Pressure of Carbon dioxide; pO$_2$: Partial Pressure of Oxygen; PSVs: Peak Systolic Velocities; RIs: Resistive Indices; sO$_2$: Oxygen Saturation; VBGs: Venous Blood Gases

Acknowledgements
We are thankful to Mr. Khalid Mahmood Anjum for statistical analysis of the data.

Funding
There was no source of funding except self-funding by the researchers.

Declaration
We have obtained proper ethical approval from institutional research board, Fatima memorial hospital, College of Medicine and Dentistry Lahore and written consent was taken from all the participants of the study

Authors' contributions
The study was designed and conceptualized by KUR, HZ, HR, ABQ, MSY, surgical procedure was performed by KUR, acquisition and interpretation of data by KUR, ABQ, AN, HR, HZ drafting of article along with intellectual input were provided by KUR, HZ, HR, ABQ, MSY, IR, AN and HR. All authors read and approved the final manuscript.

Competing interests
There are no competing interests of any author.

Author details
^{1}Department of Urology & Andrology, FMH College of Medicine & Dentistry, Shadman, Lahore, Pakistan. ^{2}Department of Anatomy and Histology, University of Veterinary and Animal Sciences, Lahore, Pakistan. ^{3}Department of Surgery, Services Institute of Medical Sciences, Lahore, Pakistan. ^{4}Department of Neurology, Services Institute of Medical Sciences, Lahore, Pakistan. ^{5}Department of Physiology, University of Veterinary and Animal Sciences, Lahore, Pakistan.

References
1. Hundeiker M. Why is the high ligation of Palomo and not the varicocele operation the therapy of choice in the treatment of fertility disorders due to varicocele? Hautarzt. 1970;21(1):37.
2. Kupriianov V. Structural dynamics of the microcirculation pathways. Arkh Patol. 1971;33(7):15–23.
3. Kim V. Pathogenesis of varicose veins in the spermatic cord. Khirurgiia. 1987;8:82.
4. Dobanovački D. Varicocele in adolescents. Med Pregl. 2010;63(11–12):741–6.
5. Gat Y, Gornish M, Navon U, Chakraborty J, Bachar GN, Ben-Shlomo I. Right varicocele and hypoxia, crucial factors in male infertility: fluid mechanics analysis of the impaired testicular drainage system. Reprod BioMed Online. 2006;13(4):510–5.
6. Reyes JG, Farias JG, Henríquez-Olavarrieta S, Madrid E, Parraga M, Zepeda AB, et al. The hypoxic testicle: physiology and pathophysiology. Oxidative Med Cell Longev. 2012;2012.
7. ur Rehman K, Shahid K, Humayun H. Hypogonadotropic hypogonadism: new identification of testicular blood flow and varicocele after treatment with gonadotropins. Fertil Steril. 2014;102(3):700–4. e1.
8. Weerasooriya TR, Yaniamoto T. Three-dimensional organisation of the vasculature of the rat spermatic cord and testis. Cell Tissue Res. 1985;241(2):317–23.
9. Sørensen H, Lambrechtsen J, Einer-Jensen N. Efficiency of the countercurrent transfer of heat and 133Xenon between the pampiniform plexus and testicular artery of the bull under in-vitro conditions. Int J Androl. 1991;14(3):232–40.
10. Ergün S, Bruns T, Soyka A, Tauber R. Angioarchitecture of the human spermatic cord. Cell Tissue Res. 1997;288(2):391–8.
11. Armellino M, Romano G, Imperato L, Rispoli G. Surgical therapy of varicocele. Technical note on the inguinal approach. Minerva Chir. 1999; 54(5):367–71.

12. Skowroński A, Jędrzejewski K. The human testicular artery and the pampiniform plexus-where is the connection? Folia Morphol (Warsz). 2003; 62(3):201–4.
13. Alexandre-Pires G, Mateus L, Martins C, Ferreira-Dias G. Seasonal changes in testes vascularisation in the domestic cat (Felis domesticus): evaluation of microvasculature, angiogenic activity, and endothelial cell expression. Anat Res Int. 2012;2012.
14. Free M, VanDemark N. Gas tensions in spermatic and peripheral blood of rams with normal and heat-treated testes. Am J Phys. 1968;214(4):863–5.
15. Donohue RE, Brown JS. Blood gases and pH determinations in the internal spermatic veins of subfertile men with varicocele. Fertil Steril. 1969;20(2):365–9.
16. Yan C. Blood gas analysis of varicocele, spermatic vein and peripheral vein. Zhonghua Wai Ke Za Zhi. 1989;27(1):37–8 62.
17. Organization WH. Comparison among different methods for the diagnosis of varicocele. Fertil Steril. 1985;43(4):575–82.
18. Hussein AF. The role of color Doppler ultrasound in prediction of the outcome of microsurgical subinguinal varicocelectomy. J Urol. 2006;176(5):2141–5.
19. Organization WH. WHO laboratory manual for the examination and processing of human semen. Switzerland: WHO press; 2010.
20. Tarhan S, Ucer O, Sahin MO, Gumus B. Long-term effect of microsurgical inguinal Varicocelectomy on testicular blood flow. J Androl. 2011;32(1):33–9.
21. Mehta A, Goldstein M. Microsurgical varicocelectomy: a review. Asian J Androl. 2013;15(1):56.
22. Ur Rehman K, Qureshi AB, Numan A, Zaneb H, Yousaf MS, Rabbani I, Rehman H. Pressure flow pattern of varicocele veins and its correlation with testicular blood flow and semen parameters. Andrologia. 2017 Aug 2. https://doi.org/10.1111/and.12856. [Epub ahead of print] PubMed PMID: 28766734.

25

Evaluation and treatment for ovotesticular disorder of sex development (OT-DSD)

Yu Mao[1], Shaoji Chen[1], Ru Wang[2], Xuejun Wang[1], Daorui Qin[1] and Yunman Tang[1*]

Abstract

Background: The aim of this study is to review and present the clinical features and process of evaluation and treatment for OT-DSD in a single center in recent years in China.

Methods: Sixteen patients with OT-DSD during the past 4 years underwent the evaluation and treatment in a single center. The clinical characteristics and outcomes of surgery were analyzed.

Results: The surgical age ranged from 17 months to 66 months with a mean age of 20 months, and the mean follow-up was 30 months (4 months to 56 months). The presentation in 11 patients was ambiguous genitalia, and the rest 5 patients were suspected to have DSD in preoperative examination before hypospadias repair. The karyotypes were 46, XX in 11 patients, 46, XX/46, XY in 3, 46, XX/47, XXY in 1, and 46, XY in 1. Initial reared sex was male in 14 patients, female in 1, and undetermined in 1. After surgery, genders were reassigned in 3 patients, while 15 patients were raised as male with testicular tissue left. Only 1 patient with ovarian tissue left was raised as female. Repair was completed in 11 males and 1 female, and stage I urethroplasty was done in 4 males. No further surgery to remove the gonads was needed for inconsonance of gender assignment. No gonadal tumors were detected.

Conclusions: OT-DSD is a rare and complex deformity with few systematic reports in China. It's important to establish a regular algorithm for evaluation and treatment of OT-DSD.

Keywords: Ovotestis, Hypospadias, Urethroplasty, Disorder of sex development

Background

The nomenclature ovotesticular disorder of sex development (OT-DSD) has replaced the obsolete one, true hermaphroditism, since 2006 [1]. It is defined by the presence of testicular tissue with well-developed seminiferous tubules and ovarian tissue with primordial follicles in the same individual. These tissues may be co-existent in the same gonad (ovotestis) or independently the ovary on one side and the testicle on the other). The incidence is rare, accounting for nearly 3 to 10% of DSD cases [2]. The external genitalia show variable phenotypes, ranging from a normal male to a normal female presentation. However, ambiguous genitalia is the most common manifestation as noted in 90% of the cases [3]. The deformed genitalia compromises psychosocial as well as physiological health of the patients and their families. In China, data are in great need on the clinical features, assessing modalities, surgical procedures and outcomes, and the prognosis in the involved patients. We share the features of OT-DSD in our recent series.

Methods

From September 2011 to December 2015, 16 patients with OT-DSD were evaluated and treated in our hospital. As shown in Fig. 1, the procedure for diagnosis and management of OT-DSD was step by step, as first collection of clinical data, second chromosomal and endocrinal assessment, third multidisciplinary team (MDT) consultation, then surgical & histopathological confirmation of gonads nature with gender assignment, gonad(s) removal and genital plastic surgery in accordance

* Correspondence: toil112@163.com
[1]Department of Pediatric Surgery of Children's Medical Center, Sichuan Academy of Medical Sciences & Sichuan Provincial People's Hospital, Chengdu, China
Full list of author information is available at the end of the article

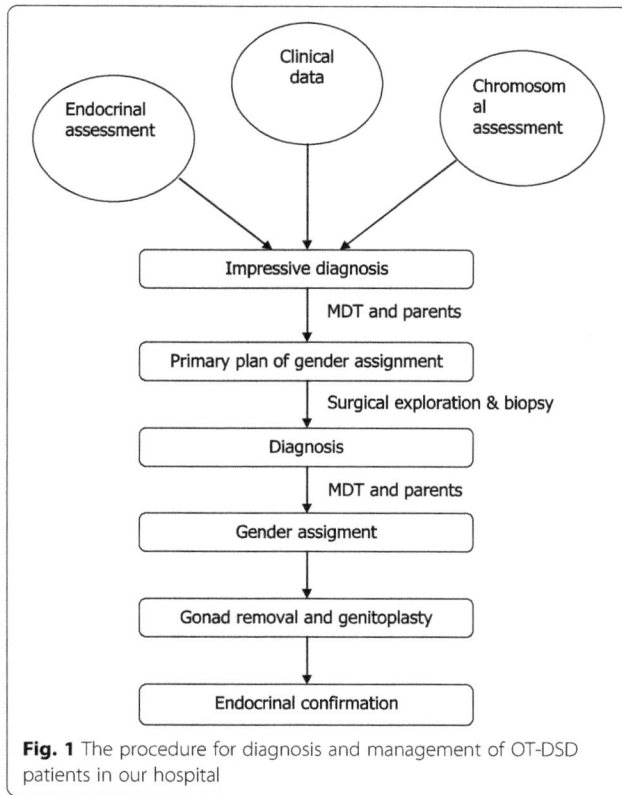

Fig. 1 The procedure for diagnosis and management of OT-DSD patients in our hospital

with assigned gender. The final diagnosis depended on gonadal histopathology.

Clinical data included age, rearing gender, medical history, physical examination, imaging and screening of associated anomalies. Prader grading of the external genitalia and palpation of gonads are of essential importance in physical examination. Although the diagnostic accuracy of the internal genital organs was unsatisfactory via ultrasonography and MRI [4, 5], we still used these imaging modalities to characterize urogenital system before surgery.

Karyotype analysis was detected from the peripheral blood in all patients.

Although the diagnosis depended on histopathological findings, we utilized biochemical examination and human chorionicgonadotropin (HCG) test to distinguish OT-DSD from other DSDs before surgery. Before HCG test, serum testosterone (T), luteinizing hormone (LH), follicle stimulation hormone (FSH), anti-müllerian hormone (AMH), InhibinB, 17-hydroxyprogesterone (17-OHP), androstenedione, and sex hormone binding globulin (SHBG) were detected. Consecutive HCG injection, a dose of 100 units/kg/day, was indicated for 3 days. At the 4th day, T, LH, FSH, androstenedione, SHBG, and dihydrotestosterone (DHT) were detected again. The T concentration after HCG stimulation of higher than 200 ng/dl was

defined as a normal response, 100 to 200 ng/dl as a borderline response, lower than 100 ng/dl as a poor response.

Patient's data were submitted to MDT, including pediatric endocrinologist, andrologist, gynecologist, pediatric urologist, geneticists, pathologist, psychologist, and medical ethics committee, for consultation. Then the parents were involved in the discussion of possible gender assignment.

Surgery included 3 parts. A cystoscopy with a 3Fr catheter was used to measure the length of urogenital sinus, water-filled vagina and the distance from the bladder neck to the vagina meatus, as well as to identify the existence of cervical orifice at the end of the vagina. The second step was gonadal detection, biopsy and selected removal. Laparoscopy was applied to confirm the components of intraperitoneal gonads and internal genital ducts combining with punctural biopsy or excisional biopsy. Parents would make final decision of gender assignment based on the results of exploration before gonad removal during the operation. Occasionally, Müllerian duct structures were removed via laparoscopy. On the basis of dominant gonads and the consensus of gender assignment, only one type of gonad was reserved, and the other was resected. The third step was genitoplasty. Clitoroplasty, vaginoplasty, and labioplasty were carried out in female gender. According to the length of urogenital sinus, we used partial urogenital mobilization (PUM) or flap vaginoplasty for vaginoplasty. Orthoplasty, urethroplasty and scrotoplasty were carried out in male gender. Plate reconstruction with two-stage tubularization urethroplasty [6] and Duckett urethroplasty-urethrostomy by stages [7] were the two-stage techniques we routinely used in severe hypospadias repairs (Fig. 2).

One month after surgery, for patient reassigned as female, human menopausal gonadotropins (HMG) test [8] with a daily intramuscular dose of 150 IU on 3 consecutive days was indicated to verify no residuary testicle tissue. While for patients reassigned as male, HCG test was carried out to confirm no residuary ovarian tissue. All the patients were followed up at 1, 3, 6, 12 months after surgery and every year thereafter.

All procedures used in the study confirmed to the tenets of the Declaration of Helsinki. The Ethics Committee of Sichuan Academy of Medical Sciences & Sichuan Provincial People's Hospital approved the protocols used. All participants have known to participate in the study. Written informed consents were obtained from all participants.

Results

As shown in Table 1, the age ranged from 17 months to 66 months with a mean age of 20 months, and the mean follow-up was 30 months (4 months to 56 months). Eleven patients came to our hospital for ambiguous

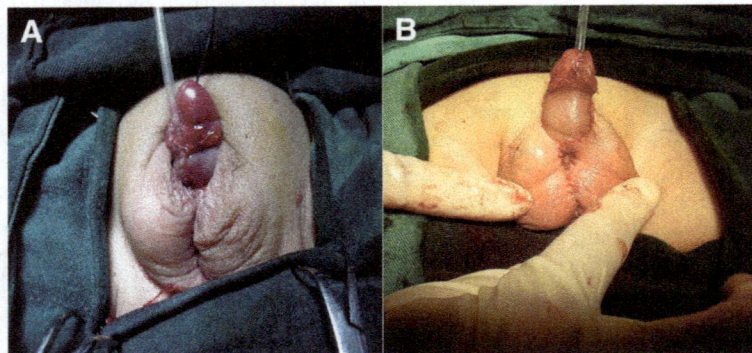

Fig. 2 The appearance after the first stage of two-stage techniques we routinely used in urethroplasty. **a** Plate reconstruction with two-stage tubularizationurethroplasty. After the first stage, the new meatus is in the shaft of the phallus. **b** Ducketturethroplasty-urethrostomy by stages. After the first stage, the urethroplasty is finished except a fistula

genitalia and 5 patients were referred to our institution for hypospadias repair. No relevant family history or associated anomalies were noted. According to Prader classification, stage II to V were recorded with stage III accounting for 62.5% (10 out of 16). Müllerian remnants were detected in 8 patients before surgery via ultrasonography or MRI.

With HCG stimulation, a normal response was noted in 13 patients, and the rest 3 patients showed a borderline response. Follow-up in puberty is important for the 3 borderline response patients. The other endocrinal indexes were normal or meaningless for considering other DSD.

In this group of patients, the karyotypes were 46, XX in 11 patients (68.75%), 46, XX/46, XY in 3 (18.75%), a rare karyotype 46, XX/47, XXY in 1 (6.25%) and 46, XY in 1 (6.25%).

The most common gonad was ovotestis (68.75%), followed with ovaries (18.75%), and the least common was testis (12.5%). Ovotestis was easily noticed in the scrotum (50%), subsequently in the inguinal canal (36.4%), then in the abdominal cavity (13.6%). All the 6

Table 1 The characteristic of these OT-DSD patients

No	Karyotype	Prader grade	MR imaging	T post HCG (ng/dl)	L gonand Position	Tissue	R gonad Position	Tissue	L duct	R duct	UVB (cm)	Uterus	Gender assignment	Complication
1	46,XX	III	+	367.5	Ing	OT	Ing	OT	Tube	Tube	3.5/4.5/2.5	+	M	No
2	46,XY	III	-	213.3	Abd	OT	Abd	OT	Tube	Tube	2/5/4	-	M	S
3	46,XX/46,XY	II	+	379.9	Abd	O	Ing	OT	Tube	Tube	3.5/5/4.5	+	M	No
4	46,XX	IV	-	416.2	Scr	OT	Abd	O	Tube	Tube	4/6/3	+	M	No
5	46,XX	III	+	209.1	Ing	OT	Ing	OT	Tube	Tube	2.5/4.5/3.5	+	M	F
6	46,XX	III	+	541.1	Scr	OT	Scr	T	Tube	Vas	1.5/6.5/5.5	+	M	No
7	46,XX	III	+	254.4	Scr	OT	Scr	T	Tube	Vas	1/6.5/5	+	M	No
8	46,XX/46,XY	III	-	322.6	Scr	OT	Abd	O	Vas	Tube	2/5.5/4.5	+	U → M	No
9	46,XX/47,XXY	III	-	186.4	Ing	T	Abd	OT	Vas	Tube	2.5/4.5/3.5	+	M	No
10	46,XX	II	+	462.8	Scr	OT	Scr	OT	Vas	Vas	2.5/5/4	+	M	No
11	46,XX/46,XY	III	-	275.4	Ing	OT	Ing	OT	Tube	Tube	3/5.5/4	+	M	[a]
12	46,XX	II	+	302.2	Abd	O	Scr	T	Tube	Vas	3.5/6/3.5	+	M	[a]
13	46,XX	III	-	166.3	Abd	O	Ing	OT	Tube	Tube	1/5.5/5.5	+	F → M	[a]
14	46,XX	III	+	532.6	Scr	OT	Scr	OT	Tube	Vas	2/5/4.5	+	M	[a]
15	46,XX	II	+	178.6	Abd	O	Scr	OT	Tube	Tube	3/5/3.5	+	M → F	No
16	46,XX	V	-	346.2	Scr	OT	Scr	OT	Vas	Vas	5/4/3.5	-	M	[a]

MR Müllerian remnant, *L* Left, *R* Right, *UVB* Length of urogenital sinus/ water-filled vagina/ the location of the vaginal confluence to the bladder neck, *Ing* Inguinal cana, *Abd* Abdominal cavity, *Scr* Scrotum, *OT* Ovotestis, *O* Ovary, *T* Testicle, *Tube* Fallopian tube, *Vas* Vas deferens, *M* Male, *F* Female, *U* Undetermined sex, *F* Fistula, *S* Urethral stricture, [a]Didn't finished the second stage

ovaries were discovered in the abdominal cavity. Three testes were found in the scrotum and the other one in the inguinal canal. Adjacent to the ovotestis, internal genital duct was verified as vas deferens on 6 lateralities via biopsy and as fallopian tube in 16. Bilateral ovotestis was the most frequent pattern of the gonads as seen in 7 patients. An ovotestis on one side and an ovary on the other side was noted in 5 patients, while an ovotestis on one side and a testis on the other side was noted in 3 patients. In only 1 patient a testis on one side and an ovary on the other was noted.

The vagina was found out in 16 patients with cystoscopy. At the end of the vagina, a cervical orifice was noted in 14 patients. The mean length of urogenital sinus (U), i.e., the length from confluence of the vagina and the urethra to the urethral meatus was 2.7 cm. The mean length of water-filled vagina (V) was 5.3 cm. The mean distance from the vaginal confluence to the bladder neck (B) was 4.1 cm. In the Table 1, we use the abbreviation UVB to describe the three distance.

During surgery, gonadal gender was determined via frozen section biopsy. In all the patients, the frozen pathological outcomes fell into anticipated possibilities of preoperative MDT consultation. Gender assignment was then decided accordingly. Initial reared sex was male in 14 patients, female in 1, and undetermined in 1. The gender was reassigned in 1 patient who was primarily reared as male, 1 as female, and the previously undetermined 1 was assigned as male. All the gonads and adjacent ducts in abdominal cavity were subjected to bipolar punctural biopsy via laparoscopy. All the ovotestes presented in a bipolar fashion. Staged urethroplasty was indicated in all the patients assigned as male. Plate reconstruction with two-stage tubularization urethroplasty (PRTU) was used in 10 patients. Stage II urethroplasty was achieved in 8 patients with urethrocutaneous fistula noted in 1 and urethral stricture in 1 as postoperative complications. Two patients just finished the first stage without complication. Duckett urethroplasty-urethrotomy

by stages was adopted in 5 patients. Three patients finished the fistula repair and 2 patients just finished the first stage of Duckett urethroplasty with a fistula left. No complications were found in the 5 cases (Table 1). Müllerian ducts were removed in 4 patients and left intact in 11. Clitoroplasty and partial urogenital mobilization (PUM) were carried out in only 1 patient who was assigned as female. No complications were noticed in this patient during the follow-up.

Histopathology was used as gold standard of final diagnosis. All the immediate outcomes of frozen section during operation were accordant with that of paraffin section after operation (Fig. 3). The testicular tissues presented numerous solid seminiferous tubules filled with immature Sertoli cells and a few primitive germ cells. The testicular interstitium contained undifferentiated spindle cells that were immature Leydig cells. In the ovarian tissue, numerous primordial follicles and a few primary and antral follicles were found in the outer cortex.

In the first month of the follow-up, HCG/HMG test was completed with no evidence of residual inconsonant gonad. No gonadal tumors were noted during the follow-up.

Discussion

Ethicists and patient support groups advocated that the genital surgery should not be warranted until the patient was able to understand the informed consent, instead of repair in infancy period [9]. However, as the appearance of bisexual phenotype and continuous anxiety of parents call for the management, it is rational and in a degree mandatory to initiate the evaluation at an early age. Ambiguous or undermasculinized genitalia of OT-DSD is easy to detect, while decision making is difficult when the genital appearance seems to be normal female or otherwise normal hypospadiac male [10]. Physical examination for the gonads is important. In 5 patients out of this series, OT-DSD was suspected as a tough nodule adjacent to the testicle or bipolar asymmetrical texture of the testicle was

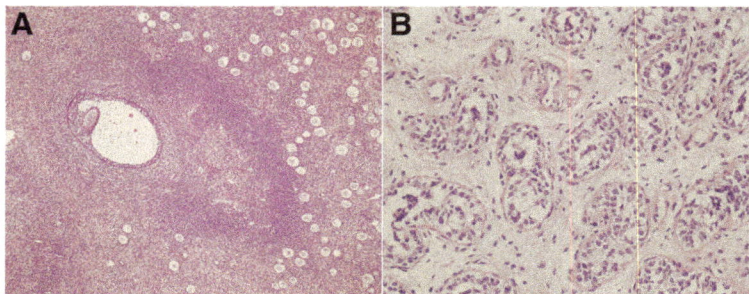

Fig. 3 Ovotestis in OT-DSD. **a** The ovarian compartment has numerous primordial and growing follicles containing primary oocytes within the ovarian cortical stroma. **b** The testicular compartment shows solid tubules filled with immature Sertoli cells and germ cells. The testicular interstitium contains immature Leydig cells

palpated in physical examination for hypospadias pre-operative evaluation. The Imaging only revealed 8 patients with internal genital ducts, however, the vagina was found out in all the 16 patients with cystoscopy. Imaging modalities to characterize urogenital system before surgery is also inaccurate.

The karyotype showed geographic variation. It was interesting that our data showed a similar pattern of karyotype in this Chinese series as that reported in Europe and North America, in contrast to that in Japan [11]. In Japan the 46, XY karyotype is more common than that in other countries [12]. The mosaicism of Klinefelter syndrome with 46,XX/47,XXY in OT-DSD is very rare with less than 10 cases reported worldwide [13]. Our patient 9 is 2 years and 5 months old with this karyotype. His manifestation as listed in Table 1 showed no difference to that with other karyotypes of OT-DSD. Though sex-determining region on the Y chromosome (SRY) is an important gene in testicular development, the implication of SRY presence in OT-DSD remains indeterminate. SRY detection is not indicated in our institution as a routine.

Ovotestis is the most common gonad in OT-DSD as reported in most articles [13, 14]. Wiersma and Ramdial [14] evaluated the gonads from 111 patients with OT-DSD in South Africa. They proposed three distinct patterns of gonad, namely the admixed pattern that was central core containing stroma and a mixture of ovarian and testicular tissue (50%), the compartmentalized pattern that was ovarian tissue in upper pole with lower pole of testicular tissue encapsulated by mantle of ovarian tissue (39%), and the bipolar pattern that was strict polar distribution of testicular and ovarian tissue (11%). In our patients, most ovotestes were of bipolar type, which was end to end fashion (Fig. 4a). Ovarian tissue located on the upper pole, was cerinous, rigid, and smaller than testicular tissue. On the contrary, the testicular tissue located on the lower pole, was buff, softer and larger than ovarian tissue. Demarcation was significant between the two parts. The demarcation

between ovarian tissue and testicular tissue in the 16th patient was not obvious on gross view (Fig. 4b). While the different texture made it evident to distinguish the boundary. This might be the type assigned as compartmentalized by Wiersma and Ramdial, except for that ovarian tissue was not found out in the mantle with microscopy. In OT-DSD, either testicular part of ovotestis or isolated testis presents maldeveloped microscopic features. On the contrary, either ovarian part of ovotestis or isolated ovary presents well-developed microstructures. In microscopy, the presence of numerous primordial follicles containing primary oocytes with or without maturing follicles is considered well developed ovarian tissue, which making a definitive diagnosis of OT-DSD. Menstruation is expected in 50% cases based on well-developed ovarian tissue [15]. The negative feedback effect of ovarian steroids suppressing gonadotropins results in tubular atrophy, poor germ cell development, Leydig cell hyperplasia, and sclerosis that finally causes infertility of the testicular tissue. As the individual gets older, the damage on the testicle in ovotesitular patient would deteriorate [15]. This is another reason why we indicate gender assignment, especially for those who with male dominance, in infancy. If the pathologists have misgivings about the nature of the gonads in the frozen section, the next step should be postponed awaiting the outcomes of hematoxylin-eosin staining.

Being the most common form of OT-DSD, ovotestis should be screened out during preoperative physical examination according to the typical morphological features. Internal genital ducts adjacent to the ovotestis are usually difficult to identify with naked eyes, and frozen biopsy is warranted in surgery.

On the basis of PVE classification system [16], we designed UVB measurement to assess the location of vagina confluence and the length of urogenital sinus and vagina. The critical factor in the vaginoplasty is not the length of the common sinus but rather the distance from the bladder neck to the location of vagina confluence. The former index is very useful in the surgical planning

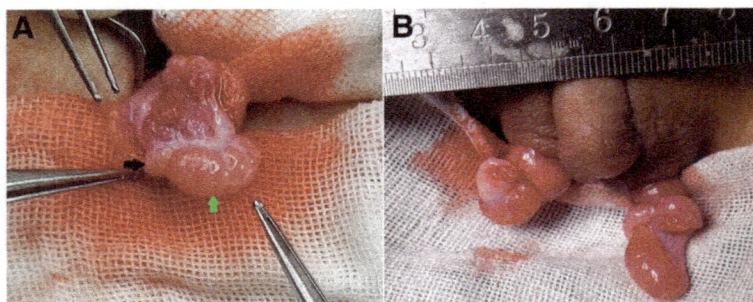

Fig. 4 Intraoperative findings of ovotestes. **a** Ovarian portion (*black* arrow) is firm and *yellow* in an upper pole, whereas testicular portion (*green* arrow) is soft and pink in a lower pole. There is a distinct line of demarcation between the two portions. **b** The demarcation between the two portions is not obvious in the 16th patient

of vaginoplasty. Partial urogenital mobilization (PUM) or flap vaginoplasty is indicated based on these evaluations.

Our multidisciplinary team and the families took part in the gender assignment. Prader grading, karyotype, nature and function of gonads, values of UVB, presence of Müllerian ducts, psychological assessment and living environment are critical factors involved in the gender assignment. However it is difficult when the decision from the MDT and that from the parents are conflicting. According to Chinese tradition that the boys carry on the family lines, most conservative families prefer male to female in OT-DSD after thorough evaluation, as well as worry about the catastrophic effect of gender reassignment on the whole family. Even with Prader II genitalia, possibility of fertility for female assignment, which lead the MDT suggesting female more appropriate, most parents still insist on male as final gender. The MDT would try to fully inform the parents with professional evaluation, but the final decision is made by the parents. All the three families accepted gender reassignment chose to move to a remote place for a new life.

Laparoscopy is widely utilized in the exploration of gonads and resection of Müllerian ducts. Resection of Müllerian duct derivatives as routine several years ago is not recommended in patients without any symptom nowadays. However, Farikullah reported 3 to 8% incidence of malignancy in Müllerian remnants [17]. Informing the parents with this incidence of malignancy, we were surprised that removal of the müllerian ducts was required in all the latest 4 asymptomatic patients for the risk of malignancy. Of course, if the gender couldn't be decided during the operation or the final gender was female, The Müllerian remnants must be retained. Bipolar and multisite punctural biopsy of gonads in abdominal cavity with laparoscopy is minimally invasive and these gonadal biopsies are enough to achieve histopathological evaluation for diagnosis. Repair of severe hypospadias is challenging and the complication rate is always high. During the recent years in our institution, plate reconstruction with two-stage tubularization urethroplasty [6] and Duckett urethroplasty-urethrotomy by stages [7] are the main two-stage techniques we routinely indicate in primary severe hypospadias repair. The complications of the two technique in primary severe hypospadias repair in our hospital are 16.7 and 9.43%, respectively [6, 7]. Both the two techniques are suitable for urethroplasty in OT-DSD.

The low incidence of Y chromosome in karyotype and young age of the patients induced no gonadal tumor to be detected. The incidence of gonadal tumors is approximately 3% in 46, XY and 46, XX/46, XY OT-DSD, though rare in 46, XX OT-DSD. Both gonadoblastoma and dysgerminoma have been described [18]. HMG/HCG test is an important content in the follow-up. The

residual gonad inconsistent with rearing sex will result in bisexual phenotype in puberty.

Conclusions

OT-DSD is a rare and complex malformation with lots of typical features. Standardized procedure of evaluation and treatment for OT-DSD is very important. MDT consultation might guarantee the high efficiency and accuracy in evaluation and treatment. Chinese parents prefer male to female when they face to the gender reassignment.

Abbreviations
17-OHP: 17-hydroxyprogesterone; AMH: Anti-müllerian hormone; DHT: Dihydrotestosterone; DSD: Disorder of sex development; FSH: Follicle stimulation hormone; HCG: Human chorionic gonadotropin; HMG: Human menopausal gonadotropins; LH: Luteinizing hormone; MDT: Multidisciplinary team; MRI: Magnetic Resonance Imaging; OT-DSD: Ovotesticular disorder of sex development; PUM: Partial urogenital mobilization; SHBG: Sex hormone binding globulin; T: Serum testosterone

Acknowledgements
We acknowledge the patients and families. We thank Mao Liu, Yue jiao Chen, Ji yun Yang and Jing Fu for making this study possible.

Funding
This study was supported by grants from the Youth Foundation of Sichuan Provincial People's Hospital (No.30305030609). The funders had no role in study design, data collection and analysis, decision to publish, or preparation of the manuscript.

Authors' contributions
YM carried out the study and drafted the manuscript. SJC, YMT designed and coordinated the study. RW helped in the laboratory work. RW, XJW,DRQ performed the data collection and statistics. All authors read and approved the final manuscript.

Competing interests
The authors declare that they have no competing interests.

Author details
[1]Department of Pediatric Surgery of Children's Medical Center, Sichuan Academy of Medical Sciences & Sichuan Provincial People's Hospital, Chengdu, China. [2]Department of Burn and Plastic Surgery, West China Hospital of Sichuan University, Chengdu, China.

References
1. Lee PA, Houk CP, Ahmed SF, Hughes IA, International Consensus Conference on Intersex organized by the Lawson Wilkins Pediatric Endocrine S, the European Society for Paediatric E. Consensus statement on management of intersex disorders. International Consensus Conference on Intersex. Pediatrics. 2006;118:e488–500.
2. Krstic ZD, Smoljanic Z, Vukanic D, Varinac D, Janjic G. True hermaphroditism: 10 years' experience. Pediatr Surg Int. 2000;16:580–3.

3. Sultan C, Paris F, Jeandel C, Lumbroso S, Galifer RB. Ambiguous genitalia in the newborn. Semin Reprod Med. 2002;20:181–8.

4. Biswas K, Kapoor A, Karak AK, Kriplani A, Gupta DK, Kucheria K, et al. Imaging in intersex disorders. J Pediatr Endocrinol Metab. 2004;17:841–5.

5. Steven M, O'Toole S, Lam JP, MacKinlay GA, Cascio S. Laparoscopy versus ultrasonography for the evaluation of Mullerian structures in children with complex disorders of sex development. Pediatr Surg Int. 2012;28:1161–4.

6. Yunman T, Shaoji C, Yu M, Xuejun W, Mao L. Plate reconstruction and tubularization urethroplasty in the repair of complicated hypospadias. Chin J Pediatr Surg. 2015;36:182–6.

7. Yunman T, Xuejun W, Yu M, Shaoji C, Mao L, Yuejiao C. Duckett urethroplasty-urethrotomy for staged hypospadias repair. Chin J Reparative Reconstr Surg. 2016;30:594–8.

8. Steinmetz L, Rocha MN, Longui CA, Damiani D, Dichtchekenian V, Setian N, et al. Inhibin A production after gonadotropin stimulus: a new method to detect ovarian tissue in ovotesticular disorder of sex development. Horm Res. 2009;71:94–9.

9. D'Alberton F. Disclosing disorders of sex development and opening the doors. Sex Dev. 2010;4:304–9.

10. Kropp BP, Keating MA, Moshang T, Duckett JW. True hermaphroditism and normal male genitalia: an unusual presentation. Urology. 1995;46:736–9.

11. Krob G, Braun A, Kuhnle U. True hermaphroditism: geographical distribution, clinical findings, chromosomes and gonadal histology. Eur J Pediatr. 1994;153:2–10.

12. Matsui F, Shimada K, Matsumoto F, Itesako T, Nara K, Ida S, et al. Long-term outcome of ovotesticular disorder of sex development: a single center experience. Int J Urol. 2011;18:231–6.

13. Paula GB, Ribeiro Andrade JG, Guaragna-Filho G, Sewaybricker LE, Miranda ML, Maciel-Guerra AT, et al. Ovotesticular disorder of sex development with unusual karyotype: patient report. J Pediatr Endocrinol Metab. 2015;28:677–80.

14. Wiersma R, Ramdial PK. The gonads of 111 South African patients with ovotesticular disorder of sex differentiation. J Pediatr Surg. 2009;44:556–60.

15. van Niekerk WA, Retief AE. The gonads of human true hermaphrodites. Hum Genet. 1981;58:117–22.

16. Rink RC, Adams MC, Misseri R. A new classification for genital ambiguity and urogenital sinus anomalies. BJU Int. 2005;95:638–42.

17. Farikullah J, Ehtisham S, Nappo S, Patel L, Hennayake S. Persistent Mullerian duct syndrome: lessons learned from managing a series of eight patients over a 10-year period and review of literature regarding malignant risk from the Mullerian remnants. BJU Int. 2012;110:E1084–9.

18. Verp MS, Simpson JL. Abnormal sexual differentiation and neoplasia. Cancer Genet Cytogenet. 1987;25:191–218.

26

Systematic review and meta-analysis of randomised trials of perioperative outcomes comparing robot-assisted versus open radical cystectomy

Zhiyuan Shen and Zhongquan Sun[*]

Abstract

Background: With the introduction of robotic surgery, whether the robot-assisted radical cystectomy (RARC) could reduce the perioperative morbidity compared with Open radical cystectomy (ORC) was unknown.

Methods: Studies reported RARC were reviewed based on all randomized controlled trials (RCTs), which focused on the efficacy of RARC versus ORC.

Results: Of the 201 studies from preliminary screening, four RCTs were included. By pooling these studies, there were significant differences in comparison of operative time ($p = 0.007$), estimated blood loss (EBL) ($p < 0.001$) and time to diet ($p < 0.001$) between the RARC group and ORC groups. There was no significant difference regarding perioperative complications (Clavien 2–5, Clavien 3–5), length of stay (LOS), positive surgical margins (PSM) and lymph node positive.

Conclusion: This meta-analysis presented evidence for a benefit of EBL, time to diet, similar perioperative complications and oncological outcomes, but a longer operative time in RARC. It is noted that RARC was considered as a comparable surgical procedure to ORC.

Keywords: Bladder cancer, Cystectomy, Meta, Robot

Background

In United States, approximately 74000 new cases of urinary bladder cancer with estimated 16000 deaths were expected in 2015 [1]. Open radical cystectomy (ORC) combined pelvic lymph node dissection (PLND) and urinary diversion (UD) is gold standard surgical intervention for high risk non-muscle invasive and muscle invasive bladder cancer, but accompanied with significant perioperative morbidity. In 2003, Menon reported the first case of robot-assisted radical cystectomy (RARC) [2]. With the introduction of robotic surgery, minimally invasive bladder cancer surgery set off a new climax with the promise of decreasing perioperative morbidity and mortality once again. Since then, a few prospective and retrospective studies had reported lower or comparable rates of complications, quicker recovery, and equivalent oncologic outcomes compared with ORC, however, which did not lead to a conclusive result [3–6]. Furthermore, these non-randomised researchs were accompanied with prominent selection bias. Although several meta-analyses regarding comparison of RARC with ORC had existed [7–11], these reviews incorporated a majority of non-randomized trials. Currently four randomized controlled trials had been publicated, therefore we conducted a systematical review of these literatures comparing surgical outcomes of RARC with those of ORC to provide powerful evidence.

Methods
Literature search
A systematic review of literatures was performed in Dec 2015. The electronic databases including PubMed, Embase, and the Cochrane Library were searched with

* Correspondence: drzhongquan@sina.cn
Department of Urology, Huadong Hospital, Fudan University, 221 West Yan'an Road, Shanghai 200040, China

restriction to English language. The following terms and their combinations were searched in [Title/Abstract]: cystectomy, cystectomies, cystoprostatectomy, bladder resection, robotic, robot, robot*, robot-assisted, and da Vinci. The related articles function was also used to broaden the search. Lists of references from the retrieved articles were manually searched to ensure as many studies as possible. When multiple reports describing the same population were published, the most recent or complete report was used.

Inclusion criteria and exclusion criteria

All available randomized controlled trials comparing RRC and ORC were considered, in addition at least one outcome of interest was mentioned. Studies as follow were excluded: (i) prospective non-randomised trials or retrospective trials comparing RARC and ORC, editorials, letters to the editor, review articles, experimental animal studies, case reports, comments, and conference abstracts, (ii) no outcomes of interest were reported.

Data extraction and outcomes of interest

Two reviewers independently selected studies for inclusion and extracted the following data: first author, year of publication, country, study interval, study design, indications for operation, number of patients who underwent RARC or ORC, rate of conversion from robot-assisted to open technique, matching criteria: age, gender, body mass index, American Society of Anesthesiologists (score), diversion type (conduit or neobladder), clinical stage, neoadjuvant chemotherapy, and outcomes of interest.

The primary outcomes were perioperative complication rates including intraoperative complications and postoperative complications classified according to the Clavien-Dindo grading system [12]. If sufficient data was available, perioperative complications were subdivided into 30d and 90d. The secondary outcome variables included operating time, estimated blood loss (EBL), number of patients receiving blood transfusion, length of stay (LOS), time to regular diet, positive margins, number of lymph nodes and pathologic stage. All disagreements were resolved by discussion until a

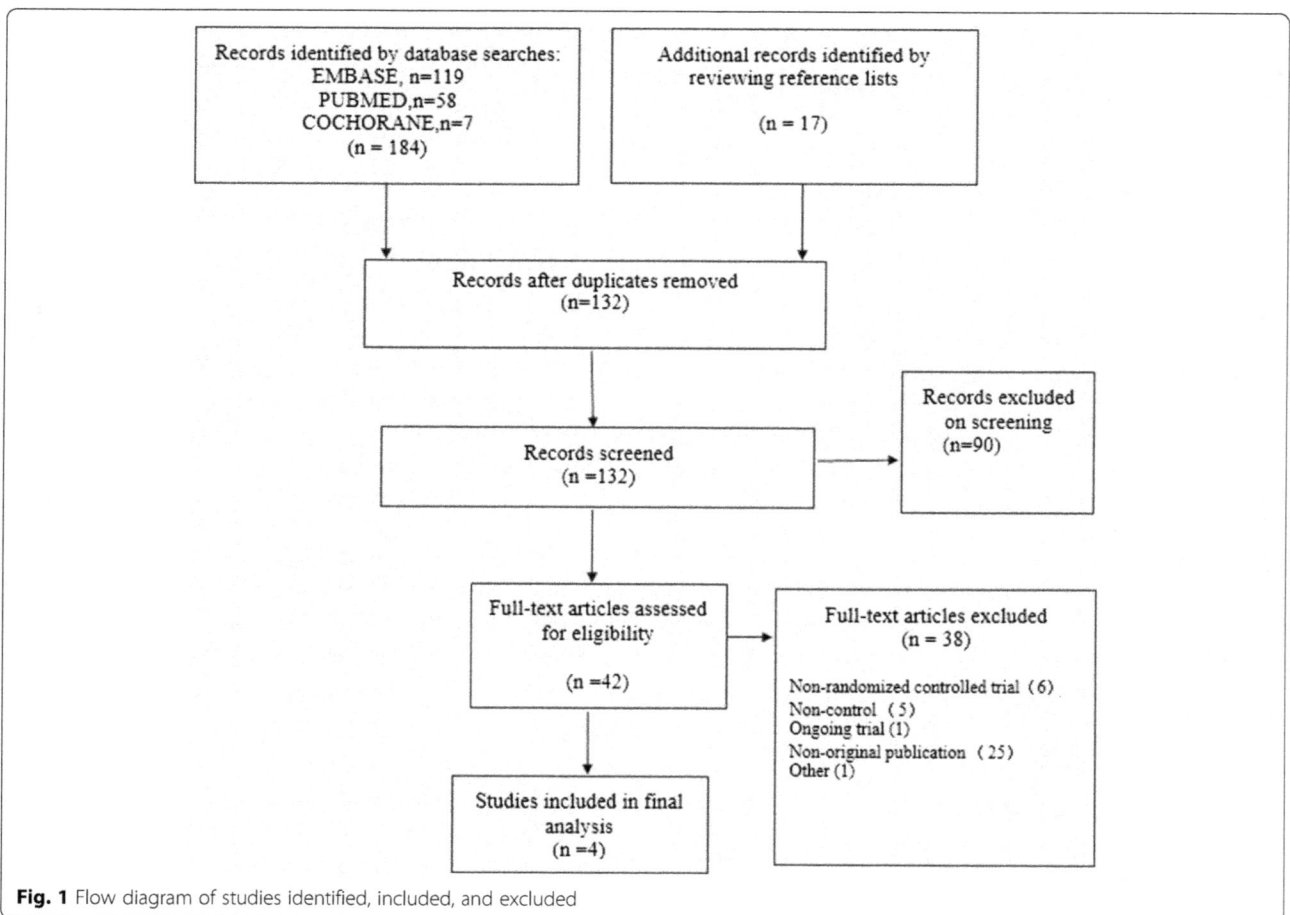

Fig. 1 Flow diagram of studies identified, included, and excluded

Table 1 Study characteristics

Publication	Country	Design	LOE	Case		Age (mean or median)		Conversion	Matching[a]	Neobladder		Urinary diversion method
				RARC	ORC	RARC	ORC			RARC	ORC	
Nix 2009	USA	RCT	2b	21	20	67.4	69.2	0	1,2,3,4,7,8	7	6	Extracorporeal
Parekh2012	USA	RCT	2b	20	20	69.5	64.5	0	1,2,3,4,6	NA	NA	NA
Bochner 2014	USA	RCT	2b	60	58	66	65	0	1,2,3,4,6,7,8	33	32	Extracorporeal
Khan 2015	UK	RCT	2b	20	20	68.6	66.6	1[b]	1,2,3,4,6,7,8	2	3	Extracorporeal

RARC robot-assisted radical cystectomy, *ORC* open radical cystectomy, *LOE* level of evidence, *RCT* randomized controlled trial, *NA* data not available
[a]Matching variables: 1 = age, 2 = gender, 3 = BMI, 4 = ASA, 5 = previous abdominal/pelvis surgery history, 6 = neoadjuvant chemotherapy, 7 = clinical stage, 8 = urinary diversion type
[b]due to equipment failure

consensus was reached. On condition that the data was incomplete, the corresponding authors were contacted.

Methodological quality

An evaluation of the methodological quality of the eligible studies was performed according to the Cochrane handbook [13]. For risk of bias assessment, the selection bias, performance bias and detection bias, attribution bias, reporting bias and other potential sources of bias were assessed in each of the included studies. The intention-to-treat analyses were described in the majority of studies.

Statistical analysis

The meta-analyses were conducted using Review Manager Version 5.3.

Dichotomous variables were presented as odds ratios (ORs) with 95 % confidence intervals (CIs), continuous variables as weighted mean differences (WMD) with 95 % CI. For studies that presented some continuous data as median and range values, the means and standard deviations were derived by statistical algorithms decribed by Wan et al. [14]. The *p*-Value was considered significant if <0.05. Statistical heterogeneity between studies was assessed using the chi-square test with $p < 0.10$ used for statistical significance. Statistical heterogeneity was also assessed using the I^2 test: I^2 values of 25 % (low), 50 % (medium), and 75 % (high). With I^2 values of 50 % or less, heterogeneity was acceptable referring to Cochrane handbook and in case that high levels of heterogeneity with I^2 values of 50 % or larger, we adopted a random-effects model.

Results

Characteristics of eligible studies

A thorough review of the potentially relevant studies resulted in 201 articles of which 4 were selected in the final analysis including 239 cases (121 cases in RARC group and 118 controls in ORC group (Fig. 1). Participant characteristics were presented as follows (Table 1). All 4 RCTs scored level 2b. 3 RCTs reported

extracorporeal urinary diversion method with the similar percentage of neobladder [15–17]. Only one patient converted to open surgery due to equipment failure [16]. Of these excluded studies, 5 lacked controls, 25 non-original publications, 6 non-randomized controlled trial, 1 ongoing trial, 1 shared overlapping populations with no outcomes of interest.

The risk of bias summary about each risk of bias item was available in Fig. 2. Nix et al. adopted

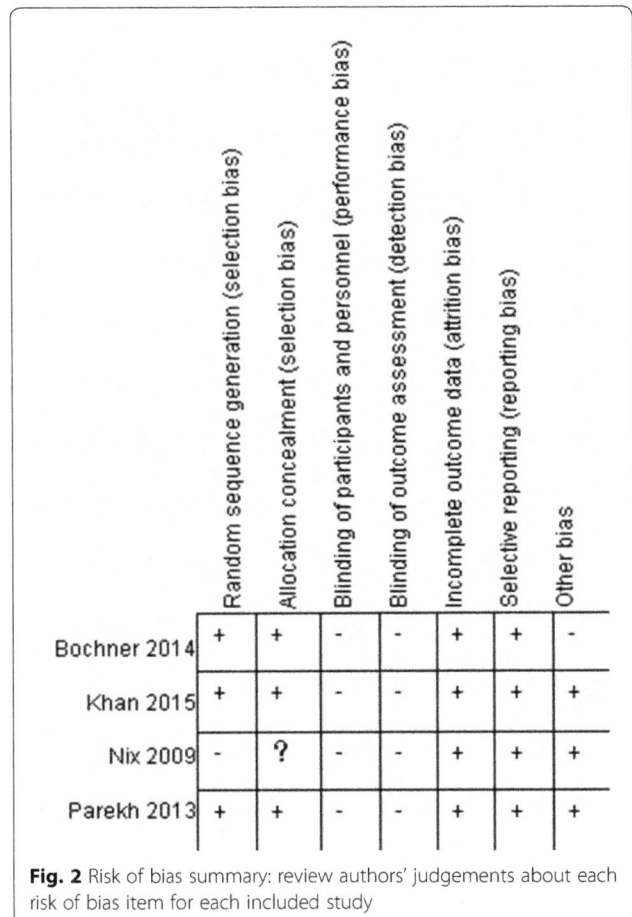

Fig. 2 Risk of bias summary: review authors' judgements about each risk of bias item for each included study

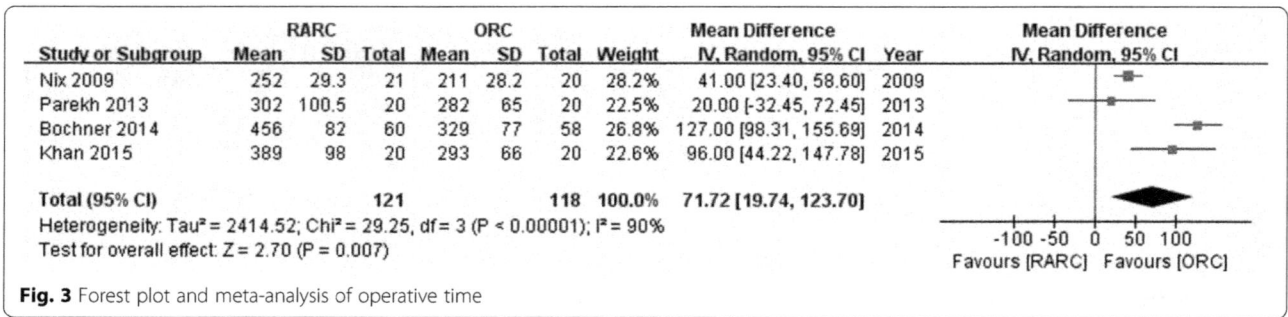

Study or Subgroup	RARC Mean	RARC SD	RARC Total	ORC Mean	ORC SD	ORC Total	Weight	Mean Difference IV, Random, 95% CI	Year
Nix 2009	252	29.3	21	211	28.2	20	28.2%	41.00 [23.40, 58.60]	2009
Parekh 2013	302	100.5	20	282	65	20	22.5%	20.00 [-32.45, 72.45]	2013
Bochner 2014	456	82	60	329	77	58	26.8%	127.00 [98.31, 155.69]	2014
Khan 2015	389	98	20	293	66	20	22.6%	96.00 [44.22, 147.78]	2015
Total (95% CI)			121			118	100.0%	71.72 [19.74, 123.70]	

Heterogeneity: Tau² = 2414.52; Chi² = 29.25, df = 3 (P < 0.00001); I² = 90%
Test for overall effect: Z = 2.70 (P = 0.007)

Fig. 3 Forest plot and meta-analysis of operative time

inappropriate randomization, and allocation conceal-ment could not be judged insufficient information. On account of different surgical approaches, blinding could not be achieved in four RCTs comparing RARC and ORC. Few data missing and ITT (intention-to-treat) analysis other than one RCT reduced attribu-tion bias. Then all preestablished outcomes were en-tirely reported. Moreover, limited cases brought out relatively weaker Statistical power.

Demographic and clinical characteristics

The mean or median age in the included studies ac-quired without sufficient standard variation for pooling data was quite close. Pooled data showed no difference in the male/female ratio or BMI. Clinical stage T4 was excluded, and no difference was found in distribution of T2-3 stage in three RCTs. There was also no difference in neochemotherapy applied in three studies. Likewise, the proportion of neobladder showed no difference in urinary conversion.

Perioperative outcomes

Pooled data from 4 studies evaluated operative time and estimated blood loss showed significantly longer OP (WMD: 71.72; 95 % CI, 19.74 to 123.70; $p = 0.007$) (Fig. 3) and less EBL (WMD:–241.99; 95 % CI,–332.55 to–151.43; $p < 0.00001$) (Fig. 4) in the RARC than the ORC group.

All RCTs compared complications using the Clavien system. Pooled data from 3 RCTs showed no significance in perioperative complications between RARC vs. ORC regarding to Clavien 2–5 (OR: 1.18; 95 % CI, 0.66 to 2.11; $p = 0.58$) (Fig. 5) or Clavien 3–5 (OR: 1.2; 95 % CI, 0.57 to 2.5; $p = 0.63$) (Fig. 6).

Data of time to flatus was extracted from 2 studies. Postoperative flatus was significantly shorter in RARC group (WMD:–0.79; 95 % CI,–1.28 to–0.30; $p = 0.002$) (Fig. 7). Likewise, time to regular diet from 3 studies was significantly shorter in RARC group (WMD:–1.14; 95 % CI,–1.71 to–0.75; $p < 0.0001$) (Fig. 8). There was no sig-nificant difference for length of stay between RARC and ORC from 4 RCTs (WMD:–0.54; 95 % CI,–1.44 to–0.35; $p = 0.23$) (Fig. 9).

Pathologic outcomes

Four studies reported the rates of positive surgical margin. There was no significant statistical difference in PSM between RARC group and ORC group (OR: 0.98; 95 % CI, 0.30 to 3.19; $p = 0.98$) (Fig. 10). Pathological stage in detail was reported in 4 studies. No significance was found in part of ≤ pT2 (OR: 1.21; 95 % CI, 0.71 to 2.05; $p = 0.49$) (Fig. 11), or ≥ pT3 (OR: 0.93; 95 % CI, 0.53 to 1.62; $p = 0.8$) (Fig. 12). Data of lymph node positive was available in 3 studies. Similarly, there was no significant statistical difference between RARC group and ORC group (OR: 0.84; 95 % CI, 0.42 to 1.72; $p = 0.64$) (Fig. 13).

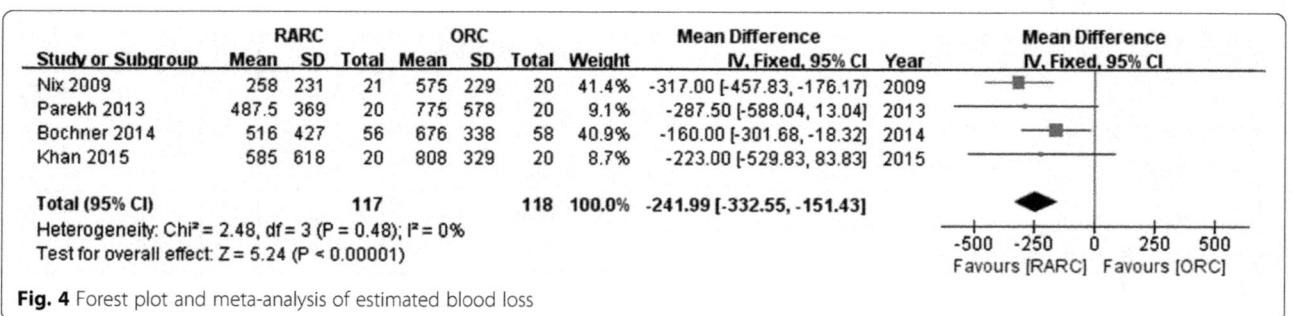

Study or Subgroup	RARC Mean	RARC SD	RARC Total	ORC Mean	ORC SD	ORC Total	Weight	Mean Difference IV, Fixed, 95% CI	Year
Nix 2009	258	231	21	575	229	20	41.4%	-317.00 [-457.83, -176.17]	2009
Parekh 2013	487.5	369	20	775	578	20	9.1%	-287.50 [-588.04, 13.04]	2013
Bochner 2014	516	427	56	676	338	58	40.9%	-160.00 [-301.68, -18.32]	2014
Khan 2015	585	618	20	808	329	20	8.7%	-223.00 [-529.83, 83.83]	2015
Total (95% CI)			117			118	100.0%	-241.99 [-332.55, -151.43]	

Heterogeneity: Chi² = 2.48, df = 3 (P = 0.48); I² = 0%
Test for overall effect: Z = 5.24 (P < 0.00001)

Fig. 4 Forest plot and meta-analysis of estimated blood loss

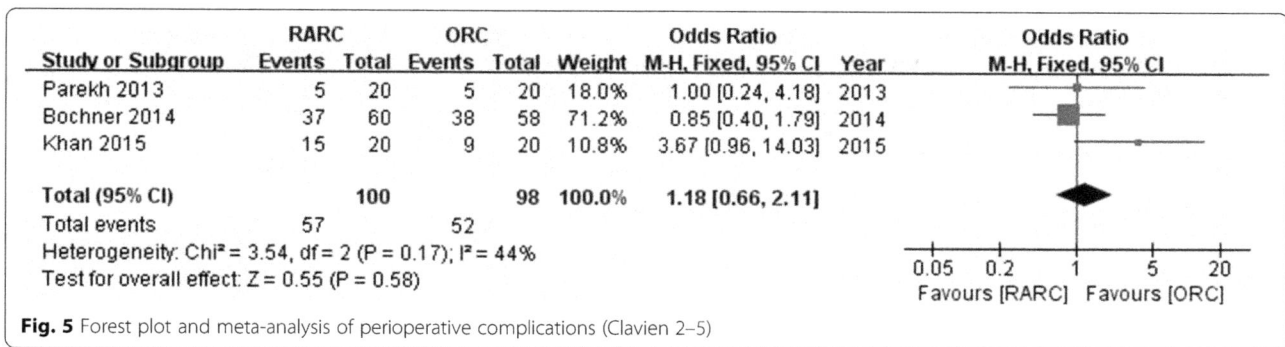

Study or Subgroup	RARC Events	Total	ORC Events	Total	Weight	Odds Ratio M-H, Fixed, 95% CI	Year
Parekh 2013	5	20	5	20	18.0%	1.00 [0.24, 4.18]	2013
Bochner 2014	37	60	38	58	71.2%	0.85 [0.40, 1.79]	2014
Khan 2015	15	20	9	20	10.8%	3.67 [0.96, 14.03]	2015
Total (95% CI)		100		98	100.0%	1.18 [0.66, 2.11]	
Total events	57		52				

Heterogeneity: Chi² = 3.54, df = 2 (P = 0.17); I² = 44%
Test for overall effect: Z = 0.55 (P = 0.58)

Fig. 5 Forest plot and meta-analysis of perioperative complications (Clavien 2–5)

Discussion

ORC with pelvic lymph node dissection still remains the gold standard approach for management of high grade non muscle-invasive and muscle-invasive bladder cancer. Notwithstanding, RARC became prevailing, especially in the U.S, which increased from 0.6 to 12.4 % of all RC cases from 2004 to 2010 [18]. Previous meta-analyses included both retrospective and prospective studies, which inevitably gave rise to selection bias. Fortunately, 4 RCTs comparing RARC and ORC could be achieved. For this reason, we conducted a meta-analysis with higher level of evidence. According to the analysis result, RARC had an advantage of less EBL and more rapid return to regular diet, but accompanied by longer operative time. Interestingly, this review showed similar rate of perioperative complications, which differed from what proposed by previous researchers. Besides, RARC was comparable with ORC in PSM, LOS.

On account of the 3 dimensional visual effect and elaborate operation, blood loss was much less in RARC group. Another important reason was the tamponade effect from the pneumoperitoneum used during RARC [19]. There is no doubt that it is the distinct advantage of RARC in terms of bleeding control, regardless of study types [5–8, 11, 15–17, 20]. Less EBL signified less blood transfusion. Unfortunately, only one RCT reported the rate of transfusion

with no statistical difference [20], therefore pooling data could not be carried out.

Pooled data of operative time showed that RARC took longer time compared with ORC as with previous results [4, 21]. No matter docking Da Vinci system or conversion to open urinary diversion adopted was time-consuming. Parekh et al. reported the similar operative time for both surgical procedures, and uniquely depicted the definition of operative time (defined as incision to closure), however, the data of urinary diversion was not available [20]. In addition, a better comparison would be drawn in case that the time of radical cystectomy, PLND and UD could be set apart. Prior studies demonstrated that learning curve was significantly associated with shorter operative time [22, 23]. In this meta-analysis, 3 RCTs reported that surgeons performed approximately 50–110 RARCs to eliminate the impact of learning curve. However, Bochner et al. only gave a vague statement that surgeons were experienced in extensive robotic pelvic surgery experience.

Previous meta-analyses demonstrated a lower complications [7–11], however no significance was found in perioperative complications between RARC and ORC in this review. Less blood loss failed to bring about lower complications in RARC groups. Moreover, the study conducted by Bochner et al. terminated, because the primary objective that the rate of grade 2–5 complications would be 20 % lower for RARC compared with

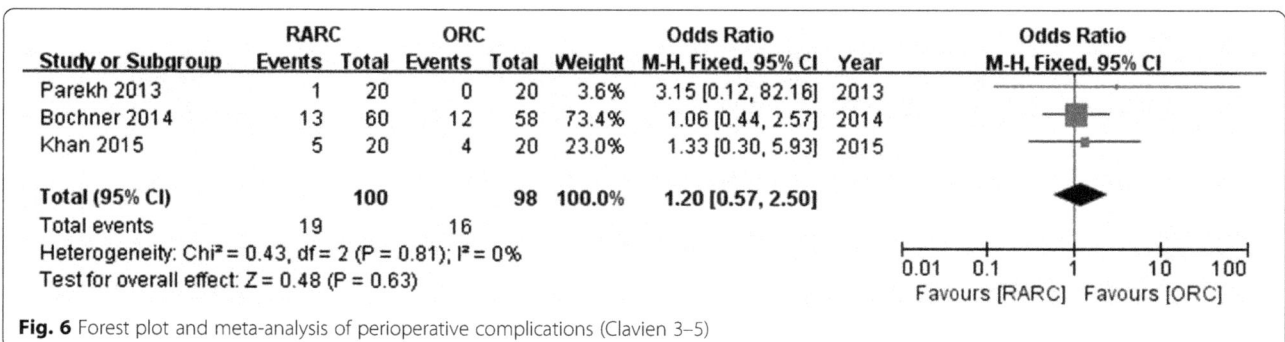

Study or Subgroup	RARC Events	Total	ORC Events	Total	Weight	Odds Ratio M-H, Fixed, 95% CI	Year
Parekh 2013	1	20	0	20	3.6%	3.15 [0.12, 82.16]	2013
Bochner 2014	13	60	12	58	73.4%	1.06 [0.44, 2.57]	2014
Khan 2015	5	20	4	20	23.0%	1.33 [0.30, 5.93]	2015
Total (95% CI)		100		98	100.0%	1.20 [0.57, 2.50]	
Total events	19		16				

Heterogeneity: Chi² = 0.43, df = 2 (P = 0.81); I² = 0%
Test for overall effect: Z = 0.48 (P = 0.63)

Fig. 6 Forest plot and meta-analysis of perioperative complications (Clavien 3–5)

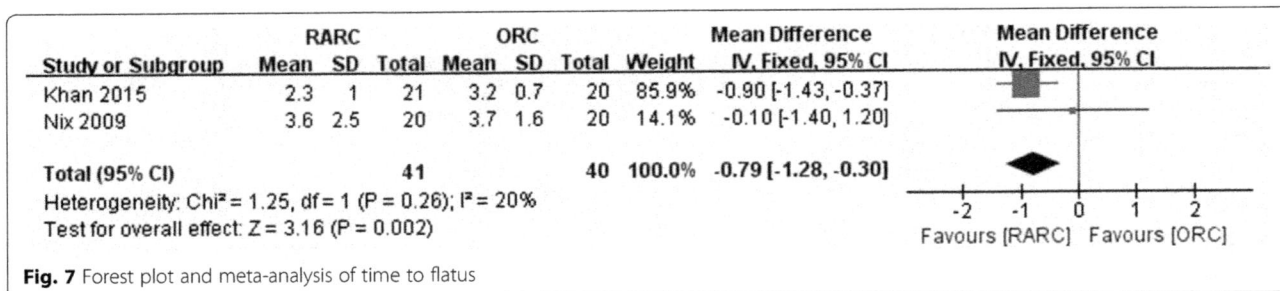

Study or Subgroup	RARC Mean	SD	Total	ORC Mean	SD	Total	Weight	Mean Difference IV, Fixed, 95% CI
Khan 2015	2.3	1	21	3.2	0.7	20	85.9%	-0.90 [-1.43, -0.37]
Nix 2009	3.6	2.5	20	3.7	1.6	20	14.1%	-0.10 [-1.40, 1.20]
Total (95% CI)			41			40	100.0%	-0.79 [-1.28, -0.30]

Heterogeneity: Chi² = 1.25, df = 1 (P = 0.26); I² = 20%
Test for overall effect: Z = 3.16 (P = 0.002)

Fig. 7 Forest plot and meta-analysis of time to flatus

ORC was not reached. Hautmann et al. reported that the majority of complications after radical cystectomy were correlated with urinary diversion [24]. Recently, totally robotic-assisted radical cystectomy with intracorporeal diversion was increasingly adopted, which brought potential benefits to the patients. Ahmed et al. demonstrated a 32 % reduction in complications at 90d comparing open with robotic urinary diversion [25]. For overall complication rates, Koupparis et al. reported a trend to lower complication rate (31 % vs 48 %) in the RARC group vs ORC group. Introducing robotic-assisted radical cystectomy with intracorporeal diversion in the future RCTs might show the potential advantage for perioperative complications. Remarkably, extracorporeal urinary diversion was adopted in 3 RCTs, which might be the reason why lower perioperative complications could not be found in RARC group.

In overall surgical margin, we draw a conclusion of an equivalent in RARC group and ORC group. The total rate of PSM in RARC groups was 5 % (range, 0–15 %), which was similar to 6.8 % raised by the International Robotic Cystectomy Consortium [26]. Higher pathological T stage was significantly correlated with an increased likelihood of a positive margin [26]. In this review, pooled data of extravesical disease (≥ pT3) showed no significance difference. However, PSM could not be detailed according to stage (<pT2 vs > pT3) for insufficient data. Only Bochner et al. reported PSM in subgroup of patients ≥ pT3 (RARC versus ORC: 12 %, 16 %, p = 0.7) [15]. PLND served as an indicator of

surgical quality of RC [27]. Parekh et al. reported an appearance of fewer median LNs in RARC with no significance. Nix et al. described a similar mean LNs between RARC and ORC. These data was insufficient for pooling data. Lymph node positive available in 3 studies was similar.

For long-term oncologic outcomes in RARC from International Robotic Cystectomy Consortium, after median follow-up of 67-months, 5 year recurrence-free survival, cancer-specific survival, and overall survival were 67 %, 75 %, and 50 %, respectively [28]. In this meta-analysis, only short term oncological outcomes were reported by Khan et al. that disease recurrence (11 %, 16 %) and disease-specific mortality (0 %, 5 %) was equivalent between RARC and ORC at 12 months.

With regard to LOS, although several retrospective studies and meta-analysis had demonstrated a significantly shorter LOS in RARC that may derive from the severe selection bias [4, 21, 29], but no significant difference was found in RARC group versus ORC group in our review, only modest trends of shorter LOS. The less bleeding and shorter time to regular diet had not brought about shorter LOS in our analysis. Above all, the similar complications might mainly contribute to longer hospital stay.

Outcomes of interest were mainly acquired, and incomplete data was depicted. The heterogeneity of variables was mostly low ($I^2 \leq 50$ %) except operative time ($I^2 = 90$ %), for which random effects were taken.

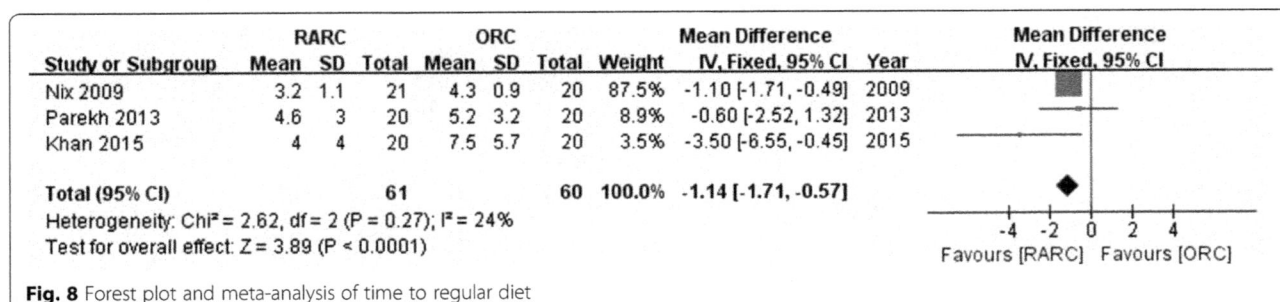

Study or Subgroup	RARC Mean	SD	Total	ORC Mean	SD	Total	Weight	Mean Difference IV, Fixed, 95% CI	Year
Nix 2009	3.2	1.1	21	4.3	0.9	20	87.5%	-1.10 [-1.71, -0.49]	2009
Parekh 2013	4.6	3	20	5.2	3.2	20	8.9%	-0.60 [-2.52, 1.32]	2013
Khan 2015	4	4	20	7.5	5.7	20	3.5%	-3.50 [-6.55, -0.45]	2015
Total (95% CI)			61			60	100.0%	-1.14 [-1.71, -0.57]	

Heterogeneity: Chi² = 2.62, df = 2 (P = 0.27); I² = 24%
Test for overall effect: Z = 3.89 (P < 0.0001)

Fig. 8 Forest plot and meta-analysis of time to regular diet

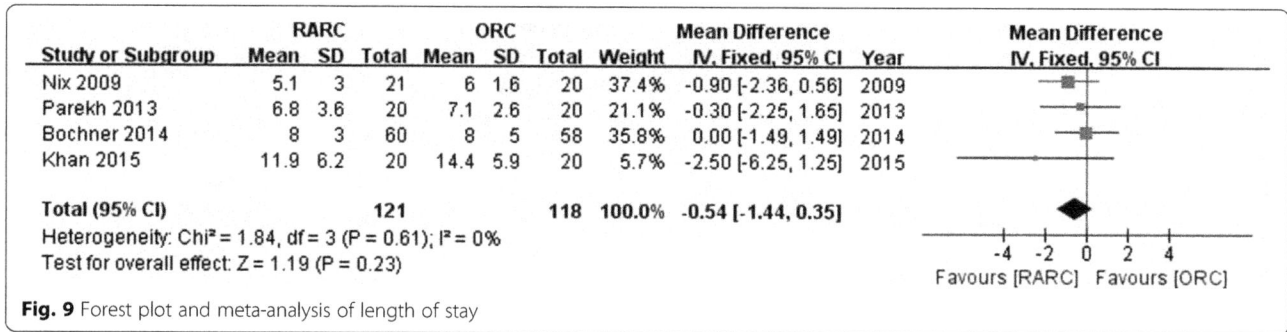

Study or Subgroup	RARC Mean	SD	Total	ORC Mean	SD	Total	Weight	Mean Difference IV, Fixed, 95% CI	Year
Nix 2009	5.1	3	21	6	1.6	20	37.4%	-0.90 [-2.36, 0.56]	2009
Parekh 2013	6.8	3.6	20	7.1	2.6	20	21.1%	-0.30 [-2.25, 1.65]	2013
Bochner 2014	8	3	60	8	5	58	35.8%	0.00 [-1.49, 1.49]	2014
Khan 2015	11.9	6.2	20	14.4	5.9	20	5.7%	-2.50 [-6.25, 1.25]	2015
Total (95% CI)			121			118	100.0%	-0.54 [-1.44, 0.35]	

Heterogeneity: Chi² = 1.84, df = 3 (P = 0.61); I² = 0%
Test for overall effect: Z = 1.19 (P = 0.23)

Fig. 9 Forest plot and meta-analysis of length of stay

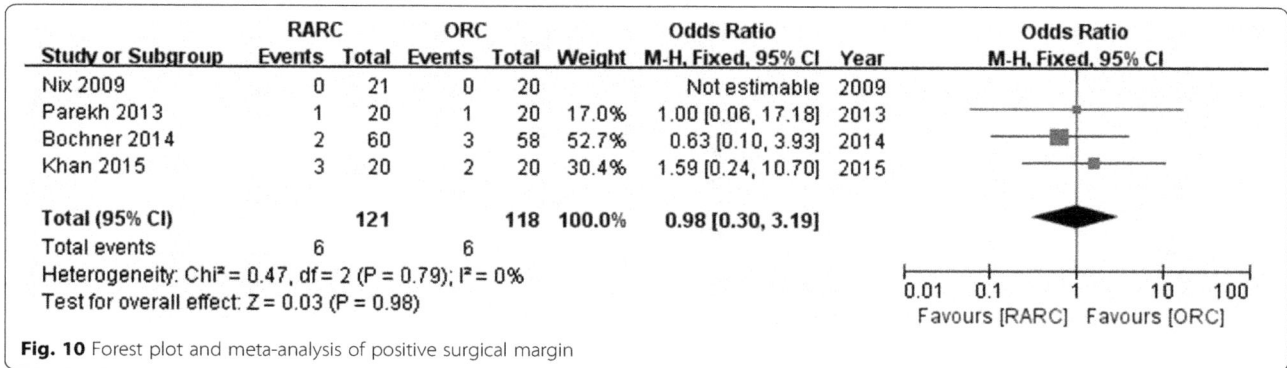

Study or Subgroup	RARC Events	Total	ORC Events	Total	Weight	Odds Ratio M-H, Fixed, 95% CI	Year
Nix 2009	0	21	0	20		Not estimable	2009
Parekh 2013	1	20	1	20	17.0%	1.00 [0.06, 17.18]	2013
Bochner 2014	2	60	3	58	52.7%	0.63 [0.10, 3.93]	2014
Khan 2015	3	20	2	20	30.4%	1.59 [0.24, 10.70]	2015
Total (95% CI)		121		118	100.0%	0.98 [0.30, 3.19]	
Total events	6		6				

Heterogeneity: Chi² = 0.47, df = 2 (P = 0.79); I² = 0%
Test for overall effect: Z = 0.03 (P = 0.98)

Fig. 10 Forest plot and meta-analysis of positive surgical margin

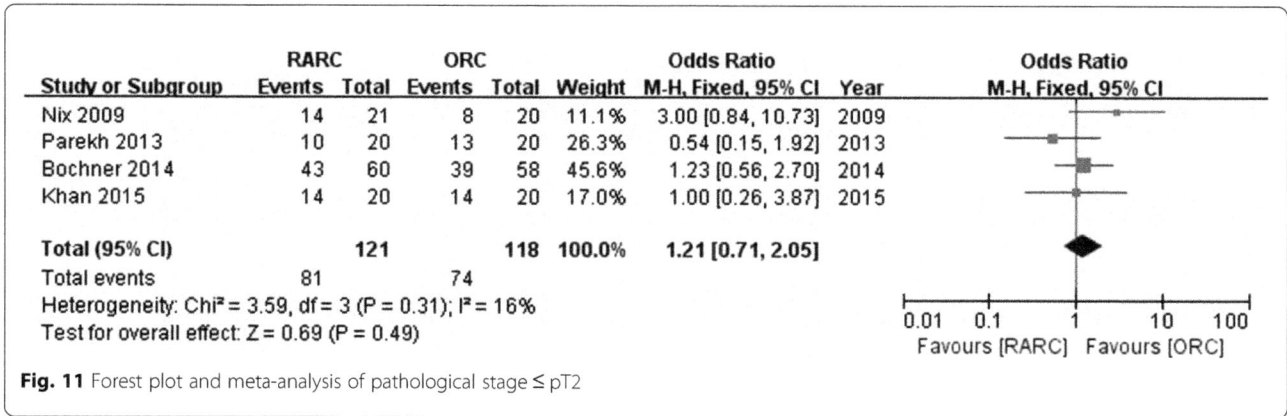

Study or Subgroup	RARC Events	Total	ORC Events	Total	Weight	Odds Ratio M-H, Fixed, 95% CI	Year
Nix 2009	14	21	8	20	11.1%	3.00 [0.84, 10.73]	2009
Parekh 2013	10	20	13	20	26.3%	0.54 [0.15, 1.92]	2013
Bochner 2014	43	60	39	58	45.6%	1.23 [0.56, 2.70]	2014
Khan 2015	14	20	14	20	17.0%	1.00 [0.26, 3.87]	2015
Total (95% CI)		121		118	100.0%	1.21 [0.71, 2.05]	
Total events	81		74				

Heterogeneity: Chi² = 3.59, df = 3 (P = 0.31); I² = 16%
Test for overall effect: Z = 0.69 (P = 0.49)

Fig. 11 Forest plot and meta-analysis of pathological stage ≤ pT2

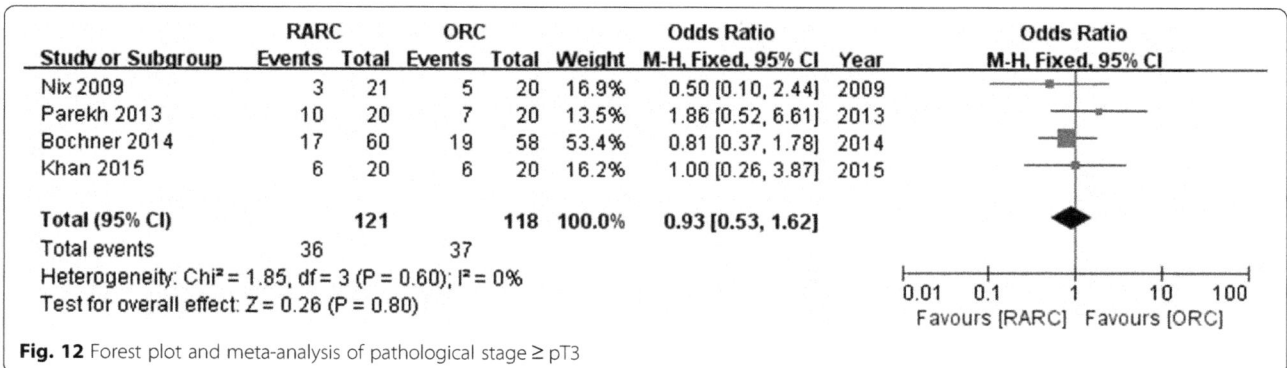

Study or Subgroup	RARC Events	Total	ORC Events	Total	Weight	Odds Ratio M-H, Fixed, 95% CI	Year
Nix 2009	3	21	5	20	16.9%	0.50 [0.10, 2.44]	2009
Parekh 2013	10	20	7	20	13.5%	1.86 [0.52, 6.61]	2013
Bochner 2014	17	60	19	58	53.4%	0.81 [0.37, 1.78]	2014
Khan 2015	6	20	6	20	16.2%	1.00 [0.26, 3.87]	2015
Total (95% CI)		121		118	100.0%	0.93 [0.53, 1.62]	
Total events	36		37				

Heterogeneity: Chi² = 1.85, df = 3 (P = 0.60); I² = 0%
Test for overall effect: Z = 0.26 (P = 0.80)

Fig. 12 Forest plot and meta-analysis of pathological stage ≥ pT3

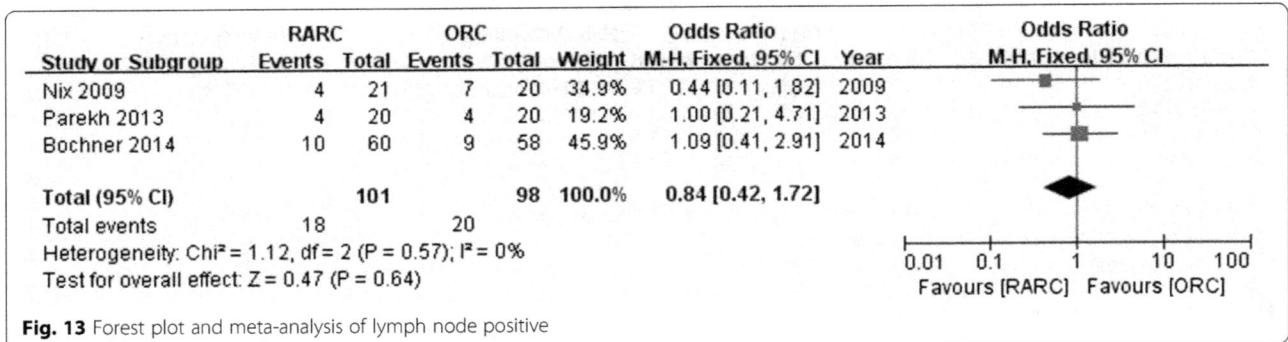

Fig. 13 Forest plot and meta-analysis of lymph node positive

Potential selection biases could be eliminated by the randomized trials, but surgeon's experience might introduce an important confounder to results. Patients unable to bear the pneumoperitoneum and steep trendelenburg position were excluded in RARC, coupled with improper randomization method applied in Nix's study. Hence, selection bias still existed.

Conclusion

Four RCTs comparing RARC and ORC were included in this meta-analysis. Based upon analysis, a benefit of less EBL, shoter time to diet, similar perioperative complications and oncological outcomes, but a longer operative time could be seen in RARC group. We might draw a conclusion that RARC was a safe and effective surgical procedure noninferior to the open approach, meanwhile randomized controlled trial comparing RARC and ORC was feasible. Despite a rigorous methodological review, restrictions were exerted to draw a straightforward conclusion for limitations of the included studies and patients. Certainly, further prospective, multicentric and large sample randomized control trials should be undertaken to confirm our findings. It's expected that Parekh et al. paved the way toward a phase III, multi-institutional, randomized trial that can offer more definitive answers.

Abbreviations

Cis: Confidence intervals; EBL: Estimated blood loss; EBL: Estimated blood loss; LOS: Length of hospital stay; LOS: Length of stay; ORC: Open radical cystectomy; ORs: Odds ratios; PLND: Pelvic lymph node dissection; PSM: Positive surgical margins; RARC: Robot-assisted radical cystectomy; UD: Urinary diversion; WMD: Weighted mean differences

Acknowledgements
Zhongquan Sun and Zhiyuan Shen conducted the conception and design of the study, acquisitionand interpretation of data, drafting the article, final approval of the version to be published.

Funding
No funding.

Authors' contributions
ZQS have made substantial contributions to conception and revisied it critically for important intellectual content. ZYS participated in acquisition of data, analysis, interpretation of data and drafting the manuscript. Both authors read and approved the final manuscript.

Competing interests
The authors declare that they have no competing interests.

References

1. Siegel RL, Miller KD, Jemal A. Cancer statistics, 2015. CA Cancer J Clin. 2015; 65(1):5–29.
2. Menon M, Hemal AK, Tewari A, et al. Nerve-sparing robot-assisted radical cystoprostatectomy and urinary diversion. BJU Int. 2003;92(3):232–6.
3. Atmaca AF, Canda AE, Gok B, Akbulut Z, Altinova S, Balbay MD. Open versus robotic radical cystectomy with intracorporeal Studer diversion. JSLS. 2015; 19(1):e2014–e00193.
4. Kader AK, Richards KA, Krane LS, Pettus JA, Smith JJ, Hemal AK. Robot-assisted laparoscopic vs open radical cystectomy: comparison of complications and perioperative oncological outcomes in 200 patients. BJU Int. 2013;112(4):E290–4.
5. Styn NR, Montgomery JS, Wood DP, et al. Matched comparison of robotic-assisted and open radical cystectomy. Urology. 2012;79(6):1303–8.
6. Sung HH, Ahn JS, Seo SI, et al. A comparison of early complications between open and robot-assisted radical cystectomy. J Endourol. 2012;26(6):670–5.
7. Fonseka T, Ahmed K, Froghi S, Khan SA, Dasgupta P, Shamim Khan M. Comparing robotic, laparoscopic and open cystectomy: a systematic review and meta-analysis. Arch Ital Urol Androl. 2015;87(1):41–8.
8. Ishii H, Rai BP, Stolzenburg JU, et al. Robotic or open radical cystectomy, which is safer? A systematic review and meta-analysis of comparative studies. J Endourol. 2014;28(10):1215–23.
9. Li K, Lin T, Fan X, et al. Systematic review and meta-analysis of comparative studies reporting early outcomes after robot-assisted radical cystectomy versus open radical cystectomy. Cancer Treat Rev. 2013;39(6):551–60.
10. Tang K, Xia D, Li H, et al. Robotic vs. open radical cystectomy in bladder cancer: A systematic review and meta-analysis. Eur J Surg Oncol. 2014; 40(11):1399–411.
11. Xia L, Wang X, Xu T, et al. Robotic versus open radical cystectomy: an updated systematic review and meta-analysis. PLoS ONE. 2015;10(3), e0121032.
12. Dindo D, Demartines N, Clavien PA. Classification of surgical complications: a new proposal with evaluation in a cohort of 6336 patients and results of a survey. Ann Surg. 2004;240(2):205–13.
13. Higgins, J. and S. Green, *Cochrane Handbook for Systematic Reviews of Interventions Version 5.1.0: The Cochrane Collaboration; 2011. Available at* http://training.cochrane.org/handbook.
14. Wan X, Wang W, Liu J, Tong T. Estimating the sample mean and standard deviation from the sample size, median, range and/or interquartile range. BMC Med Res Methodol. 2014;14:135.

15. Bochner BH, Dalbagni G, Sjoberg DD, et al. Comparing Open Radical Cystectomy and Robot-assisted Laparoscopic Radical Cystectomy: A Randomized Clinical Trial. Eur Urol. 2015;67(6):1042–50.
16. Khan MS, Gan C, Ahmed K, et al. A Single-centre Early Phase Randomised Controlled Three-arm Trial of Open, Robotic, and Laparoscopic Radical Cystectomy (CORAL). Eur Urol. 2016;69(4):613–21.
17. Nix J, Smith A, Kurpad R, Nielsen ME, Wallen EM, Pruthi RS. Prospective randomized controlled trial of robotic versus open radical cystectomy for bladder cancer: perioperative and pathologic results. Eur Urol. 2010;57(2):196–201.
18. Leow JJ, Reese SW, Jiang W, et al. Propensity-matched comparison of morbidity and costs of open and robot-assisted radical cystectomies: a contemporary population-based analysis in the United States. Eur Urol. 2014;66(3):569–76.
19. Farnham SB, Webster TM, Herrell SD, Smith Jr JA. Intraoperative blood loss and transfusion requirements for robotic-assisted radical prostatectomy versus radical retropubic prostatectomy. Urology. 2006;67(2):360–3.
20. Parekh DJ, Messer J, Fitzgerald J, Ercole B, Svatek R. Perioperative outcomes and oncologic efficacy from a pilot prospective randomized clinical trial of open versus robotic assisted radical cystectomy. J Urol. 2013;189(2):474–9.
21. Musch M, Janowski M, Steves A, et al. Comparison of early postoperative morbidity after robot-assisted and open radical cystectomy: results of a prospective observational study. BJU Int. 2014;113(3):458–67.
22. Hayn MH, Hellenthal NJ, Seixas-Mikelus SA, et al. Is patient outcome compromised during the initial experience with robot-assisted radical cystectomy? Results of 164 consecutive cases. BJU Int. 2011;108(6):882–7.
23. Richards KA, Kader K, Pettus JA, Smith JJ, Hemal AK. Does initial learning curve compromise outcomes for robot-assisted radical cystectomy? A critical evaluation of the first 60 cases while establishing a robotics program. J Endourol. 2011;25(9):1553–8.
24. Hautmann RE, De Petriconi RC, Volkmer BG. Lessons learned from 1,000 neobladders: the 90-day complication rate. J Urol. 2010;184(3):990–4. quiz 1235.
25. Ahmed K, Khan SA, Hayn MH, et al. Analysis of intracorporeal compared with extracorporeal urinary diversion after robot-assisted radical cystectomy: results from the International Robotic Cystectomy Consortium. Eur Urol. 2014;65(2):340–7.
26. Hellenthal NJ, Hussain A, Andrews PE, et al. Surgical margin status after robot assisted radical cystectomy: results from the International Robotic Cystectomy Consortium. J Urol. 2010;184(1):87–91.
27. Buscarini M, Josephson DY, Stein JP. Lymphadenectomy in bladder cancer: a review. Urol Int. 2007;79(3):191–9.
28. Raza SJ, Wilson T, Peabody JO, et al. Long-term oncologic outcomes following robot-assisted radical cystectomy: results from the International Robotic Cystectomy Consortium. Eur Urol. 2015;68(4):721–8.
29. Khan MS, Challacombe B, Elhage O, et al. A dual-centre, cohort comparison of open, laparoscopic and robotic-assisted radical cystectomy. Int J Clin Pract. 2012;66(7):656–62.

Laparoscopic radical cystectomy with pelvic re-peritonealization: the technique and initial clinical outcomes

Qiang Cao[†][*], Pengchao Li[†], Xiao Yang[†], Jian Qian, Zengjun Wang, Qiang Lu[*] and Min Gu[*]

Abstract

Background: Delayed bowel function recovery and postoperative ileus are relatively serious complications of laparoscopic radical cystectomy (LRC). Our study aimed to determine whether performing pelvic re-peritonealization reduces the incidence of these complications.

Methods: Clinical data of 78 patients who had undergone LRC with pelvic re-peritonealization from August 2015 to December 2017 were retrospectively collected and compared with those of 92 patients who had undergone LRC alone between January 2013 and July 2015 in our institution. Differences in duration of surgery, estimated blood loss, time to recovery of bowel function, the complications of intestinal and blood vessel injury, and incidence of postoperative ileus between the two groups were analyzed.

Results: Baseline characteristics such as age, sex and BMI were balanced between the two groups. There were no significant differences in duration of surgery ($P = 0.072$), estimated blood loss ($P = 0.717$), or incidence of intestinal obstruction ($P = 0.225$) between the two groups. Interestingly, patients who had undergone pelvic re-peritonealization recovered bowel function more rapidly than those had not (2.79 d vs. 3.72 d, $P = 0.001$). Additionally, hospitalization stay was significantly shorter for patients with re-peritonealization than for those without (5.46 d vs. 6.68 d, $P = 0.029$).

Conclusions: Compared with LRC alone, LRC with pelvic re-peritonealization as described in the present study had comparable perioperative complications, but was associated with more rapid gastrointestinal recovery and shorter hospitalization stay.

Keywords: Laparoscopic radical cystectomy, Bowel function recovery, Re-peritonealization, Postoperative ileus

Background

Bladder carcinoma (BC), which is characterized by high risks of recurrence and mortality, is among the fifth most common malignancies worldwide [1] . Open radical cystectomy (ORC) with pelvic lymphadenectomy and subsequent urinary diversion remains the standard treatment for muscle-invasive and high-grade non-invasive bladder carcinoma [2, 3]. However, ORC is considered one of the most invasive of urological surgeries and has significant perioperative complications [4, 5]. Before 1970, the perioperative complication rate was approximately 35%

with a mortality rate of nearly 20% [6]. With medical advances, the mortality rate has decreased significantly, however, the postoperative morbidity of this surgery remains as high as 30% [7, 8]. Laparoscopic radical cystectomy (LRC), a minimally invasive treatment for bladder cancer, has achieved surgical outcomes that are comparable to those of ORC, but with fewer perioperative complications. Therefore, it has been widely substituted for ORC by urologists.

Perioperative complications related to the gastrointestinal tract are among the most common complications following radical cystectomy and urinary diversion [9]. Delayed recovery of bowel function and bowel obstruction may occur in the early postoperative period, the latter resulting from either paralytic ileus or mechanical obstruction [9]. Even in patients undergoing LRC, these complications are still problematic. Additionally, adhesive

---
* Correspondence: doctorlvqiang@sina.com; lancetgu@aliyun.com
[†]Qiang Cao, Pengchao Li and Xiao Yang contributed equally to this work.
Department of Urology, the First Affiliated Hospital of Nanjing Medical University, 300 Guangzhou Road, Nanjing 210029, China

ileus may occur at an early stage after surgery as a result of the intestinal tract adhering to the wound in the pelvic cavity. Figure 1 shows a typical example in which the intestinal tract adhered to the pelvic wound surface leading to angulation of the bowel followed by mechanical obstruction four days postoperatively, which may have been prevented if the pelvic peritoneum had been preserved. Although possible risk factors such as age, BMI and various perioperative variables have been suggested, as have preventive techniques for early postoperative paralytic ileus [10], there are few reports of techniques for minimizing the incidence of gastrointestinal complications. Here, we introduce a technique of pelvic re-peritonealization following LRC with pelvic lymphadenectomy and subsequent urinary diversion aimed at enhancing recovery of bowel function and reducing the incidence of postoperative ileus, report our preliminary experience with this procedure in 78 patients, and retrospectively compare the outcomes with those of 92 patients who had undergone LRC alone.

Methods

From August 2015 to December 2017, 78 consecutive patients with muscle invasive bladder cancer underwent LRC with pelvic re-peritonealization (LRC-PR) and standard lymph node dissection in our department. For comparison with these patients, another 92 patients who had undergone LRC between January 2013 and July 2015 in our center were identified and matched to the LRC-PR group by age, sex and BMI. All patients had undergone pelvic magnetic resonance/enhanced computed tomography, cystoscopy, and biopsy preoperatively. The clinical characteristics of these patients are presented

in Table 1. The study was approved by the Institutional Review Board of the first affiliated hospital of Nanjing Medical University. Written informed consent was obtained from all the participants.

All the patients were administered general anesthesia and placed in the supine position with the head tilted down at an angle of 30°. Laparoscopic ports were introduced as previously described [11]. In the LRC alone group, only the peritoneum covering the iliac blood vessels was preserved. In the LRC-PR group, the procedure was conducted as follows. During the operation, the superficial peritoneum of the external iliac vessel was incised, dissected medially along the vas deferens to the seminal vesicle, and preserved. The contralateral vas deferens and seminal vesicle were dissected using the same procedure. The peritoneum was then incised transversely at the dome of bladder (Fig. 2a), after which it was separated from the dome in a posterolateral direction (Fig. 2c-e). The peritoneum covering the dome of bladder was removed with the bladder if it was difficult to separate it from the bladder (Fig. 2f). The bladder was then dissected dorsally from the dome. During the dissection, the seminal vesicle could be easily identified. Denonvilliers' fascia was then incised, followed by dissection of the lateral ligaments of the bladder. A standard pelvic lymphadenectomy was performed after removal of the bladder. If the preserved peritoneum covering the anterior wall of the bladder blocked the surgical field during the procedure, a Hem-o-lok clip

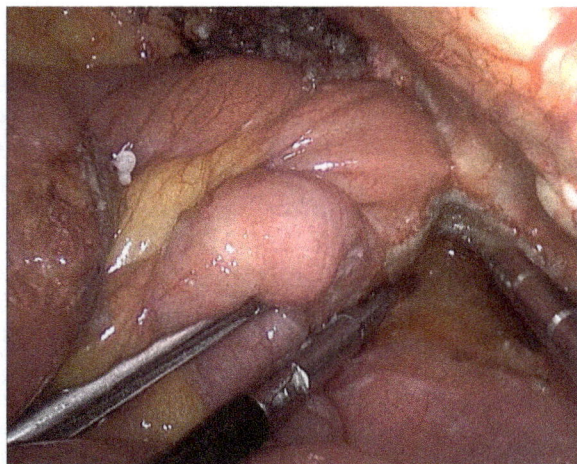

Fig. 1 An illustrative case of a 65-year-old woman who developed ileus four days postoperatively. Laparoscopic examination revealed that the intestinal tract had adhered to the pelvic wound surface, creating angulation of the bowel

Table 1 The clinical characteristics and perioperative parameters of patients received LRC with or without pelvic re-peritonealization

Variables	LRC-PR	LRC	p [#]
Patients, n	78	92	
Age	58.1 ± 8.35	57.5 ± 7.29	0.709
Gender			
Male	56 (71.8%)	68 (73.9%)	0.757
Female	22 (29.2%)	24 (26.1%)	
BMI (kg/m^2)	23.05 ± 3.48	24.34 ± 3.13	0.149
Total operative time	263.5 ± 36.5	244.1 ± 41.2	0.072
Estimated blood loss	312.3 ± 120.1	301.8 ± 91.3	0.717
Major Complications [*]	–	–	–
Bowel recovery time	2.79 ± 1.07	3.72 ± 0.93	0.001
Bowel obstruction	4 (5.1%)	9 (9.8%)	0.225
Hospitalization stay, d	5.46 ± 1.82	6.68 ± 2.21	0.029

[*] No major complications such as intestinal and blood vessels injury was observed in both groups
[#] Student t test for continuous variables; the chi-square test for categorical variables
LRC-PR laparoscopic radical cystectomy with pelvic re-peritonealization, LRC laparoscopic radical cystectomy

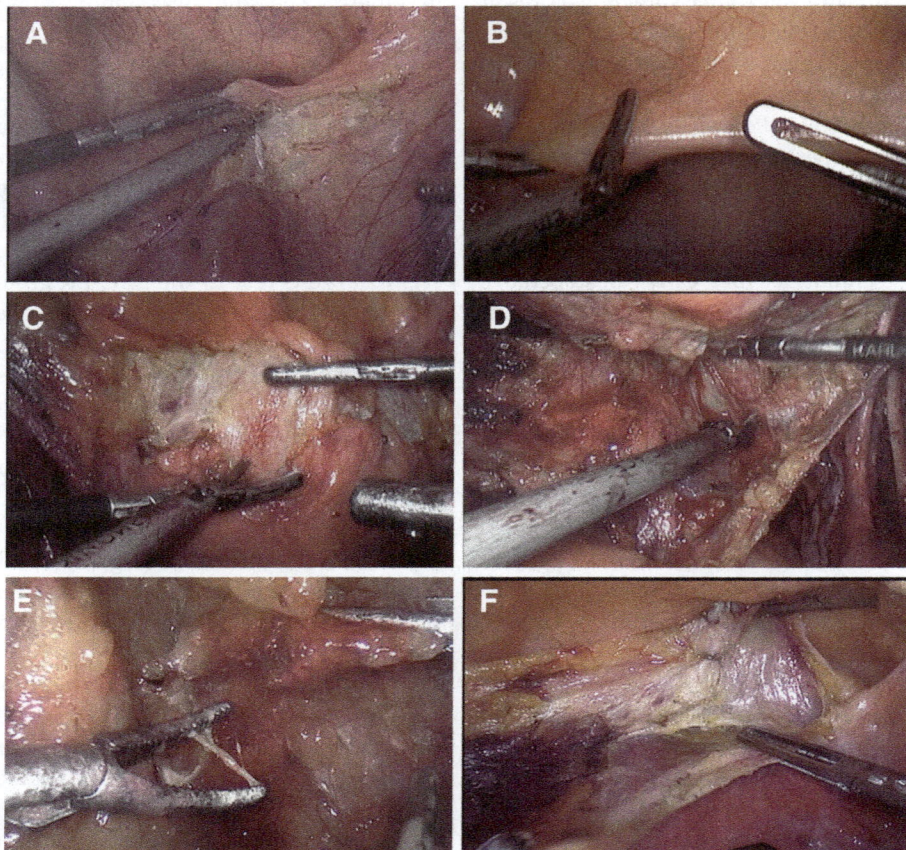

Fig. 2 The procedure for dissection of the peritoneum: (**a**) The peritoneum is incised transversely at the dome of the bladder. (**b**) The peritoneum is incised longitudinally. (**c–e**) Dissection of the peritoneum from the dome of the bladder in a posterolateral direction. (**f**) Removal of the peritoneum covering the dome of bladder because of difficulty in separating it from the bladder

was used to temporarily fix it to the ipsilateral abdominal wall.

Another way of preserving the peritoneum was to incise the peritoneum covering the bladder longitudinally from the ventral to the dorsal side (Fig. 2b). The peritoneum at the dome of the bladder was not preserved if it was difficult to dissect (Fig. 2f). During the dissection, careful attention was paid to avoiding incising the muscle layer of bladder. When dissecting the left part, the surgeon lifted the peritoneum to the left, using an ultrasonic scalpel to isolate the peritoneum along the adipose tissue while the assistant pulled the bladder to the opposite side to maintain tension. The same principles were adopted as for dissection of the right side of peritoneum.

After performing cystectomy and lymphadenectomy, the reperitonealization was achieved as follows (Fig. 3). First, the lateral peritoneum was closed along the external iliac vessels using a Hem-o-lok or titanium clip from the cranial to the caudal end (Fig. 3a, b). The pelvic peritoneum was then continuously sutured using barbed surgical

thread to seal the pelvic cavity (Fig. 3c). In patients who had undergone ureterocutaneostomy, a drainage tube was inserted into the pelvic cavity though a space between the peritoneal stitches (Fig. 3e). In patients who had had an orthotopic ileal neobladder constructed, the preserved peritoneum was sewn with interrupted sutures to the neobladder to seal the pelvic space (Fig. 3d-f) with the aim of reducing the risk of internal herniation.

All operations were performed by the same laparoscopic surgical team (QL, PL and QC). The following perioperative data were collected: duration of operation, time to bowel recovery, estimated blood loss, hospital stay, incidence of bowel and vessel injury, and incidence of bowel obstruction. Because few patients had ileal conduits or orthotopic ileal neobladders constructed, only patients who had undergone LRC with ureter–abdominal ostomies were included in the present study. Statistical analysis was performed using Student's t-test for continuous variables and the χ^2 test for categorical variables. All data are reported as means and ranges,

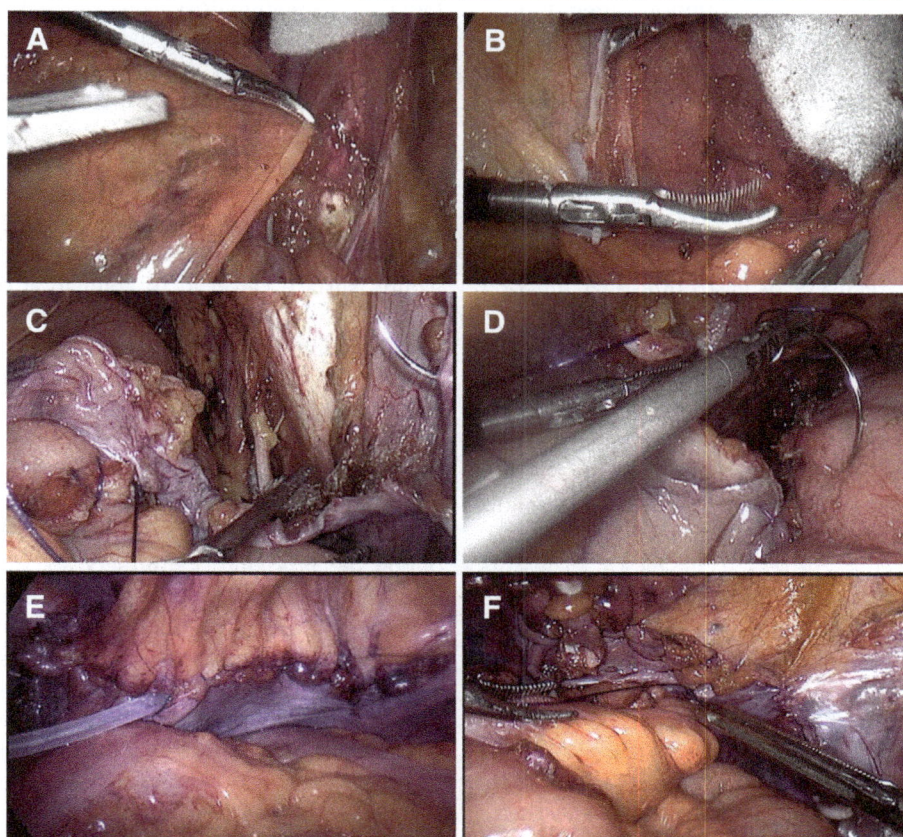

Fig. 3 Closing of the preserved peritoneum. (**a**, **b**) Closing of the lateral peritoneum. (**c**) Barbed surgical thread is used to continuously suture the pelvic peritoneum. (**d**) In patients undergoing construction of an orthotopic ileal neobladder, the preserved peritoneum is sewn using interrupted sutures to the neobladder. (**e**, **f**). The end result of pelvic peritonealization during laparoscopic radical cystectomy with ureterocutaneostomy (**e**) and construction of an orthotopic ileal neobladder (**f**)

with *P* values less than 0.05 considered to denote statistical significance.

Results

All procedures were successfully performed laparoscopically without the need for open conversion. Relevant clinical characteristics of the two groups are presented in Table 1. There were no significant differences in the distribution of age, sex or BMI between the two groups (all *P* > 0.05). At 263.5 mins, the mean duration of surgery was slightly longer in the LRC–PR than the LRC group (244.1 mins); however this difference is not statistically significant (*P* = 0.072). The mean estimated blood loss was 312.3 mL and 301.8 mL in the LRC-PR and LRC groups, respectively; these values are comparable (*P* = 0.717). No major complications such as bowel or vessel injury occurred in either group. The time to bowel recovery was 2.79 days in the LRC-PR group, which is significantly shorter than that in the LRC group (3.72 days) (*P* = 0.001). The incidence of bowel obstruction

was 5.1% (four patients) in the LRC–PR and 9.8% (nine patients) in the LRC group; this difference is not significant (*P* = 0.225). The four patients with bowel obstruction in the LRC–PR group recovered with conservative treatment, whereas six of the nine patients with bowel obstruction in the LRC group underwent laparoscopic surgery for adhesive ileus; an example is shown in Fig. 1. Additionally, hospital stay was significantly shorter in the group with re-peritonealization than in the group with LRC alone (5.46 d vs.6.68 d, *P* = 0.029).

Discussion

We here report our experience of the first clinical use of a novel technique for laparoscopic radical cystectomy with pelvic re-peritonealization. We demonstrated that the patients who underwent this procedure had more rapid postoperative recovery of gastrointestinal function and shorter hospital stay than those who underwent LRC alone.

Intestinal complications are common after radical cystectomy. The most frequent of these complications is postoperative ileus, which is often responsible for extended hospital stays and delayed recovery after surgery. The pathophysiology of postoperative ileus is complex and not yet fully understood. The many factors that have been recognized to be associated with postoperative ileus can be categorized as preoperative, intra-operative, and postoperative [10]. Several factors that may be associated with postoperative recovery of gastrointestinal function have been addressed in enhanced recovery after surgery (ERAS) protocols, which include evidence-based steps to optimize postoperative recovery and shorten hospital stay, mainly through expediting recovery of gastrointestinal function.

The incidence of paralytic ileus is reportedly significantly reduced by implementing ERAS protocols in patients undergoing radical cystectomy [9, 12]. However, most items addressed in ERAS protocols are pre- or post-operative; there are few reports on improving surgical techniques to reduce the incidence of gastrointestinal complications. For instance, Rivas et al. [12] reported a study using an ERAS protocol in patients with bladder cancer undergoing laparoscopic radical cystectomy. Of the 17 items included in their protocol, only four were intra-operative, namely using short-acting anesthetic agents, epidural anesthesia/analgesia, normothermia, and maintenance of normovolemia. Although none of these items involve modification of surgical technique, they found the complication of paralytic ileus occurred significantly less frequently in patients undergoing the ERAS protocol. In a review of gastrointestinal complications in patients subjected to enhanced recovery protocols, Djaladat et al. found that general anesthesia, opiate use, surgical trauma and bowel manipulation, bowel preparation, postoperative nasogastric tube, perioperative goal-directed fluid therapy, and chewing gum to be associated with reduced time to recovery of gastrointestinal function and a lower rate of paralytic ileus [9]. However, none of these items are related to surgical technique.

In the present study, during the procedure, we performed pelvic peritonealization after the cystectomy and lymphadenectomy. Patients who underwent this modified technique had significantly earlier bowel recovery, a lower incidence of paralytic ileus, and shorter hospital stays than those who did not. It has been suggested that neutrophil infiltration of the muscularis mucosae and subsequent ileus are related to the presence of inflammatory mediators released in response to surgical stimulation [13]. Additionally, exposure of the bowel to urine or transudation during intra- or post-operatively also induce an inflammatory reaction in the muscularis. In patients who undergo pelvic re-peritonealization, the pelvic space is sealed by peritonealization, confining intra- and post-operative exudates such as urine, blood, interstitial fluid, and lymphatic fluid to the pelvic cavity and thus facilitating their drainage through a drainage tube, reducing irritation of the intestines and possibly expediting recovery of bowel function. As previously mentioned, adhesion of the intestinal tract to the pelvic wound surface can lead to angulation of the bowel and consequent mechanical obstruction; this occurs relatively frequently in clinical practice (Fig. 1). Theoretically, pelvic re-peritonealization may also reduce the risk of intestinal adhesion and late adhesive intestinal obstruction. Additionally, without pelvic re-peritonealization, the intestine may prolapse into the pelvic cavity, which can also result in intestinal angulation and consequently obstruction. However, there is a risk of cutting bladder muscle during the procedure for preservation of the peritoneum. Therefore, we consider this procedure contraindicated in patients with greater than T2 disease and in slender patients with insufficient extraperitoneal adipose tissue.

The initial procedure for constructing an ileal conduit included closure of all mesenteric and peritoneal defects to minimize potential internal herniation; however, recent advances in laparoscopic and robotic techniques have often resulted in these defects being left open [14] [15]. Such defects can lead to small bowel entrapment and consequently obstruction, which carries a significant morbidity and mortality. The incidence of internal herniation is reportedly not affected by prior abdominal radiation or peritonitis; however, sewing the cut peritoneal edge to the conduit to reperitonealize it [14, 15] and closure of any mesenteric defects may prevent internal herniation [16]. In the present study, we used interrupted sutures to sew the preserved peritoneum to the conduit in patients undergoing construction of an orthotopic ileal neobladder; these patients' bowel function recovered rapidly and none of them developed postoperative paralytic ileus. However, the incidence of late intestinal complications requires further investigation.

Several limitations of the present study need to be addressed. First, this was a small study, especially regarding patients who underwent construction of an orthotopic ileal neobladder. Second, this was a single-center trial and would thus inevitably have been subject to selection bias. Third, the duration of follow-up was relatively short, allowing investigation of perioperative complications only. Late complications such as adhesive intestinal obstruction occur frequently in patients who have undergone LRC; long-term follow-up is therefore needed.

Conclusions

We here introduce a new technique for pelvic re-peritonealization during LRC. We found that this procedure is feasible and safe. Although, the procedure was slightly time consuming, it could effectively promote the bowel function recovery and may facilitate the ERAS program for patients with bladder cancer. Therefore, we suggest that LRC with pelvic re-peritonealization should be considered in suitable patients if surgically available available. However, larger studies and a multicenter prospective randomized controlled trial are required to confirm our results.

Abbreviations

BC: Bladder carcinoma; BMI: Body Mass Index; EBL: Estimated blood loss; ERAS: Enhanced recovery after surgery; LRC: Laparoscopic radical cystectomy; LRC-RP: LRC with pelvic re-peritonealization; ORC: Open radical cystectomy

Acknowledgements

The authors would like to thank all our participants in this study.

Funding

This work was supported by the National Natural Science Foundation of China (grants No. 81772711, 81602235 and 81272832), Jiangsu Province's Key Provincial Talents Program (ZDRCA2016006), the "333" project of Jiangsu Province (LGY2016002), the Provincial Initiative Program for Excellency Disciplines of Jiangsu Province (grant no. BE2016791), the Priority Academic Program Development of Jiangsu Higher Education Institutions (grant no. JX10231801) and Six Talent Peak Project in Jiangsu province (2015-wsw-033).

Authors' contributions

QL and MG participated in the conception and design of the study; QC, PCL, JQ, ZJW and XY participated in the acquisition, analysis and interpretation of data; QL, QC and XY drafted the manuscript of the study. All authors gave final approval for the manuscript and agree to be accountable for all aspects of the work herein.

Competing interests

The authors declare that they have no competing interests.

References

1. Zhang M, Li H, Zou D, Gao J. Ruguo key genes and tumor driving factors identification of bladder cancer based on the RNA-seq profile. OncoTargets and therapy. 2016;9:2717–23.
2. Ng CK, Kauffman EC, Lee MM, Otto BJ, Portnoff A, Ehrlich JR, Schwartz MJ, Wang GJ, Scherr DS. A comparison of postoperative complications in open versus robotic cystectomy. Eur Urol. 2010;57(2):274–81.
3. Hautmann RE. Urinary diversion: ileal conduit to neobladder. J Urol. 2003; 169(3):834–42.
4. Tang K, Xia D, Li H, Guan W, Guo X, Hu Z, Ma X, Zhang X, Xu H, Ye Z. Robotic vs. open radical cystectomy in bladder cancer: a systematic review and meta-analysis. Eur J Surg Oncol. 2014;40(11):1399–411.
5. Mansur RB, Rizzo LB, Santos CM, Asevedo E, Cunha GR, Noto MN, Pedrini M, Zeni M, Cordeiro Q, McIntyre RS, et al. Impaired glucose metabolism moderates the course of illness in bipolar disorder. J Affect Disord. 2016;195:57–62.
6. Khan MS, Elhage O, Challacombe B, Rimington P, Murphy D, Dasgupta P. Analysis of early complications of robotic-assisted radical cystectomy using a standardized reporting system. Urology. 2011;77(2):357–62.
7. Stein JP, Lieskovsky G, Cote R, Groshen S, Feng AC, Boyd S, Skinner E, Bochner B, Thangathurai D, Mikhail M, et al. Radical cystectomy in the treatment of invasive bladder cancer: long-term results in 1,054 patients. J Clin Oncol. 2001;19(3):666–75.
8. Studer UE, Burkhard FC, Schumacher M, Kessler TM, Thoeny H, Fleischmann A, Thalmann GN. Twenty years experience with an ileal orthotopic low pressure bladder substitute--lessons to be learned. J Urol. 2006;176(1):161–6.
9. Djaladat H, Daneshmand S. Gastrointestinal complications in patients who undergo radical cystectomy with enhanced recovery protocol. Current urology reports. 2016;17(7):50.
10. Maffezzini M, Campodonico F, Canepa G, Gerbi G, Parodi D. Current perioperative management of radical cystectomy with intestinal urinary reconstruction for muscle-invasive bladder cancer and reduction of the incidence of postoperative ileus. Surg Oncol. 2008;17(1):41–8.
11. Shao P, Meng X, Li J, Lv Q, Zhang W, Xu Z, Yin C. Laparoscopic extended pelvic lymph node dissection during radical cystectomy: technique and clinical outcomes. BJU Int. 2011;108(1):124–8.
12. Rivas JG, Sergio Alonso Y, JCL G, Orejón RU, Doslada PU, Sebastián JD, Gómez ÁT, de la Peña Barthel JJ. Early recovery protocol in patients undergoing laparoscopic radical cystectomy. Urological Science. 2015;28(1):2–5.
13. Kalff JC, Carlos TM, Schraut WH, Billiar TR, Simmons RL, Bauer AJ. Surgically induced leukocytic infiltrates within the rat intestinal muscularis mediate postoperative ileus. Gastroenterology. 1999;117(2):378–87.
14. Gill IS, Fergany A, Klein EA, Kaouk JH, Sung GT, Meraney AM, Savage SJ, Ulchaker JC, Novick AC. Laparoscopic radical cystoprostatectomy with ileal conduit performed completely intracorporeally: the initial 2 cases. Urology. 2000;56(1):26–9 discussion 29-30.
15. Murphy DG, Challacombe BJ, Elhage O, O'Brien TS, Rimington P, Khan MS, Dasgupta P. Robotic-assisted laparoscopic radical cystectomy with extracorporeal urinary diversion: initial experience. Eur Urol. 2008;54(3):570–80.
16. Gause CD, Casamassima MG, Yang J, Hsiung G, Rhee D, Salazar JH, Papandria D, Pryor HI 2nd, Stewart D, Lukish J, et al. Laparoscopic versus open inguinal hernia repair in children </=3: a randomized controlled trial. Pediatr Surg Int. 2017;33(3):367–76.

Transperineal ultrasound-guided prostate biopsy is safe even when patients are on combination antiplatelet and/or anticoagulation therapy

Kimitoshi Saito[1]*, Satoshi Washino[1], Yuhki Nakamura[1], Tsuzumi Konishi[1], Masashi Ohshima[1], Yoshiaki Arai[2] and Tomoaki Miyagawa[1]

Abstract

Background: To assess whether hemorrhagic complications associated with transperineal prostate biopsy increased in patients on antiplatelet and/or anticoagulant therapy.

Methods: In total, 598 consecutive patients underwent transperineal prostate biopsy. The medication group comprised patients who took anti-thromboembolic agents, and the control group comprised those who did not take these agents. No anti-thromboembolic agent was stopped before, during, or after prostate biopsy in the medication group. Complications developing in both groups were compared and classified using the modified Clavien classification system. Subgroup analyses to compare complications in patients taking single antiplatelet, single anticoagulant, and dual antiplatelet and/or anticoagulant agents, and multivariate analyses to predict bleeding risk were also performed.

Results: Of the 598 eligible patients, 149 comprised the medication group and 449 comprised the control group. Hematuria (Grade I) developed in 88 (59.1%) and 236 (52.5%) patients in the medication and control group, respectively (p = 0.18). Clot retention (Grade I) was more frequently observed in the medication group than the controls (2.0% versus 0.2%, respectively, p < 0.05). Hospitalization was more frequently prolonged in the medication than the control group (4.0% versus 0.4% of patients, respectively). No complication of Grade III or higher developed in either group. Hematuria was more frequent in patients taking a single anticoagulant (p = 0.007) or two anti-thromboembolic agents (p = 0.04) compared with those taking a single antiplatelet agent. Other complications were generally similar among the groups. In the multivariate analysis, taking more than two anti-thromboembolic agents was the only significant risk factor for bleeding events.

Conclusion: No severe complication developed after the transperineal biopsies in either group, although minor bleeding was somewhat more frequent in the medication group. It may not be necessary to discontinue anticoagulant and/or antiplatelet agents when transperineal prostate biopsy is contemplated.

Keywords: Anticoagulant, Antiplatelet, Complication, Dual antiplatelet therapy, Transperineal prostate biopsy

* Correspondence: k.saito@jichi.ac.jp
[1]Department of Urology, Jichi Medical University Saitama Medical Center, 1-847, Amanuma-cho, Omiya-ku, Saitama 330-8503, Japan
Full list of author information is available at the end of the article

Background

Systematic prostate biopsy is routinely performed on patients with suspected prostate cancer, to obtain tissue cores [1]. Certain hemorrhagic complications including hematuria, hematospermia, and rectal and perineal bleeding, have been reported [2]. Recently, urologists are increasingly encountering patients with multiple comorbidities including coronary arterial disease that earlier required percutaneous coronary arterial intervention with angioplasty, together with placement of bare metal or drug-eluting stent (DES). Other patients have cardiac dysrhythmias such as atrial fibrillation, valvular heart disease, or deep vein thrombosis. In others, inferior vena cava filters have been placed [3]. These comorbidities are managed using an increasing array of oral antiplatelet (AP) and anticoagulant (AC) drugs; such patients require comprehensive management to mitigate the risk of complications after urological interventions. DESs are often placed in patients with coronary artery disease; such patients cannot simply stop taking AP drugs in the perioperative period surrounding prostate biopsy.

When patients taking such drugs require surgical intervention, including transrectal ultrasound (TRUS)-guided prostate biopsy, one of the following three medication options must be chosen after detailed discussion between doctor and patient and the giving of informed consent: drug continuation, interruption, or use of a heparin bridge. Several studies have shown that aspirin increases the incidence of minor but not severe bleeding events during TRUS-guided biopsy [4–7]. An International Consultation on Urological Disease/American Urological Association (ICUD/AUA) review reported that prostate biopsy is safe for patients taking low-dose aspirin; the risk of minor bleeding is only approximately one-third higher than in controls [3]. However, these studies featured transrectal, not transperineal biopsy. Furthermore, it has been but seldom studied whether patients on AC therapy, dual antiplatelet therapy (DAPT), or combination AP and AC therapy, can safely undergo prostate biopsy while remaining on these drugs.

This study evaluated whether transperineal prostate biopsy could be performed safely on patients taking Aps or ACs, without discontinuing the drugs.

Methods

Patients

This was a retrospective observational study approved by our local institutional review board. A total of 598 eligible patients underwent prostate biopsy (with collection of more than 14 tissue cores from each), on suspicion of prostate cancer, at Jichi Medical University Saitama Medical Center, from July 2011 to December 2015. The AP/AC group comprised patients taking APs or ACs, and the remainder constituted the control group. The APs were aspirin, cilostazol, clopidogrel, and ticlopidine. The ACs were warfarin, rivaroxaban, dabigatran, and apixaban. No AP or AC drug was stopped before, during, or after the prostate biopsy.

Biopsy protocol

All of the biopsies were performed via the transperineal approach, using an 18-gauge needle (Tru-Core II Automatic Biopsy Instrument, ARGON MEDICAL DEVICES, Athens, TX, USA) under general or spinal anesthesia. Each TRUS-guided systematic biopsy typically yielded 14 cores, eight from the peripheral lobe and six from the transitional lobe. In patients with suspicious lesions evident on magnetic resonance imaging (MRI), two additional targeted cores were collected for each lesion. All targeted biopsies were performed using a cognitive registration technique, as described previously, with some modification [8]. As perioperative antimicrobial prophylaxis, levofloxacin 500 mg was prescribed once daily for 3 days. The patients were discharged the next morning.

Evaluation of comorbidities

All of the patients were evaluated about 2 weeks after the prostate biopsy at the first outpatient visit. They were asked about the incidence of bleeding-associated events and other complications. Bleeding-associated events were gross hematuria, perineal hematoma, and clot retention. Events observed at least once were included. Gross hematuria was defined as passing blood or red urine. Perineal hematoma was defined as a non-pulsatile mass > 1.5 cm in diameter diagnosed by visual examination and palpation of the perineum. Clot retention was defined as acute urinary retention due to clot. Hematospermia was not evaluated. Other complications were acute urinary retention and infection. Prolonged hospitalization was defined as a patient who was not discharged the next morning. Comorbidities were classified using the modified Clavien classification system [9].

Statistical analysis

The types and proportions of complications between the AP/AC and control groups were compared. Subgroup analysis was performed among groups taking single APs, single ACs, and dual APs and/or ACs. Statistical analysis was performed with the aid of GraphPad Prism ver. 5.0 or SPSS ver. 19.0. Data were compared using Student's t-test, the Mann–Whitney U-test, or the chi-square test. Multivariate analysis was performed using logistic regression analysis to determine significant predictors of bleeding events. The hazard ratio and 95% confidence interval were determined. All data shown are means and standard deviations, or medians with interquartile ranges (IQR). Statistical significance was set at $p < 0.05$.

Results

Patient characteristics and biopsy outcomes

A total of 598 eligible patients underwent prostate biopsies: 149 took APs or ACs (AP/AC group), while 449 did not take APs or ACs (control group). Table 1 shows the patient characteristics and biopsy outcomes. Patients in the AP/AC group were significantly older than those in the control group (71.6 ± 6.7 vs. 68.7 ± 7.5 years; $p < 0.0001$). The prostate-specific antigen (PSA) level, prostate volume, number of biopsy cores collected, and cancer detection rate did not significantly differ between the two groups.

AP and AC therapy

Of the 149 patients in the AP/AC group, 80, 34, 19, and 16 were on single AP, single AC, DAPT, and combination AP and AC therapy, respectively (Table 2). Most patients in the single AP and single AC subgroups were taking aspirin (65/80 patients) or warfarin (25/34 patients). The daily dosage of aspirin, cilostazol, clopidogrel, and ticlopidine was 100 mg, 75 mg, 100–200 mg, and 100–200 mg, respectively. The daily dosage of warfarin, rivaroxaban, dabigatran, and apixaban was 0.56–4.75 mg, 10–15 mg, 150–300 mg, and 5 mg, respectively. The median (IQR) prothrombin time- international normalized ratio in patients taking warfarin was 1.735 (1.420–2.053).

Reasons for taking APs or ACs

Table 3 shows the reasons for taking APs or ACs. Ischemic heart disease, atrial fibrillation, and cerebral infarction were the first (34.9%), second (30.9%), and third (17.4%) most common reasons.

Complications in the AP and/or AC group *versus the control group*

Complications after prostate biopsy in the two groups are shown in Table 4. Grade I complications: the frequency of hematuria was similar in both groups (59.1% in the AP/AC vs. 52.5% in the control group; $p = 0.18$); three patients (2.0%) of the AP/AC group experienced clot retention, the incidence of which was significantly higher than in the control group (one [0.2%] patient; $p = 0.049$); two (1.3%) and three patients (0.7%) of the

AP/AC and control groups, respectively, experienced perineal hematoma ($p = 0.60$); four (2.7%) and seven (1.6%) patients in the AP/AC and control groups, respectively, experienced acute urinary retention ($p = 0.48$). Grade II complications: two (1.3%) and one (0.2%) patient in the AP/AC and control groups, respectively, experienced urinary tract infection ($p = 0.15$). No Grade III or higher complication developed in either group. Six AP/AC patients required prolonged hospitalization, the incidence of which was significantly higher than in the control group (two patients [0.4%]; $p = 0.01$). The causes of prolonged hospitalization in AP/AC group patients were clot retention in three, perineal hematoma in one, acute urinary retention in one, and aspiration pneumonitis in

Table 2 Details of the antiplatelet and anticoagulant therapies

		n = 149	(%)
Single	Antiplatelet		
	Aspirin	65	(43.6)
	Cilostazol	7	(4.7)
	Clopidogrel	5	(3.4)
	Ticlopidine	3	(2.0)
	Total	80	(53.7)
	Anticoagulant		
	Warfarin	25	(16.8)
	Rivaroxaban	4	(2.7)
	Dabigatran	4	(2.7)
	Apixaban	1	(0.7)
	Total	34	(22.8)
Dual	Dual antiplatelet therapy		
	Aspirin + Clopidogrel	14	(9.4)
	Aspirin + Ticlopidine	3	(2.0)
	Aspirin + Cilostazol	2	(1.3)
	Total	19	(12.8)
	Antiplatelet + Anticoagulant		
	Aspirin + Warfarin	10	(6.7)
	Other combinations	6	(4.0)
	Total	16	(10.7)

Table 1 Patient characteristics and cancer detection rate

	Control, n = 449	AP/AC, n = 149	
	mean (SD)	mean (SD)	p value
Age	68.7 (7.5)	71.6 (6.7)	< 0.0001
PSA, ng/mL	10.3 (8.5)	11.4 (15.4)	0.44
Prostate volume, cm³	50.2 (24.3)	51.1 (27.8)	0.75
Biopsy cores, median (range)	16 (14–22)	16 (14–22)	0.67
Cancer detection, n (%)	254 (56.6)	93 (62.4)	0.21

PSA Prostate specific antigen, *AP* Antiplatelet, *AC* Anticoagulant

Table 3 Reason for taking antiplatelet or anticoagulant therapy

	n = 149	(%)
Ischemic heart disease	52	(34.9)
Atrial fibrillation	46	(30.9)
Cerebral infarction	26	(17.4)
Heart valve replacement surgery	13	(8.7)
Arteriosclerosis obliterans or cervical arterial stenosis	8	(5.4)
Primary prophylaxis	11	(7.4)
Others/Unknown	6	(4.1)

Table 4 Complications in the antiplatelet/anticoagulant group versus the control group

Modified Clavien-Dindo Classification	Complications	Control n = 449	AP/AC n = 149	
		n (%)	n (%)	p value
I	Hematuria	236 (52.5)	88 (59.1)	0.18
	Perineal hematoma	3 (0.7)	2 (1.3)	0.60
	Acute urinary retention	7 (1.6)	4 (2.7)	0.48
	Clot retention	1 (0.2)	3 (2.0)	< 0.05
II	Urinary tract infection	1 (0.2)	2 (1.3)	0.15
	Prolonged hospitalization	2 (0.4)	6 (4.0)	< 0.05

AP Antiplatelet, *AC* Anticoagulant

one; both control group patients had perineal hematomas. No patient of either group required re-admission.

Complications in the single AP vs. the single AC vs. the dual therapy subgroups

The complications among subgroups taking single APs, single ACs, and dual antithrombotic agents are compared in Table 5. Hematuria was more frequent in the single AC ($p = 0.007$) and dual antithrombotic subgroups ($p = 0.04$) than the single AP subgroup. No other complication, nor the need for prolonged hospitalization, differed significantly among subgroups.

Risk factors for bleeding events

We performed a multivariate analysis to predict which patients were more likely to have bleeding events by comparing patients who experienced bleeding events, such as hematuria, perineal hematoma, and clot retention ($n = 302$), with those who did not ($n = 257$). Patients who had missing data were excluded from this analysis ($n = 39$). The results are shown in Table 6. Taking more than two

Table 5 Complications in the single antiplatelet or single anticoagulant versus the dual therapy subgroups

Modified Clavien Classification	Complications	Single, n = 114		Dual, n = 35
		AP, n = 80 n (%)	AC, n = 34 n (%)	n (%)
I	Hematuria	38 (47.5)	26 (76.5)*	24 (68.6)*
	Perineal hematoma	0	2 (5.9)	0
	Acute urinary retention	1 (1.3)	2 (5.9)	1 (2.9)
	Clot retention	3 (3.8)	0	0
II	Urinary tract infection	0	0	2 (5.7)
	Prolonged hospitalization	4 (5.0)	1 (2.9)	1 (2.9)

* $p < 0.05$ vs. AP group, *AP* Antiplatelet, *AC* Anticoagulant

Table 6 Multivariate analysis to predict the risk factors for bleeding events

	Variable	N	Hazard ratio	95% CI	p value
Age	< 70	294	-	-	
	≥ 70	265	0.931	0.657–1.319	0.687
PSA, ng/ml	< 6.0	158	-	-	
	6.0–9.9	214	0.839	0.551–1.277	0.413
	≥ 10	187	0.696	0.450–1.076	0.103
Number of biopsy cores	< 16	204	-	-	
	≥ 16	355	0.974	0.683–1.389	0.883
Prostate volume, cm³	< 45.0	278	-	-	
	≥ 45.0	281	1.135	0.805–1.600	0.470
No. of AP/AC agents	0	420	-	-	
	1	105	1.339	0.863–2.076	0.193
	≥ 2	34	2.230	1.028–4.839	0.042

PSA Prostate specific antigen, *AP* Antiplatelet, *AC* Anticoagulant, *CI* Confidence interval

APs/ACs was a significant predictor of bleeding events (Hazard ratio [95% CI]: 2.230 [1.028–4.839], $p = 0.042$), while age, PSA levels, number of biopsy cores, and prostate volume were not significant.

Discussion

In the study, we found the following that complications arising after transperineal biopsy were generally similar in patients who were or were not taking AP/AC, although clot retention was somewhat more frequent in patients taking AP/AC agents (Table 4). In addition, patients who were taking more than two AP/AC agents were more likely to experience bleeding events (Table 6), and no complication of grade III or higher were noted in any group.

It has been suggested that 10–12 systematic biopsy cores are required for a histopathological diagnosis of prostate cancer [1]. Recently, targeted biopsies of suspicious MRI lesions have improved prostate cancer detection. However, biopsy of not only targeted lesions but also systematic prostate biopsy is required [10–12]. As the number of biopsy cores increases, possible hemorrhagic complications must be considered.

In this study, we examined the safety of transperineal prostate biopsy in patients taking APs/ACs compared with controls (not on APs or ACs). The frequency of hematuria was similar in the AP/AC and control groups (Table 4). However, hemorrhagic events requiring treatment, such as clot retention and transperineal hematoma, were somewhat more frequent in the AP/AC than the control group, which might increase the frequency of prolonged hospitalization in the AP/AC group.

Halliwell et al. reported that 72% of patients taking aspirin experienced hematuria after transrectal biopsy;

this value was significantly higher than the control value of 62% [5]. By contrast, Chowdhury et al. found that hematuria developed after transrectal biopsy in 28, 34, and 37% of patients on warfarin, aspirin, and controls, respectively; these proportions did not significantly differ [6]. The meta-analysis of Carmignani et al. [13] showed that hematuria was significantly more frequent among patients taking aspirin than controls (odds ratio [OR] of 1.36). However, the increased risk was for minor bleeding only. The ICUD/AUA have stated that prostate biopsy can be performed safely on patients on low-dose aspirin; the risk of minor bleeding is only approximately one-third higher than in the controls [3]. However, this suggestion held only for transrectal, and not transperineal, biopsy. Recently, Asano et al. [14] studied whether it was safe to continue antithrombotic agents in patients undergoing transperineal biopsy and found that the frequencies of hemorrhagic complications after transperineal biopsy were similar among control, continued drug administration, and interrupted drug administration groups; no severe hemorrhagic complications occurred, consistent with our results.

Patients on DAPT are increasing in line with the popularization of DESs in patients with coronary artery disease. Other patients take AP/AC combinations to treat various conditions. However, it has been unclear whether prostate biopsy was safe when patients were on two antithrombotics. Recently, Raheem et al. found that patients taking APs and/or ACs (5 and 11% of all patients studied were on aspirin-plus-warfarin or aspirin-plus-clopidogrel, respectively) had fewer hematuria episodes than controls [15]. We found that the frequency of complications did not generally differ among subgroups taking single APs, single ACs, or dual anti-thromboembolic agents, although hematuria was more frequent in the single AC and dual anti-thromboembolic subgroups than in the single AP subgroup (Table 5). In the multivariate analysis, the number of AP/AC agents was the only significant predictor of bleeding events (Table 6). No complication of grade III or higher was encountered in any group. Therefore, patients who are taking two APs or ACs may experience minor bleeding events more frequently, but will not experience severe complications after transperineal prostate biopsy.

Aspirin non-adherence/withdrawal is associated with a three-fold higher risk of major adverse cardiac events (OR 3.14) [16]. This risk is magnified in patients with intracoronary stents; discontinuation of AP treatment was associated with an even higher risk of adverse events (OR 89.78). Furthermore, aspirin interruption increases the incidence of ischemic stroke/transient ischemic attack (OR 3.4) [17].

In 493 patients who stopped continuous anticoagulation therapy to allow the performance of dental procedures, 5

(1%) developed severe embolic complications, including four deaths [18]. Discontinuation of ACs might increase the risk of severe embolic complications. When warfarin is discontinued, a heparin bridge is recommended [19]. However, heparin bridging is controversial because it was recently demonstrated that a heparin bridge did not decrease the risks of ischemic stroke or systemic embolism in stable non-valvular atrial fibrillation [20]. Overall, discontinuation of APs/ACs is associated with severe thrombotic events; thus, the continuation of these drugs is ideal. When patients taking anti-thromboembolic agents are scheduled to undergo transperineal TRUS-guided prostate biopsy, clinicians and patients can select one of two following plans: to continue these agents with the risk of minor bleeding or to interrupt these agents with the risk of rare severe thromboembolic complications. We believe that it is more reasonable to continue anti-thromboembolic agents than to refuse to accept the slight risk of a mild bleeding event.

There were several limitations in this study. First, the retrospective nature of the work increased the risk of patient selection bias. Second, we did not assess the extent or duration of hematuria; thus, we do not know if they differed among groups. However, no Grade III or higher complication developed in any group.

Conclusions

No Grade III or higher complication developed after transperineal biopsy in either the medication or control group, although clot retention was observed somewhat more frequently in the medication group. It may not be necessary to discontinue anticoagulant or antiplatelet agents when transperineal prostate biopsy is performed.

Abbreviations

AC: Anticoagulant; AP: Antiplatelet; AUA: American Urological Association; DAPT: Dual antiplatelet therapy; DES: Drug-eluting stent; ICUD: International Consultation on Urological Disease; IQR: Interquartile range; MRI: Magnetic resonance imaging; OR: Odds ratio; PSA: Prostate specific antigen; TRUS: Transrectal ultrasound

Acknowledgments

Not applicable.

Funding

None.

Authors' contributions

KS was a major contributor to the conception and design of the study and in drafting the manuscript. SW and MT analyzed and interpreted the patient data. YN, TK, MO, and YA provided administrative and technical support, including data acquisition. All of the authors read and approved the final manuscript.

Competing interests

The authors declare that they have no competing interests.

Author details

[1]Department of Urology, Jichi Medical University Saitama Medical Center, 1-847, Amanuma-cho, Omiya-ku, Saitama 330-8503, Japan. [2]Department of Urology, Nishi-Omiya Hospital, 1-1173, Mihashi, Omiya-ku, Saitama 330-0856, Japan.

References

1. EAU guidelines on prostate cancer. European Association of Urology. http://uroweb.org/guideline/prostate-cancer. Accessed 30 Sep 2016.
2. Kakehi Y, Naito S, Japanese Urological Association. Complication rates of ultrasound-guided prostate biopsy: a nation-wide survey in Japan. Int J Urol. 2008;15:319–21.
3. Culkin DJ, Exaire EJ, Green D, Soloway MS, Gross AJ, Desai MR, et al. Anticoagulation and antiplatelet therapy in urological practice: ICUD/AUA review paper. J Urol. 2014;192:1026–34.
4. Giannarini G, Mogorovich A, Valent F, Morelli G, De Maria M, Manassero F, et al. Continuing or discontinuing low-dose aspirin before transrectal prostate biopsy: results of a prospective randomized trial. Urol. 2007;70:501–5.
5. Halliwell OT, Yadegafar G, Lane C, Dewbury KC. Transrectal ultrasound-guided biopsy of the prostate: aspirin increases the incidence of minor bleeding complications. Clin Radiol. 2008;63:557–61.
6. Chowdhury R, Abbas A, Idriz S, Hoy A, Rutherford EE, Smart JM. Should warfarin or aspirin be stopped prior to prostate biopsy? An analysis of bleeding complications related to increasing sample number regimes. Clin Radiol. 2012;67:e64–70.
7. Vasudeva P, Kumar N, Kumar A, Singh H, Kumar G. Safety of 12 core transrectal ultrasound guided prostate biopsy in patients on aspirin. IBJU. 2015;41:1096–100.
8. Kasivisvanathan V, Dufour R, Moore CM, Ahmed HU, Abd-Alazeez M, Charman SC, et al. Transperineal magnetic resonance image targeted prostate biopsy versus transperineal template prostate biopsy in the detection of clinically significant prostate cancer. J Urol. 2013;189:860.
9. Mamoulakis C, Efthimiou I, Kazoulis S, Christoulakis I, Sofras F. The modified Clavien classification system: a standardized platform for reporting complications in transurethral resection of the prostate. World J Urol. 2011;29:205–10.
10. Rooij M, Hamoen EHJ, Fütterer JJ, Barentsz JO, Rovers MM. Accuracy of multiparametric MRI for prostate cancer detection: a meta-analysis. AJR. 2014;202:343–51.
11. Kumar V, Jagannathan NR, Thulkar S, Kumar R. Prebiopsy magnetic resonance spectroscopy and imaging in the diagnosis of prostate cancer. Int J Urol. 2012;19:602–13.
12. Miyagawa T, Ishikawa S, Kimura T, Suetomi T, Tsutsumi M, Irie T, et al. Real-time virtual sonography for navigation during targeted prostate biopsy using magnetic resonance imaging data. Int J Urol. 2010;17:855–60.
13. Carmignani L, Picozzi S, Bozzini G, Negri E, Ricci C, Gaeta M, et al. Transrectal ultrasound-guided prostate biopsies in patients taking aspirin for cardiovascular disease: a meta-analysis. Transfus Apher Sci. 2011;45:275.
14. Asano T, Kobayashi S, Yano M, Otsuka Y, Kitahara S. Continued administration of antithrombotic agents during transperineal prostate biopsy. In Braz J Urol. 2015;41:116–23.
15. Raheem OA, Casey RG, Galvin DJ, Manecksha RP, Varadaraj H, McDermott T, et al. Discontinuation of anticoagulant or antiplatelet therapy for transrectal ultrasound-guided prostate biopsies: a single-center experience. Korean J Urol. 2012;53:234–9.
16. Biondi-Zoccai GG, Lotrionte M, Agostoni P, Abbate A, Fusaro M, Burzotta F, et al. A systematic review and meta-analysis on the hazards of discontinuing or not adhering to aspirin among 50,279 patients at risk for coronary artery disease. Eur Heart J. 2006;27:2667–74.
17. Maulaz AB, Bezerra DC, Michel P, Bogousslavsky J. Effect of discontinuing aspirin therapy on the risk of brain ischemic stroke. Arch Neurol. 2005;62:1217–20.
18. Wahl MJ. Dental surgery in anticoagulated patients. Arch Intern Med. 1998; 158:1610–6.
19. Kristensen SD, Knuuti J, Saraste A, Anker S, Bøtker HE, Hert SD, et al. 2014 ESC/ESA guidelines on non-cardiac surgery: cardiovascular assessment and management: the joint task force on non-cardiac surgery: cardiovascular assessment and management of the European Society of Cardiology (ESC) and the European Society of Anaesthesiology (ESA). Eur Heart J. 2014;35:2383–431.
20. Bouillon K, Bertrand M, Boudali L, Ducimetiere P, Dray-Spira R, Zureik M. Short-term risk of bleeding during heparin bridging at initiation of vitamin K antagonist therapy in more than 90000 patients with nonvalvular atrial fibrillation managed in outpatient care. J Am Heart Assoc. 2016;31:5–15.

Bilateral benign renal oncocytomas and the role of renal biopsy

Andrew R. Leone[*†], Laura C. Kidd[†], Gregory J. Diorio, Kamran Zargar-Shoshtari, Pranav Sharma, Wade J. Sexton and Philippe E. Spiess

Abstract

Background: The goal was to assess the natural history and management of patients with pathologically proven bilateral (synchronous) RO after undergoing initial partial nephrectomy (PN).

Methods: All patients underwent either robotic/laparoscopic or open PN by two experienced genitourinary oncologists from 2005–2013. Final pathology was determined by surgical excision, CT-guided percutaneous core biopsy (CT-biopsy) or fine needle aspiration (FNA). Patient demographics, tumor characteristics (pathologic data, location, size) type of surgery, pre/post estimated glomerular filtration rate (eGFR) and surgical complications were recorded.

Results: Twelve patients were identified with bilateral RO. Median age at the time of surgery was 68 years (46–77) (Table 1). The median size of the largest tumor(s) resected was 2.75 cm (1.5–5.5 cm) and second largest tumor(s) was 1.75 cm (1.0–4.0 cm). Four patients underwent bilateral staged PN and one patient underwent simultaneous bilateral PN (horseshoe kidney). Two patients underwent RFA at the time of biopsy of the contralateral mass after PN. Five patients underwent CT-bx/FNA (5/5) of the contralateral mass followed by active surveillance.
Mean follow up was 34 months. There was no significant change in median creatinine pre- and post-operatively. One patient was lost to follow up and one patient died of unknown causes 5 years post-operatively. eGFR decreased an average of 16.96% post-operatively, including a single patient whose eGFR increased by 7.8% after surgery and a single patient whose eGFR did not change (Table 2).

Conclusions: Patients with bilateral renal masses and pathologically proven RO can be safely managed with active surveillance after biopsy confirmation of the contralateral mass.

Keywords: Bilateral, Biopsy, Oncocytoma, Renal cell carcinoma, Synchronous

Background

Renal oncocytoma (RO) is the second most common benign renal neoplasm which arises from the intercalated collecting duct cells in the kidney [1, 2]. It has an estimated incidence of 3 to 7% of all primary renal masses [3, 4] and comprises 10 to 15% of enhancing small renal masses (≤4 cm in diameter) [5]. It commonly presents in men in the seventh decade of life and is often diagnosed incidentally [3]. RO can be unilateral or bilateral (4 to 14% of cases), solitary or multifocal (2 to 12% of cases) and can exist concurrently with malignant components, specifically renal cell carcinoma (RCC) [6], frequently chromophobe RCC (chRCC) [7]. Oncocytosis has been used to describe numerous discrete oncocytic nodules, usually with the presence of a larger primary nodule [7].

In clinical practice, RO often represents a diagnostic challenge, due to its similarity in appearance to renal cell carcinoma on both pathology and imaging, [2] specifically chromophobe RCC. RO and chromophobe RCC share a common cellular origin from intercalated cells [8]. Recent research has attempted to distinguish the two tumors. The radiologic finding of "segmental

---

* Correspondence: Andrew.leone@moffitt.org
[†]Equal contributors
Department of Genitourinary Oncology, H. Lee Moffitt Cancer Center and Research Institute, 12902 Magnolia Drive Office 12538, Tampa, FL 33612, USA

Table 1 Demographic and outcomes data

Parameter	
Number of patients	12
Mean Age (yrs.)	66.8
Gender	
Male	10
Female	2
Mean BMI (kg/m^2)	32.1
Median largest tumor size (cm)	2.75
Median next largest tumor (cm)	1.75
Mean Pre-operative Creatinine (mg/dL)	0.95
Pre-operative CKD[b]	16.7%
Post-operative CKD[b]	33.3%
Post-operative Creatinine (mg/dL) at 1 month	1.01
Median follow-up after PN (months)	33.5
Alive at follow-up	91.7%[a]
Underwent RFA	8.3%

[a]Excludes one patient lost to follow-up
[b]CKD defined as eGFR <60 mL/min/1.73 m^2

enhancement inversion" on computerized tomography (CT) has shown acceptable specificity, but tends to be reliable in a size-dependent matter [2]. Also, this finding has shown low sensitivity, ranging from 15 to 21% in magnetic resonance imaging (MRI) and CT respectively, and only fair inter-observer agreement [9]. One recent study showed a high sensitivity (receiver-operating characteristic area under the curve 0.817, $p < 0.001$) of predicting RO versus chRCC with the combined presence of a central stellate scar and higher Hounsfield Units (HUs) on multiphase CT [8]. Despite these and other studies, there is an inability to clinically accurately

distinguish between RCC and RO based on imaging alone. Thus, enhancing suspicious small renal masses (SRMs) are treated as probable malignancy and managed via surgical excision (partial or radical nephrectomy (RN)), ablation, or surveillance [10, 11]. Recently, the role of renal mass biopsy (RMB) has experienced resurgence in popularity in managing patients with SRMs. In an effort to avoid the morbidity associated with treatment modality, and possibly avoid overtreatment in patients with bilateral renal masses, some have even advocated for all patients with SRM to undergo RMB preoperatively [12].

The efficacy and practical role of biopsy in the diagnosis of renal oncocytoma has been a focus of study in recent years. There have been variable data to both support and refute the use of a core or FNA prior to deciding upon management. Depending on the adequacy of the tissue obtained, pathology can result as either a specific subtype of RCC, RO, or a mix of both, called hybrid oncocytic/chromophobe tumors (HOCT). When pathologists cannot discriminate between chRCC and oncocytoma, the designation of "oncocytic neoplasm" is used [13]. Again, this contributes to a clinical dilemma in how to manage these patients.

Despite the risk of concurrent malignancy, however, there is a shift toward more conservative management of SRMs. This study sought to investigate the use of renal biopsy following unilateral partial nephrectomy in the setting of primary bilateral synchronous renal oncocytomas. This subset has been previously observed in a case series of three patients in 2010 [14]. Our cohort of patients represents the largest presenting with bilateral renal oncocytomas. We propose that an approach involving partial nephrectomy proven diagnosis of

Table 2 Follow-up Characteristics

Patient	Age*	Pre-op Creatinine (mg/dL)	Pre-op eGFR[†]	Pre-op CKD (Category)[†]	Follow-up after PN (months**)	Follow-up Creatinine (mg/dL)	Follow-up eGFR[†]	Post-op CKD (Category)[†]	Change in eGFR[†]
1	55–60	0.7	104	G1	3.9	0.8	100	G1	-3.8%
2	65–70	0.8	75	G2	24.0	0.9	64	G2	-14.7%
3	65–70	1.0	77	G2	19.6	1.1	68	G2	-11.7%
4	70–75	0.8	88	G2	49.3	0.8	86	G2	-2.3%
5	65–70	0.9	87	G2	69.2*	1.6	42	G3b	-51.7%
6	60–65	0.7	102	G1	55.1	1.2	63	G2	-38.2%
7	75–80	0.9	62	G2	64.7	1.3	38	G3b	-38.7%
8	65–70	1.4	51	G3a	19.4	1.3	55	G3a	+7.8%
9	45–50	1.0	90	G1	125.3*	1.0	84	G2	-6.7%
10	65–70	1.0	79	G2	43.0	1.2	61	G2	-22.8%
11	75–80	1.3	53	G3a	2.5	1.3	53	G3a	0%
12	65–70	0.9	87	G2	0.2	1.1	69	G2	-20.7%

* range provided to ensure no identifying information
** follow-up period from first partial nephrectomy
[†] eGFR calculated using CKD-EPI equation, definitions of CKD per KDIGO guidelines

oncocytoma with bilateral masses undergo renal mass biopsy. In the case of confirmation of oncocytoma or oncocytic neoplasm, patients can be safely followed on active surveillance protocols.

Methods

After institutional review board approval MCC 15666, we searched our nephrectomy database between 2005 and 2013 for all patients with bilateral oncocytoma. Twelve patients were identified who had also undergone either a robotic/laparoscopic or open partial nephrectomy by two surgeons (PES, WJS) at Moffitt Cancer Center in Tampa, Florida. Further record provided the final pathology, which was determined by surgical specimen and correlated with CT-guided percutaneous core biopsy or fine needle aspirate. Size of biopsy needle, as well as biopsy technique was variable and performed at the discretion of the radiologist. Additional patient information was gathered retrospectively, including: age, gender, BMI, largest and next largest tumor sizes, number of tumors per patient, pre-operative creatinine, the presence of absence of pre-operative chronic kidney disease (CKD), post-operative creatinine at one month, percent of patients surviving to follow-up, median follow-up time and percent undergoing radiofrequency ablation (RFA). Management decisions were based on surgeon discretion, based on factors such as linear growth rate kinetics, size of the contralateral tumor, patient comorbidities and patient preference.

Patient demographic data was listed and pathological characteristics were reported based on phrasing used in the patients' charts. Renal function pre- and postoperatively was also recorded. Estimated GFR (eGFR) was calculated via the CKD-EPI equation with CKD classifications per KDIGO practice guidelines [15]. Follow-up was determined on an individual basis at the discretion of the two surgeons listed above. Patients were generally followed in clinic with labs and imaging every three to six months for two years, with increasing intervals after that. All statistics were performed using IBM SPSS software version 22.

Results

Of the 583 patients in our database from 2005 to 2013, twelve were found who were diagnosed with synchronous bilateral renal oncocytoma and had undergone unilateral partial nephrectomy. Nine of these patients had also undergone subsequent CT-guided biopsy or FNA of the contralateral kidney. Table 1 summarizes patient demographics. The patient median age at time of surgery was 68 years (46–77). The median size of the largest tumor(s) resected was 2.75 cm (1.5–5.5 cm). Median size of the second largest tumor(s) was 1.75 cm (1.0–4.0 cm). Four patients underwent bilateral staged PN and one

patient underwent simultaneous bilateral partial nephrectomy for horseshoe kidney. Two patients underwent radiofrequency ablation at the time of biopsy of the contralateral mass following PN. Five patients underwent CT-guided biopsy ($n = 5$) and FNA ($n = 5$) of the contralateral mass after PN, followed by active surveillance with routine imaging. There were no reported complications secondary to FNA or core biopsy collection. No patients required repeat intervention for suspected malignancy at a mean follow-up time of 34 months. There was no significant change in median creatinine pre- and post-operatively (0.95 mg/dL and 1.01 mg/dL, respectively). Two patients (16.7%) demonstrated CKD (defined as eGFR <60 mL/min/1.73 m^2) pre-operatively, which doubled after the surgeries to four patients with CKD (33.3%). One patient was lost to follow up and one patient died of unknown causes five years after PN. Of the five followed by active surveillance, three showed no growth at one year via CT scan and two had minimal growth, 3 mm and 1 mm.

Estimated GFR was calculated via the CKD-EPI equation and definitions of CKD were per KDIGO [15] guidelines. Pre-operative and post-operative CKD category, creatinine (mg/dL) and eGFR are all listed in Table 2, as well as percent change in eGFR after surgery at follow-up. Three of 12 patients (25%) were at stage G1, 7 of 12 (58.3%) at stage G2 and 2 patients (16.7%) were at G3a prior to surgery. After surgery, one of the 12 patients (8.3%) was at stage G1, 7 of 12 (58.3%) were at G2, 2 of 12 (16.7%) were at G3a, likewise for G3b, with no patients falling into G4 and G5 ranges. eGFR decreased an average of 16.96%, including a single patient whose eGFR increased by 7.8% after surgery and a single patient whose eGFR did not change post-operatively.

Table 3 details the procedure performed (PN vs. RN, FNA vs. core biopsy) and laterality, surgical pathology and sizes of tumors, as well as biopsy pathology. Two patients who underwent bilateral PN, also had either FNA or core biopsy performed. In one of the two cases, initial right FNA showed "oncocytic neoplasm, favor oncocytoma", while right PN surgical pathology confirmed oncocytoma. In the second case, left core biopsy showed "renal neoplasm with oncocytic features", confirmed as oncocytoma after left PN, as well as right FNA demonstrative of "cytologic change consistent with oncocytoma" and right PN surgical pathology affirmed the diagnosis of oncocytoma.

Discussion

Despite the relative rarity and benign nature of renal oncocytoma ad compared to other renal tumors, the possibility of co-existence with RCC warrants further evaluation when suspected on incidental imaging. Although scarce, there have been few cases of development

Table 3 Pathological Characteristics

	Left Kidney				Right Kidney			
Patient	# of Tumors	Tumor Sizes (cm)	Management	Pathology	# of Tumors	Tumor Sizes (cm)	Management	Pathology
1	–	–	Core bx + AS	"renal oncocytic neoplasm"	1	1.6	PN	"oncocytoma"
2	–	–	PN	"oncocytoma"	1	1.5	PN	"oncocytoma"
3	1	4.0	PN	"oncocytoma"	–	–	FNA + AS	"oncocytic neoplasm"
4	4	1.6, 1.5, 1.5, 0.7	PN	"oncocytoma"	–	–	FNA + PN	"oncocytic neoplasm (favor oncocytoma)"
5	1	4.8	PN	"oncocytoma"	1	2.0	PN	"oncocytoma"
6	–	–	Core bx + AS	"oncocytoma"	1	2.3	PN	"oncocytoma"
7	1	3.0	PN	"oncocytoma"	–	–	FNA + AS	"oncocytic neoplasm (favor oncocytoma)"
8	2	2.5, 2.0	PN	"oncocytoma"	–	–	Core bx + AS	"oncocytic neoplasm (c/w oncocytoma)"
9	6	3.1, 3.0, 2.7, 0.8, 0.4, 0.1	Core bx + PN	"oncocytoma" (surgical pathology); "renal neoplasm with oncocytic features" (biopsy)	6	5.5, 4.0, 2.8, 2.8, 2.2, 0.7	FNA + PN	"cytologic changes c/w oncocytoma"
10	4	1.5, 1.0, 1.0, 0.4	PN	"oncocytoma"	–	–	Core bx + RFA	"renal oncocytoma"
11	–	–	FNA + RFA	"cytologic changes c/w oncocytoma"	1	3.5	PN	"oncocytoma"
12	1	1.5	PN	"renal oncocytic neoplasm"	1	3.2	RN*	"oncocytoma"

PN partial nephrectomy; *RN* radical nephrectomy (patient with horseshoe kidney); *bx* biopsy; *FNA* fine needle aspiration; *RFA* radiofrequency ablation; *AS* active surveillance

of contralateral RCC in patients with RO, with chromophobe carrying the best prognosis [7]. In the case of renal oncocytosis, besides hybrid tumors, chRCC has been shown to be both the most common malignant dominant tumor type (26%; 6 of 23 specimens) as well as secondary tumor type (70%; 16 of 53 specimens) found on histology.

Childs et al. investigated metachronous renal tumors following PN of primary RO, showing that these newly arising tumors were more likely to be benign compared to patients presenting with a newly diagnosed SRM; of 12 patients with either surgical or biopsy pathology, 8 were RO versus 4 RCC (of various types). They also determined that the risk of metachronous RCC after PN of renal oncocytoma was similar to that of the general population, and utilized a less aggressive surveillance approach with ultrasound (US) versus CT [16].

Other studies have confirmed the benign nature of oncocytoma by showing no evidence of metastasis in patients both undergoing active surveillance and/or nephrectomy. Bhatt et al. published 36 patients with RO, 34 of whom underwent nephrectomy, none of whom developed metastases at a median follow-up time of 84 months after surgery [17]. Similar results were obtained in a cohort of 20 patients with oncocytosis, who showed no metastases at a median follow-up of 35 months, although CKD was a major morbidity, with 50% affected prior to surgery and 25% developing CKD after nephrectomy [7]. One consideration in that case is

the presence of multiple oncocytic nodules which have been shown to intersperse between the nephrons and affect nearby tubules in oncocytosis [7]. Familial syndromes can also play a role in the clinical and pathologic presentation of oncocytoma, which is associated with the autosomal dominant Birt-Hogg-Dubé (BHD) syndrome. The most common tumor type found in these patients is a hybrid mixed histology, containing features of both oncocytoma and RCC, [7] often termed "oncocytic neoplasms" by pathologists [13].

Recent investigation has also elucidated more about the growth rates of renal oncocytoma. These rates have been cited at 0.14 to 0.20 cm per year [5, 18], compared to small renal masses in general, at 0.28 cm per year,, according to a meta-analysis [18], and 0.38 cm/yr for chRCC [5].

Renal mass biopsy has shown to have promising utility. Diagnostic yield on first biopsy has been shown to be 80.6 to 93% [13, 19, 20] with overall improvement in yield with a subsequent biopsy [13, 19]. Core biopsy sensitivity and specificity are 99.1 and 99.7%, respectively, while FNA is 93.2 and 89.8%, respectively [19]. In addition, complications have not been found to be a major morbidity in RMB, with studies quoting complication rates between 8.5 and 10.4%, most of which were minor and self-limited [13, 20]. Both the high rate of diagnostic accuracy of RMB, as well as the low rate of complications, argues in favor of biopsy and subsequent implementation of an active surveillance protocol.

A single-institution study of 15 patients diagnosed with renal oncocytoma via CT-guided biopsy was followed to better elucidate the course of RO with watchful waiting. Mean follow-up time was 30 months and showed that 6 of the 15 underwent surgery (2 partial and 4 total nephrectomies) for rapid growth (0.5 cm/yr.), tumor burden or patient preference. All surgical pathologies were confirmed RO except for a single case of oncocytoma associated with chRCC (T2 Fuhrman grade 3). Nine of the 15 patients underwent biannual ultrasound imaging and were asymptomatic at a mean follow-up time of 49.7 months. Those who underwent surgery were younger and had a significantly higher tumor growth velocity than the non-operative patients (2.4 ± 2.1 mm/yr versus 0.7 ± 0.5 mm/yr., $P = 0.008$) [21].

This possibility of harboring malignant histology was demonstrated in a study of 20 patients with oncocytosis. After either partial or radical nephrectomies, 13 patients had dominant tumor hybrid histology, followed by 6 chRCC, 3 pure oncocytoma and 1 with clear cell RCC. Multiple secondary nodules were examined and were also varied in histology, including hybrid, chRCC, pure RO, conventional RCC and clear cell papillary RCC [7].

One essential consideration in patients diagnosed with SRMs is that of preserving renal function. In our single institution review, 2 of 12 patients had baseline CKD with 2 more developing it after surgery (bilateral PN and left PN). Lane et al. showed that medically-induced CKD (versus surgically-induced CKD) was associated with greater rate of progressive decline in renal function, all-cause mortality and non-renal cancer mortality, with non-renal mortality and GFR stability being similar in the surgically-induced CKD and non-CKD cohorts. Another study of 1928 patients showed male gender (odds ratio (OR) 3.55), older age at diagnosis of SMR (OR 1.04), hypertension (OR 0.46), serum calcium (OR 2.06) and lower serum albumin (OR 0.23) to be significantly correlated with pre-operative CKD. Additionally, radical nephrectomy, as compared to partial nephrectomy, was shown to have the strongest association with post-operative CKD (OR 11.89). Hence, the authors of that paper suggested consideration of elderly men with hypertension as candidates for PN versus radial nephrectomy to avoid development of CKD [22].

Although the latter study only addressed RCC patients, these are certainly still factors to be considered in the setting of patients with bilateral RO. Taken together, they suggest the importance of careful screening of patients for risk factors pre-operatively, which may compel intervention instead of surveillance.

In summary, renal mass biopsy followed by active surveillance has been considered safe [5, 23], reliable, cost-effective, with no change in survival overall. Use of renal mass biopsy has increased and should also be applied to the unique subset of patients suspected of having bilateral renal oncocytoma. Biopsy plus active surveillance is also of benefit because it does not preclude the patient from future urologic interventions, such as partial nephrectomy or ablation [23].

Limitations of this study include its retrospective nature and one patient lost to follow-up. We also had a small sample size, due to the rarity of bilateral synchronous oncocytoma. Our median time to follow-up was 34 months, which could perhaps not be long enough to capture development of new tumors or other complications in the disease course after partial nephrectomy. Also, we recommend the use of confirmatory biopsy in diagnosing the contralateral tumor, but not every patient in our cohort underwent biopsy and/or FNA (only 9 out of 12). Another limitation is the fact that all patients in our cohort underwent partial nephrectomy, denying us the ability to observe these masses free of intervention.

Conclusion

From our single institution experience we believe that patients with unilateral renal oncocytoma with contralateral mass who have undergone unilateral partial nephrectomy of the RO should undergo confirmatory biopsy of the contralateral mass and can be safely managed with active surveillance imaging protocols. Future prospective multi-institutional trials are needed to determine optimal management of bilateral renal masses in the setting of prior unilateral oncocytoma.

Abbreviations
AS: Active surveillance; chRCC: Chromophobe type, renal cell carcinoma; FNA: Fine needle aspiration; RCC: Renal cell carcinoma; RMB: Renal mass biopsy; RO: Renal Oncocytoma; SRM: Small renal mass

Acknowledgements
None.

Funding
None.

Authors' contribution
AL: acquisition of data, analysis and interpretation of data, drafting manuscript, critical revision of the manuscript and statistical analysis. Co-first author. LK: acquisition of data, analysis and interpretation of data, drafting manuscript, critical revision of the manuscript and statistical analysis. Co-first author. GD analysis and interpretation of data, drafting manuscript, critical revision of the manuscript and statistical analysis. KZ analysis and interpretation of data, drafting manuscript, critical revision of the manuscript and statistical analysis. PS analysis and interpretation of data, drafting manuscript, critical revision of the manuscript and statistical analysis. WS drafting manuscript, critical revision of the manuscript and statistical analysis. PS acquisition of data, analysis and interpretation of data, drafting manuscript, critical revision of the manuscript and statistical analysis. All authors read and approved the final manuscript.

Competing interests

Co-authors Dr. Kamran Zargar-Shoshtari and Dr. Pranav Sharma are Associate Editors and Dr. Philippe Spiess is a Section Editor for this journal. The authors have nothing to disclose.

References

1. Vernadakis S, Karaolanis G, Moris D, Zavvos V, Liapis G, Zavos G. Multiple bilateral oncocytomas of the native kidneys following renal transplantation: report of a rare case and review of the literature. World J Surg Oncol. 2013; 11:119.
2. Woo S, Cho JY. Imaging findings of common benign renal tumors in the era of small renal masses: differential diagnosis from small renal cell carcinoma - current status and future perspectives. Korean J Radiol. 2015; 16(1):99–113.
3. Biswas B, Wahal S, Gulati A. Renal oncocytoma: A diagnostic dilemma on cytology. J Cytol. 2014;31:59–60.
4. Campbell MF, Walsh PC, Wein AJ, Kavoussi LR. Campbell-Walsh Urology. Philadelphia, PA: Saunders; 2012.
5. Richard PO, Jewett MA, Bhatt JR, Evans AJ, Timilsina N, Finelli A. Adult Urology: Active Surveillance for Renal Neoplasms with Oncocytic Features is Safe. J Urol. 2016;195(3):581–587.
6. Wentzel SW, Vermeulen LP. Bilateral multifocal renal oncocytoma in pregnancy. Rare Tumors. 2012;4(4):e54.
7. Adamy A, Lowrance WT, Yee DS, Chong KT, Bernstein M, Tickoo SK, Coleman JA, Russo P. Adult urology: renal oncocytosis: management and clinical outcomes. J Urol. 2011;185:795–801.
8. Jae Hyeok C, Jong Won K, Joo Yong L, Woong Kyu H, Koon Ho R, Young Deuk C, Sung Joon H, Young Eun Y. Comparison of computed tomography findings between renal oncocytomas and chromophobe renal cell carcinomas. Korean J Urol. 2015;56(10):695–702.
9. Schieda N, Al-Subhi M, Flood TA, El-Khodary M, McInnes MDF. Diagnostic accuracy of segmental enhancement inversion for the diagnosis of renal oncocytoma using biphasic computed tomography (CT) and multiphase contrast-enhanced magnetic resonance imaging (MRI). Eur Radiol. 2014;11:2787.
10. Ljungberg B, Bensalah K, Canfield S, Dabestani S, Hofmann F, Hora M, Kuczyk MA, Lam T, Marconi L, Merseburger AS, et al. Guidelines: EAU guidelines on renal cell carcinoma: 2014 update. Eur Urol. 2015;67:913–24.
11. Campbell SC, Novick AC, Belldegrun A, Blute ML, Chow GK, Derweesh IH, Faraday MM, Kaouk JH, Leveillee RJ, Matin SF, et al. Adult urology: guideline for management of the clinical T1 renal mass. J Urol. 2009;182:1271–9.
12. Richard PO, Jewett MAS, Bhatt JR, Kachura JR, Evans AJ, Zlotta AR, Hermanns T, Juvet T, Finelli A. Renal tumor biopsy for small renal masses: a single-center 13-year experience. Eur Urol. 2015;68:1007–13.
13. Delahunt B, Samaratunga H, Martignoni G, Srigley JR, Evans AJ, Brunelli M. Percutaneous renal tumour biopsy. Histopathology. 2014;65(3):295–308.
14. Ivey BS, Devarajan K, Sundaram CP. Bilateral oncocytoma and the value of needle biopsy. Can J Urol. 2010;17(2):5131–4.
15. Stevens PE, Levin A: Evaluation and Management of Chronic Kidney Disease: Synopsis of the Kidney Disease: Improving Global Outcomes 2012 Clinical Practice Guideline. ANNALS OF INTERNAL MEDICINE 2013, 158(11):825 − +.
16. Childs MA, Breau RH, Umbreit EC, Lohse CM, Cheville JC, Thompson RH, Blute ML, Leibovich BC. Metachronous renal tumours after surgical management of oncocytoma. BJU Int. 2011;108(6):816–9.
17. Bhatt NR, Davis NF, Flynn R, McDermott T, Thornhill JA, Manecksha RP. Dilemmas in diagnosis and natural history of renal oncocytoma and implications for management. Can Urol Assoc J. 2015;9:E709–12.
18. Chawla SN, Crispen PL, Hanlon AL, Greenberg RE, Chen DYT, Uzzo RG. Review article: the natural history of observed enhancing renal masses: meta-analysis and review of the world literature. J Urol. 2006;175:425–31.
19. Marconi L, Dabestani S, Lam TB, Hofmann F, Stewart F, Norrie J, Bex A, Bensalah K, Canfield SE, Hora M, Kuczyk MA et al. Platinum Priority – Review – Kidney Cancer: Systematic Review and Meta-analysis of Diagnostic Accuracy of Percutaneous Renal Tumour Biopsy. Eur Urol. 2016;69(4):660–673.
20. Volpe A, Kachura JR, Geddie WR, Evans AJ, Gharajeh A, Saravanan A, Jewett MAS. Review article: techniques, safety and accuracy of sampling of renal tumors by fine needle aspiration and core biopsy. J Urol. 2007;178:379–86.
21. Neuzillet Y, Lechevallier E, Andre M, Daniel L, Nahon O, Coulange C. Follow-up of renal oncocytoma diagnosed by percutaneous tumor biopsy. Urology. 2005;66(6):1181–5.
22. Kim SH, Lee SE, Hong SK, Jeong CW, Park YH, Kim YJ, Kang SH, Hong SH, Choi WS, Byun SS. Incidence and risk factors of chronic kidney disease in Korean patients with T1a renal cell carcinoma before and after radical or partial nephrectomy. Jpn J Clin Oncol. 2013;43(12):1243–8.
23. Bahouth Z, Halachmi S, Meyer G, Avitan O, Moskovitz B, Nativ O. The natural history and predictors for intervention in patients with small renal mass undergoing active surveillance. Adv Urol. 2015;2015:692014.

Surgical management of large adrenal tumors: impact of different laparoscopic approaches and resection methods on perioperative and long-term outcomes

Wei Chen[1], Yong Liang[1], Wei Lin[1], Guang-Qing Fu[1] and Zhi-Wei Ma[2]* 🆔

Abstract

Background: The indication of retroperitoneal laparoscopic adrenalectomy (RLA) was extended with the retroperitoneal approach and has been wildly accepted and technologically matured. However, the management of large adrenal tumors via this approach still remains controversial. The aim of this study was to perform a comprehensive analysis on the minimally invasive surgical management of larger adrenal tumors.

Methods: A total of 78 patients with large adrenal tumors (> 5 cm) and 97 patients with smaller adrenal tumors (< 5 cm) were enrolled in this study. The patient characteristics were preferentially analyzed. The intra-operative and postoperative indicators were compared between those who underwent RLA and those who underwent transperitoneal laparoscopic adrenalectomy (TLA); the intra-operative and postoperative indicators were also compared between the large tumor group and smaller tumor group of those who underwent RLA. Furthermore, the analyses of partial RLA were focused on the perioperative indicators and follow-up results.

Results: RLA was superior to TLA in terms of operation time (98.71 ± 32.30 min vs. 124.36 ± 34.62 min, respectively, $P = 0.001$), hospitalization duration (7.43 ± 2.82 days vs. 8.91 ± 3.40 days, respectively, $P = 0.04$), duration of drain (4.83 ± 0.37 days vs. 3.94 ± 2.21 days, respectively, $P = 0.02$), first oral intake (2.82 ± 0.71 days vs. 1.90 ± 0.83 days, respectively, $P < 0.001$) and time to ambulation (3.89 ± 1.64 days vs. 2.61 ± 1.42 days, respectively, $P < 0.001$). Further analyses of the RLA patients demonstrated that the larger tumor (> 5 cm) group showed superior results for the intraoperative indicators than the smaller tumor (< 5 cm) group ($P < 0.05$), while the results for the postoperative indicators between the two tumor size groups were similar ($P > 0.05$). Data confirmed that the partial resection method was superior to the total resection method from the perspective of the hormone supplement (0% vs. 48.15%, $P = 0.002$). The 2-year recurrence-free rates were 92.60 and 92.86% for the total and partial RLA resection methods, respectively ($P = 0.97$). The partial RLA resection method had a similar complete remission rate as the total RLA resection method (96.30% vs. 100%, respectively, $P = 0.47$).

Conclusion: Both RLA and TLA seem to provide similar effects for the surgical management of large adrenal tumors. However, partial RLA resection should be considered for the management of benign tumors to reduce the hormone supplement.

Keywords: Retroperitoneal laparoscopic adrenalectomy, Minimally invasive surgery, Adrenal tumor

* Correspondence: csssmu@163.com
[2]Department of Urology, Sichuan Academy of Medical Sciences & Sichuan Provincial People's Hospital, No.32 West Second Section First Ring Road, Chengdu 641000, Sichuan, China
Full list of author information is available at the end of the article

Background

Laparoscopic adrenalectomy, which includes both the retroperitoneal and transperitoneal approaches, has been regarded as the gold standard for the management of adrenal tumors. In a previous study, we demonstrated that the retroperitoneal approach was superior to the transperitoneal method in terms of the perioperative indicators [1]. However, it is known that the tumor diameter is an important factor in the surgical management of adrenal tumors using the retroperitoneal laparoscopic technique. Satisfactory clinical results of lateral retroperitoneal laparoscopic adrenalectomy (RLA) for small adrenal tumors have been reported [2–4]. Scholars have also reported that the largest adrenal benign tumor managed by the transperitoneal approach was 15 cm in diameter, and the largest adrenal benign tumor managed by the retroperitoneal method was 6 cm in diameter. Since the retroperitoneal approach has been wildly accepted and technologically matured, its indication has been extended. However, the management of large adrenal tumors, which are often defined as tumors larger than 5 cm, via this approach still remains controversial. There were approximately 800 cases of adrenal tumors that underwent operation in Sichuan Provincial People's Hospital and Zigong Fourth People's Hospital during 2011–2015. The percentage of large adrenal tumors was approximately 9.7%. The aim of this study was to perform a comprehensive analysis of the surgical management of larger adrenal tumors based on patient information from the databases of the abovementioned hospitals.

Methods

The present study was designed as an observational study and approved by the hospital ethics committee of Zigong Fourth People's Hospital and Sichuan Provincial People's Hospital. All of the patients gave informed consent to participate in the study before the operation. A prospectively maintained urology database in the Department of Urology at Zigong Fourth People's Hospital and Sichuan Provincial People's Hospital was retrospectively reviewed to collect data on the large diameter complicated adrenal tumor patients who underwent an RLA or transperitoneal laparoscopic adrenalectomy (TLA) procedure. The present study adheres to the STROBE reporting guidelines (Additional file 1).

The inclusion criteria for our study were as follows: (i) the patient was confirmed as having an adrenal tumor by imaging examination and underwent minimally invasive surgery treatment, (ii) the baseline indicators and perioperative parameters were completely recorded, and (iii) a large adrenal tumor was defined as an adrenal tumor with a diameter larger than 5 cm. The exclusion

criteria were as follows: (i) there were no measurable data reported, (ii) the tumor was operated on via open surgery, and (iii) a hand-assisted laparoscopic method was adopted during the surgery. From January 2011 to June 2015, there were 78 patients with an adrenal tumor larger than 5 cm. Of these 78 patients, 41 (26 males and 15 females) patients underwent RLA, and the other 37 (23 males and 14 females) patients underwent the TLA procedure. All of the patients received a complete laboratory examination, which included 17-keto-steroid, 17-hydroxycorticosteroids, vanilmandelic acid, aldosterone/renin ratio, aldosterone, renin and plasma metanephrines measurements. Image evaluations, such as computed tomography, were used to determine the localization and diameter of the adrenal mass. All of the patients were provided operative informed consent, which mentioned the benefits and potential risks of the proposed operation method. We also informed all of the patients that open conversion might occur if any difficulties were encountered during the operation.

Surgical technique

The patients were divided into the RLA group and TLA group according to the approach of the laparoscopic technique that they underwent. Subgroups were formed in the RLA group based on the diameter or resection method used.

A lateral position was selected for these patients. A 30-degree laparoscope was used as an observation mirror though a 10-mm trocar, and the other two trocars were located in the anterior axillary line and posterior axillary line of the subcostal space at a diameter of 5 mm or 10 mm, respectively. The operation sequence was performed according to the steps shown in Fig. 1. Ultrasonic shears were used to divided and identify the edge of the adrenal gland. The central adrenal vein was divided between hem-o-lok clips. After the adrenal gland was completely dissected, a homemade bag was used to dress up the adrenal gland via a 10-mm trocar placed into the peritoneal cavity. The mass was cut and examined on the operation table to ensure the involvement of the entire tumor. After the adrenal area was exposed, special attention was given to the evaluation of the tumor location and determination of whether there was periadrenal involvement. The TLA method was administered as it is referred to in the paper reported by Mohammadi-Fallah et al. [5].

In both the RLA and TLA groups, the main principle of the procedure was a resection with as much periadrenal tissue as possible to ensure that the highest negative margin rate in malignant tumors was obtained. A drainage tube was routinely placed before the operation completed. All of the procedures were performed

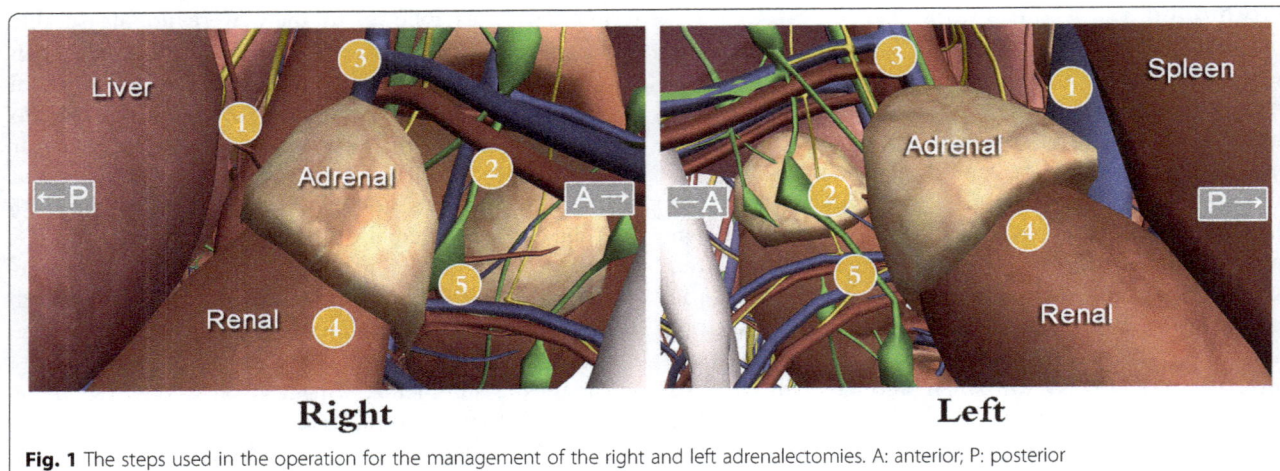

Fig. 1 The steps used in the operation for the management of the right and left adrenalectomies. A: anterior; P: posterior

by an experienced senior laparoscopic surgeon to reduce the selective bias.

Postoperative management

We routinely put the patients in the post-anesthesia care unit until their blood pressure and heart rate were stable and they regained consciousness after the surgery. Patients with significant bleeding or an unstable blood pressure would be transferred to the intensive care unit (ICU). After approximately 30 min of postoperative monitoring in the post-anesthesia care unit, the patients were transferred to the urology department for a half day to 1 day for electrocardiograph monitoring. A fasting period of 24 h to 2 days was implemented to help the bowel function recovery of the patients. During this period, postoperative intravenous fluid supplementation was used in all of the patients. Postoperative hypotension, which might have been caused by bleeding or an inadequate intravenous fluid supplementation during the intraoperative or postoperative period, was corrected in a timely manner. Fortunately, none of the patients required this management. The patients were discharged after an adequate pain control was achieved and after the drainage tube was extubated. In addition, patients could receive a regular diet and normal ambulation based on the requirement of the condition for achieving a discharge standard.

Outcome definition

The basic characteristics of the patients were preferentially analyzed to assess the balance and comparability between the two groups. These characteristics included the mean age, gender, body mass index (BMI), tumor size, tumor side, previous abdominal surgery, resection method and pathology type of the patients.

To evaluate the efficacies of the RLA and TLA procedures, both the intra-operative terms and postoperative terms were required. The intra-operative terms included the operation time (OT), estimated blood loss (EBL), number of complications, and number of ICU conversions. The postoperative terms included hospitalization, duration of the draining, hormone supplementation, the time to first oral intake and the time to first ambulation. The follow-up indicators included the two-year recurrence-free rate (RFR) and complete remission (CR). RFR was defined as the detection of no new tumors and was based on clinical and imagology evidence. CR was defined as a complete disappearance of the manifestations of disease, which included hypertension, central obesity, osphyalgia, etc.

Statistical analysis

All of the continuous data were expressed as the mean ± standard deviation, while the discontinuous data were presented as the percentage. The statistical analyses were performed using SPSS version 20.0 (SPSS Inc., Chicago, IL). Two independent-sample t tests were used to compare the continuous variables between the groups, and Chi-square tests were used to compare the discontinuous variables between the two groups. Curve estimations were used to explore the correlation between the tumor diameter and other potential factors. The estimation model included linear, logarithmic, inverse, quadratic, cubic, compound, power, s curve, growth curve and exponential analyses. $P < 0.05$ was used to indicate statistically significant differences between the groups.

Results

Patient characteristics

During January 2011 and June 2015, a total of 78 adrenalectomies were performed at Zigong Fourth People's Hospital and Sichuan Provincial People's Hospital. Of these procedures, the RLA approach was used in 41 patients (27 with a total excision and 14 with a partial excision), and the TLA approach was used in 37 patients (17 with a total excision and 20 with a partial excision). The groups consisted of 49 (62.82%) male patients and 29 (37.18%) female patients who had an age range of 21–67 years (mean age: 46.59 ± 35.60 years). The mean tumor diameter was 5.78 ± 1.29 cm, and there were no statistically significant differences between the groups ($P = 0.86$). The tumor localization and peritoneal invasion of each patient was previously evaluated by a computed tomography scan. There were 57 (69.23%) left-side and 3 (2.99%) bilateral-sided surgeries. Of the total patient population, 38 patients (48.72%) had the diagnosis of aldosterone-producing adenoma or adrenocortical hyperplasia, while 8 patients (10.26%) had the diagnosis of pheochromocytoma. There were 4 patients (5.13%) with hematoma and an adrenal cyst. In the patient population, there were 2 patients with adrenocortical carcinoma who received LRA and 4 patients with ACC who received TLA. Total adrenal resection was performed

in 44 of the patients (56.41%). All of the basic characteristics showed no significant differences between the two groups ($P > 0.05$). The disease and patient characteristics are shown in Table 1.

Retroperitoneal procedure versus Transperitoneal procedure

There were no significant differences in numbers of intra-operative estimated blood loss, conversions to the ICU and postoperative complications between the RLA and TLA groups ($P > 0.05$). The RLA group had a shorter operation time (98.71 ± 32.30 min vs. 124.36 ± 34.62 min, $P = 0.001$) and shorter hospitalization duration (7.43 ± 2.82 days vs. 8.91 ± 3.40 days, $P = 0.04$) compared to the TLA group. The TLA group had a longer duration of draining (4.83 ± 0.37 days vs. 3.94 ± 2.21 days, $P = 0.02$), longer time to first oral intake (2.82 ± 0.71 days vs. 1.90 ± 0.83 days, $P < 0.001$) and longer time to ambulation (3.89 ± 1.64 days vs. 2.61 ± 1.42 days, $P < 0.001$) than the RLA group (Table 2).

Table 1 A comparison of the basic characteristics between the two groups

	Overall	RLA	TLA	P value
No. of patients	78	41	37	
Mean age (yrs)	46.59 ± 35.60	44.41 ± 38.90	47.92 ± 29.61	0.65
BMI (kg/m^2)	23.58 ± 2.07	23.52 ± 2.46	23.60 ± 2.92	0.89
Tumor size (cm)	5.78 ± 1.29	5.81 ± 1.17	5.76 ± 1.34	0.86
Gender				0.90
Male	49	26	23	
Female	29	15	14	
Localization				0.79
Left	54	29	25	
Right	21	11	10	
Bilateral	3	1	2	
Previous abdominal surgery	3	1	2	0.49
Resection				0.07
Total	44	27	17	
Partial	34	14	20	
Pathology				0.47
Adrenocortical hyperplasia	18	10	8	
Aldosterone-producing adenoma	38	18	20	
Adrenal medullary hyperplasia	3	1	2	
Adrenal myelolipoma	1	1	0	
Adrenocortical carcinoma	6	2	4	
Adrenal cyst	3	3	0	
Hematoma	1	1	0	
Pheochromocytoma	8	5	3	

BMI body mass index, *RLA* retroperitoneal laparoscopic adrenalectomy, *TLA* transperitoneal laparoscopic adrenalectomy

Table 2 A comparison of the operative and postoperative outcomes between RLA and TLA groups

	Overall	RLA	TLA	P value
No. of patients	78	41	37	
Convert to ICU	5	3	2	0.73
Complication	1	0	1	0.29
Operation time (min)	103.96 ± 32.09	98.71 ± 32.30	124.36 ± 34.62	0.001
Estimated blood loss (cc)	33.72 ± 21.34	31.93 ± 20.01	36.34 ± 19.83	0.33
Hospitalization (d)	8.09 ± 2.67	7.43 ± 2.82	8.91 ± 3.40	0.04
Duration of drain (d)	4.18 ± 2.92	3.94 ± 2.21	4.83 ± 0.37	0.02
First oral intake (d)	2.31 ± 0.75	1.90 ± 0.83	2.82 ± 0.71	< 0.001
Time to ambulation (d)	2.99 ± 1.68	2.61 ± 1.42	3.89 ± 1.64	< 0.001

ICU intensive care unit, *RLA* retroperitoneal laparoscopic adrenalectomy, *TLA* transperitoneal laparoscopic adrenalectomy

Retroperitoneal approach for the management of tumors larger than 5 cm versus tumors smaller than 5 cm

During the same period of this study, there were 97 patients with a tumor of a diameter smaller than 5 cm who received retroperitoneal adrenal surgeries. Comparing between the larger tumor and smaller tumor groups, there were no significant differences in the number of conversions to the ICU, number of postoperative complications, time to first oral intake and time to ambulation. However, a longer operation time and higher intra-operative estimated blood loss were detected in the larger tumor group compared to the smaller tumor group (OT: 98.71 ± 32.30 min vs. 42.63 ± 18.51 min, $P < 0.001$; EBL: 31.93 ± 20.01 cm^3 vs. 10.29 ± 6.04 cm^3, $P << 0.001$). Moreover, the larger tumor group experienced a longer hospitalization duration (7.43 ± 2.82 days vs. 2.07 ± 0.36 days, $P < 0.001$) and longer duration of draining (3.94 ± 2.21 days vs. 0.98 ± 0.07 days, $P < 0.001$) compared to the smaller tumor group (Table 3).

Retroperitoneoscopic total resection versus retroperitoneoscopic partial resection in large adrenal tumors

According to the tumor characteristics, a total of 14 of the 41 patients (34.15%) received partial adrenalectomy via the retroperitoneoscopic procedure. All of the 14 patients had benign tumors, which was confirmed by a careful postoperative pathological examination. The operation time for partial resection was 102.68 ± 30.92 min, whereas the operation time for total resection was 79.64 ± 28.39 min ($P = 0.02$). Partial resection was associated with a higher EBL than was total resection (45.19 ± 18.63 cm^3 vs. 28.60 ± 21.75 cm^3, $P = 0.02$). However, there were zero hormone supplements in the partial resection group, while this number in the total patient population was 13. The partial resection method was superior to the total resection method from the perspective of hormone supplementation (0% vs. 48.15%, $P = 0.002$) (Table 4).

Follow-up results of retroperitoneal laparoscopic adrenalectomy

The 2-year RFR was 92.60% for the total resection RLA and was 92.86% for the partial resection RLA ($P = 0.97$). The rate of CR in the partial resection RLA group was similar to that of the total resection RLA group (26 (96.30%) vs. 14 (100%), $P = 0.47$).

Table 3 A comparison of the perioperative indicators between the patients in the larger adrenal tumor and smaller adrenal tumor groups who underwent RLA

	Overall	> 5 cm	< 5 cm	P value
No. of patients	138	41	97	
Convert to ICU	3	3	2	0.13
Complication	1	0	1	0.52
Operation time	63.28 ± 28.91	98.71 ± 32.30	42.63 ± 18.51	< 0.001
Estimated blood loss	19.61 ± 12.50	31.93 ± 20.01	10.29 ± 6.04	< 0.001
Hospitalization	4.63 ± 1.95	7.43 ± 2.82	2.07 ± 0.36	< 0.001
Duration of drain	1.84 ± 1.52	3.94 ± 2.21	0.98 ± 0.07	< 0.001
First oral intake	1.16 ± 0.58	1.90 ± 0.83	1.72 ± 0.31	0.07
Time to ambulation	2.03 ± 1.07	2.61 ± 1.42	2.32 ± 0.48	0.08

ICU intensive care unit

Table 4 A comparison of the perioperative indicators between the different resection methods use in the RLA procedure for adrenal tumors with a diameter larger than 5 cm

	Overall	Total Resection	Partial Resection	P value
No. of patients	41	27	14	
Conversions to ICU	3	3	0	0.20
Hormone supplements	13	13	0	0.002
Tumor size (cm)	5.81 ± 1.17	5.92 ± 1.54	5.63 ± 1.08	0.49
Operation time	98.71 ± 32.30	79.64 ± 28.39	102.68 ± 30.92	0.02
Estimated blood loss	31.93 ± 20.01	28.60 ± 21.75	45.19 ± 18.63	0.02
Hospitalization	7.43 ± 2.82	7.05 ± 0.69	7.68 ± 1.52	0.07
Duration of draining	3.94 ± 2.21	3.60 ± 2.07	4.53 ± 2.78	0.23
First oral intake	1.90 ± 0.83	1.58 ± 0.61	2.06 ± 0.97	0.06
Time to ambulation	2.61 ± 1.42	2.14 ± 1.07	2.81 ± 0.96	0.05

Discussion

Adrenal surgery is a type of high-risk operation that has been used in urology for a long time. In the past, even adrenal tumors with a small diameter needed a large incision and high position in the operation due to the special location of the adrenal gland [6]. This method not only causes great trauma to the patient but also significantly increases the numbers of pleural lesions and surgical complications. Most importantly, adrenal vasculature can only be ligated through blind separation and hand feeling because most adrenal tumors could show difficulties, thereby causing the probability of tissue injury and hemorrhage [7]. Laparoscopic adrenal surgery has gained widespread popularity, and this procedure could own a more fine and convenient operation that could clearly separate the important vessels under direct vision. This technique can significantly decrease the number of postoperative complications [8].

There are many methods of minimally invasive surgeries in the management of adrenal tumors. According to the surgical approach used, the methods can be divided into transperitoneal and retroperitoneal laparoscopy adrenalectomies [1]. Advantages and disadvantages have been reported for transperitoneal and retroperitoneal adrenalectomies. The transperitoneal approach benefits from more visibility and a larger working space, as well as involving the most familiar anatomy for surgeons. Previous opinions show that TLA is better than RLA in the treatment of large adrenal tumors (> 5 cm). However, TLA disturbs intra-abdominal structures and organs, which produces a high risk for organ or vascular injury. The complications of TLA also include a prolonged ileus and the risk for adhesion formation. In patients who received previous abdominal surgery, TLA is especially difficult to perform. While RLA owns obvious advantages, it has a more direct route and cannot interfere with the intra-abdominal organs. In our previous research, we

identified that the operative time of RLA is shorter than that of TLA [1]. With the development of minimally invasive surgery, scholars constantly show that large adrenal tumors also benefit from the RLA approach.

Different positions, such as lateral, posterior or anterior, could be considered by surgeons when performing RLA. Since Zhang et al. [9] promoted and standardized lateral retroperitoneoscopic adrenalectomy (LRA), it has been the most commonly used method for treating adrenal tumors in China. In this position, we can rapidly and directly separate the adrenal tumor, which leads to a shorter operation time and less blood loss, as well as less postoperative complications. In our experience, even though the retroperitoneal approach is difficult, it is beneficial to the postoperative recovery of patients. Since the improvement of laparoscopic instruments and proficiency of operation skill, the tumor diameter may not be a major restricted factor [10] even though scholars have reported the successful use of the partial resection method in large adrenal tumors [11]. However, the opinions on the application of laparoscopy in the management of large (> 5 cm) adrenal tumors are controversial [12, 13].

In the present study, we performed a comprehensive analysis of minimally invasive surgery methods used in the management of large adrenal tumors, which included perioperative and long-term follow-up results. The results revealed that LRA was superior to TLA in terms of operation time, hospitalization duration, time to first oral intake and time to ambulation. Further analyses focusing on RLA for tumors with different diameters demonstrated that the intraoperative indicators in larger adrenal tumors (> 5 cm) showed superior results to those of smaller adrenal tumors (< 5 cm), while the postoperative indicators between the two groups showed similar results. On the other hand, we further analyzed the different resection methods in the RLA group. The results confirmed that the partial resection method was superior to the total resection method from the perspective of hormone supplementation. There were three patients in the RLA group and 2 patients in the TLA group who were converted to the ICU. Among these patients, four of them had pheochromocytoma (PHEO) with unstable blood pressure after the operation, which could be potentially caused by the over-secretion of catecholamines during the tumor disturbance [14]. Abnormal blood vessels and huge blood volumes were found in all of the PHEO patients. Both of these features could lead to sharp fluctuations in the blood pressure and heart rate of patients, as well as to the increase in bleeding.

The complication rate of RLA was usually approximately 11.5%, and the complications include adrenal cataclastic, peritoneal injury, vena cava injury and renal vein injury [15]. In addition, hypercapnia and pneumoderm, which are caused by the high pressure of CO_2 or by a shallow insertion of the trocar, can also occur [16]. According to our experience, the CO_2 insufflation pressure was usually between 12 cmH_2O and 15 cmH_2O. Studies have shown that these complications are mainly related to the different learning curves among surgeons [17, 18].

The inevitable bleeding from RLA will be less severe with only slight tissue injury when a small incision is made. Our experience suggested that we can inject approximately 350 ml normal saline or air into a homemade gasbag to expand the potential peritoneal cavity. Three minutes of compression was needed following this in order to prevent the bleeding caused by the rupture of small blood vessels. In addition, an ultrasonic knife could be used in the solidification of small blood vessels during the separation of the renal fascia and adipose capsule. However, open surgery hemostasis would be chosen without any hesitation when the operating vision was influenced by adrenal cataclastic or unmanageable vascular injury [19].

There were certain limitations of the RLA procedure that need to be taken into consideration. First, the restricted potential cavity has limited the diameter of the removable portion of the tumor. The interaction of surgical instruments could also affect the ease of the operation. Many scholars have reported that retroperitoneal laparoscopy could just be used for small-sized to medium-sized benign adrenal tumors [20]. However, the evidence from our present study has extended this restriction. Secondly, the normal anatomic marks of the peritoneal cavity would be disturbed by the use of a gasbag, which was usually used to expand the peritoneal cavity. This method may also enhance the difficulty of the operation. Third, the effect of gasbag extrusion could

also make the tumor over-secrete catecholamines in PHEO patients; therefore, the preoperative control of blood pressure and sphygmus is very important [21].

It is well-known that there are potential limitations and biases of a retrospective analysis design that may affect the results. On one hand, the number of patients in the groups in the *RLA* vs. *TLA* and *partial resection* vs. *total resection of RLA* comparisons were not equal, which could lead to a potential bias of the results. However, we analyzed the baseline characteristics and measurements between the groups in this study. The results confirmed that there were no statistically significant differences in the basic characteristics between the groups, which could be used in further analyses of outcome indicators. On the other hand, the further subgroups analyses, which included the variables of obesity and adhesion, were not completed due to a lack of sufficient data. Moreover, due to the lack of a sufficient number of patients with malignant tumors, we cannot further perform a survival analysis to determine the overall survival and progression-free survival of adrenocortical carcinoma patients during the follow-up period.

Conclusions
Based on our analyses, both RLA and TLA seem to provide similar effects for the surgical management of large adrenal tumors. However, for benign tumors, partial RLA should be considered to reduce the need for hormone supplementation. Our results have strengthened the opinion that RLA is an efficacious surgical intervention for the treatment of adrenal tumors larger than 5 cm in diameter.

Abbreviations
BMI: Body mass index; CR: Complete remission; EBL: Estimate blood loss; ICU: Intensive care unit; OT: Operation time; RFR: Recurrence-free rate; RLA: Retroperitoneal laparoscopic adrenalectomy; TLA: Transperitoneal laparoscopic adrenalectomy

Acknowledgements
We would like to express our deepest gratitude to all of the staff in the Urology Department of Zigong Fourth People's Hospital and Sichuan Provincial People's Hospital who assisted us with this research.

Funding
This study was funded by the Key Research Base of Humanistic and Social Sciences of the Sichuan Department of Education- Sichuan Hospital Management and Development Research Center (SCYG2017–32).

Availability of data and materials
The information supporting the conclusions of this article is included within the article.

Authors' contributions

WC participated in the design of the study and performed the statistical analysis. GQF and WL conceived the study, participated in its design and helped collect the peri-operative data. YL and ZWM participated in the surgical operations of the adrenal tumors. All of the authors read and approved the final manuscript.

Competing interests

The authors declare that they are no competing interest.

Author details

[1]Department of Urology, Zigong No.4 People's Hospital, Sichuan 643000, China. [2]Department of Urology, Sichuan Academy of Medical Sciences & Sichuan Provincial People's Hospital, No.32 West Second Section First Ring Road, Chengdu 641000, Sichuan, China.

References

1. Chen W, Li F, Chen D, Zhu Y, He C, Du Y, Tan W. Retroperitoneal versus transperitoneal laparoscopic adrenalectomy in adrenal tumor: a meta-analysis. Surg Laparosc Endosc Percutan Tech. 2013;23(2):121–7.
2. Tobias-Machado M, Rincon Rios F, Tulio Lasmar M, Tristao R, Herminio Forseto P Jr, Vaz Juliano R, Wroclawski ER. Laparoscopic retroperitoneal adrenalectomy as a minimally invasive option for the treatment of adrenal tumors. Archivos Espanoles de Urologia. 2006;59(1):49–54.
3. Suzuki K. Laparoscopic adrenalectomy: retroperitoneal approach. Urol Clin North Am. 2001;28(1):85–95.
4. Gasman D, Droupy S, Koutani A, Salomon L, Antiphon P, Chassagnon J, Chopin DK, Abbou CC. Laparoscopic adrenalectomy: the retroperitoneal approach. J Urol. 1998;159(6):1816–20.
5. Mohammadi-Fallah MR, Mehdizadeh A, Badalzadeh A, Izadseresht B, Dadkhah N, Barbod A, Babaie M, Hamedanchi S. Comparison of transperitoneal versus retroperitoneal laparoscopic adrenalectomy in a prospective randomized study. J Laparoendosc Adv Surg Tech A. 2013; 23(4):362–6.
6. Eichhorn-Wharry LI, Talpos GB, Rubinfeld I. Laparoscopic versus open adrenalectomy: another look at outcome using the Clavien classification system. Surgery. 2012;152(6):1090–5.
7. Wang HS, Li CC, Chou YH, Wang CJ, Wu WJ, Huang CH. Comparison of laparoscopic adrenalectomy with open surgery for adrenal tumors. Kaohsiung J Med Sci. 2009;25(8):438–44.
8. Boylu U, Oommen M, Lee BR, Thomas R. Laparoscopic adrenalectomy for large adrenal masses: pushing the envelope. J Endourol. 2009;23(6):971–5.
9. Zhang X, Fu B, Lang B, Zhang J, Xu K, Li HZ, Ma X, Zheng T. Technique of anatomical retroperitoneoscopic adrenalectomy with report of 800 cases. J Urol. 2007;177(4):1254–7.
10. Karanikola E, Tsigris C, Kontzoglou K, Nikiteas N. Laparoscopic adrenalectomy: where do we stand now? Tohoku J Exp Med. 2010; 220(4):259–65.
11. Xu T, Xia L, Wang X, Zhang X, Zhong S, Qin L, Zhang X, Zhu Y, Shen Z. Effectiveness of partial adrenalectomy for concomitant hypertension in patients with nonfunctional adrenal adenoma. Int Urol Nephrol. 2015; 47(1):59–67.
12. Dalvi AN, Thapar PM, Thapar VB, Rege SA, Deshpande AA. Laparoscopic adrenalectomy for large tumours: single team experience. J Minimal Access Surg. 2012;8(4):125–8.
13. Elfenbein DM, Scarborough JE, Speicher PJ, Scheri RP. Comparison of laparoscopic versus open adrenalectomy: results from American College of Surgeons-National Surgery Quality Improvement Project. J Surg Res. 2013; 184(1):216–20.
14. Hisano M, Vicentini FC, Srougi M. Retroperitoneoscopic adrenalectomy in pheochromocytoma. Clinics (Sao Paulo, Brazil). 2012;67(Suppl 1):161–7.
15. Gaujoux S, Bonnet S, Leconte M, Zohar S, Bertherat J, Bertagna X, Dousset B. Risk factors for conversion and complications after unilateral laparoscopic adrenalectomy. Br J Surg. 2011;98(10):1392–9.
16. Lombardi CP, Raffaelli M, De Crea C, Sollazzi L, Perilli V, Cazzato MT, Bellantone R. Endoscopic adrenalectomy: is there an optimal operative approach? Results of a single-center case-control study. Surgery. 2008; 144(6):1008–14. discussion 1014-1005
17. Fiszer P, Toutounchi S, Pogorzelski R, Krajewska E, Ciesla W, Skorski M. Laparoscopic adrenalectomy - assessing the learning curve. Polski Przeglad Chirurgiczny. 2012;84(6):293–7.
18. Dalvi AN, Thapar PM, Shah NS, Menon PS. Has experience changed the scenario in laparoscopic adrenalectomy? Indian J Surg. 2009;71(2):78–83.
19. Tiberio GA, Baiocchi GL, Arru L, Agabiti Rosei C, De Ponti S, Matheis A, Rizzoni D, Giulini SM. Prospective randomized comparison of laparoscopic versus open adrenalectomy for sporadic pheochromocytoma. Surg Endosc. 2008;22(6):1435–9.
20. Castillo O, Sanchez-Salas R, Vidal I. Laparoscopic adrenalectomy. Minerva Urol e Nefrol. 2008;60(3):177–84.
21. Zaki FM, Osman SS, Abdul Manaf Z, Mahadevan J, Yahya M. The value of pre-operative embolisation in primary inferior vena cava paraganglioma. Malays J Med Sci. 2011;18(2):70–3.

Preoperative lipiodol marking and its role on survival and complication rates of CT-guided cryoablation for small renal masses

Fumiya Hongo[1*], Yasuhiro Yamada[1], Takashi Ueda[1], Terukazu Nakmura[1], Yoshio Naya[1], Kazumi Kamoi[1], Koji Okihara[1], Yusuke Ichijo[2], Tsuneharu Miki[1], Kei Yamada[2] and Osamu Ukimura[1]

Abstract

Background: Partial nephrectomy for small renal masses (SRM) may be useful for preserving renal function, but is technically more difficult than radical nephrectomy. Cryoablation may be performed under local anesthesia. The objective of the present study is to assess the safety and therapeutic efficacy of cryoablation with lipiodol marking for SRM.

Methods: Cryoablation therapy was performed on 42 patients under local anesthesia. Their median age was 74 years (31–91). The median tumor diameter was 21 mm (10–42). Responses to the treatment were evaluated using modified Response Evaluation Criteria in Solid Tumors (mRECIST) by contrast-enhanced CT. In six patients (14.3%) for whom it was not possible to use contrast medium, plain CT findings were assessed according to Response Evaluation Criteria in Solid Tumors (RECIST).

Results: Twenty-nine (69%) and five (12%) patients achieved complete responses (CR) and partial responses (PR), respectively, while four (10%) and four (10%) patients each had stable disease (SD) and progressive disease (PD) after the first course of therapy. A second course of cryoablation therapy with lipiodol marking was performed on three out of four patients with PD after the first course of therapy, and resulted in a total of 32 patients achieving CR (76%). Four (36.4%) out of 11 patients for whom lipiodol marking was not conducted had PD, whereas none of the 31 patients for whom lipiodol marking was conducted had PD. All grade complications were reported in 11 (24.4%) patients while grade 3 in two (4.4%) patients. 11 (24.4%) A significant difference was observed in postoperative hemorrhagic events in all grades (18% in patients undergoing cryoablation without lipiodol marking vs. 0% in patients undergoing cryoablation without lipiodol marking).

Conclusions: Although further studies involving more patients are needed in order to evaluate long-term results, cryoablation therapy appears to be a useful treatment option for SRM. Preoperative marking with lipiodol was helpful for improving complication and survival rates with cryoablation.

Keywords: Ablation, Cryoablation, Lipiodol marking, Renal cell cancer, Small renal mass

Background

Renal function-preserving surgery has recently been recommended as a treatment for small renal cancer [1–3]. Percutaneous cryoablation therapy, which includes thermal ablation, for humans was initially reported by Uchida [4]. Laparoscopic cryoablation was subsequently conducted, and favorable outcomes were reported [5]. In Japan, cryoablation has been covered by national health insurance since 2011. We started to perform percutaneous cryoablation therapy for SRM in March 2013, and herein report our initial experience with this procedure.

Computed tomography (CT)- or magnetic resonance imaging (MRI)-guided puncture is conducted in cryoablation therapy. One of the advantages of CT-guided puncture is that it provides a broader space for puncture than MRI-guided puncture; however, it is more difficult

* Correspondence: fhongo@koto.kpu-m.ac.jp
[1]Department of Urology, Kyoto Prefectural University of Medicine, 465 Kajii-cho, Kamigyo-ku, Kyoto 602-8566, Japan
Full list of author information is available at the end of the article

to recognize tumor margins with CT-guided puncture than with MRI-guided puncture. Plain CT-guided puncture is performed in our hospital. In some patients with submerged tumors or tumor margins that are difficult to recognize, marking with lipiodol is conducted prior to cryoablation therapy.

Lipiodol is a lipid-soluble contrast material that is used for lymphangiography [6], hysterosalpingography [7], and transcatheter arterial chemoembolization (TACE) of hepatocellular carcinoma [8]. Since lipiodol remains in place for several days, it is easy to localize nodules using X-ray or CT fluoroscopy during surgery. In the present study, we examined the efficacy of cryoablation therapy for SRM and the usefulness of preoperative lipiodol marking.

Methods

Patients

In March 2013, our hospital started to perform cryoablation therapy on patients who were not indicated for radical surgery under general anesthesia because of active double cancer or complications or on those who did not wish to undergo surgery due to the presence of only one kidney or for some other reason. A preoperative staging imaging evaluation (chest to abdominal CT) was routinely performed on all patients. We retrospectively examined the efficacy of this procedure, adverse events, and post-treatment changes in renal function. Pre- and postoperative serum creatinine levels and adverse events in patients aged 75 years or older were compared with those in patients aged 74 years or younger. The present study was conducted in accordance with the Principles of Helsinki. This study protocol was approved by Institutional Review Board of Kyoto Prefectural University of Medicinw. The Ethics board approval number was ERB-C-54-1. All patients included in this study provided informed consent for cryosurgery, accompanying standard care and the use of their data in research.

Cryoablation methods

The treatment plan was made by performing CT before ablation. A CryoHit® device (Galil Medical USA; Hitachi Medical Corporation, Japan) was employed. IceSeed® or IceRod® needles were used in accordance with the tumor diameter. One to three needles were used for ablation as one IceSeed® for less than 10 mm, 2 IceSeeds® for 10–12 mm, 3 IceSeeds® or 2 IceRods® for 13–20 mm, 3 IceRods® for 21–30 mm, and 4 IceRods® for 31–40 mm. The cryoprobe was introduced under CT fluoroscopic guidance (Vigor Laudator, Toshiba Medical System, Tokyo, Japan) after local anesthesia had been administered by a subcutaneous injection of 1% lidocaine.

The tumor site was cooled with argon gas and thawed with helium gas. The cryoablation area was monitored at appropriate times during puncture or cryoablation. Two cycles of cryoablation were then performed, with the first cycle typically lasting 10–15 min and the second 10 min. Passive thaw was performed between the ablation cycles, and active thaw was performed after the second cycle.

When the tumor was adjacent to peripheral organs, such as the intestinal tract, hydrodissection with physiological saline was performed in order to avoid injury. Transdiaphragmatic puncture with an artificial pneumothorax was conducted for transthoracic puncture. When the tumor was adjacent to the renal pelvis, a ureteral catheter was inserted in some patients, and the tumor site was perfused with warm physiological saline to avoid injury to the renal pelvic mucosa.

As a rule, percutaneous tumor biopsy using 18-gauge Max-Core® (BARD, USA) was performed for a histopathological diagnosis before or at the time of cryoablation because the tumor histology and grade of preoperative biopsy predicted the oncological outcomes of renal cryoablation [9]. Local anesthesia and the prophylactic administration of antibiotics were permitted as combined and supportive therapies.

Transarterial lipiodol marking was performed 1–3 days before cryoablation therapy when difficulties were associated with identifying the tumor location on plain CT. Transfemoral visceral arteriography was conducted using a standard angiographic approach. Selective catheterization of the tumor-feeding arteries was performed under fluoroscopic guidance. After confirming the presence of the catheter tip in the branches of the renal arteries feeding the tumor, lipiodol (Laboratoire Guerbet, Roissy, France) was manually injected (range, 0.2–0.4 mL) under fluoroscopy to make a lipiodol spot.

Evaluation of efficacy

Responses to the treatment were evaluated by performing contrast-enhanced CT after 6 months. Efficacy was evaluated based on the tumor response rate, namely, a complete response (CR) or partial response (PR), using the modified Response Evaluation Criteria in Solid Tumors (mRECIST) criteria [10, 11]. The mRECIST criteria incorporate amendments to the original RECIST criteria. Tumor responses were defined as: (i) CR: the disappearance of any intratumoral arterial enhancement in all target lesions; (ii) PR: at least a 30% decrease in the sum of diameters of viable (enhancement in the arterial phase) target lesions, taking the baseline sum of the diameters of target lesions as the reference; (iii) stable disease (SD): any cases that do not qualify for either PR or progressive disease (PD); (iv) PD: An increase of at least 20% in the sum of the diameters of viable (enhancing) target lesions, taking the smallest sum of the diameters of viable (enhancing) target lesions recorded since the treatment started as the reference.

Efficacy was evaluated based on the tumor response rate, namely, CR or PR, using the mRECIST criteria.

Complications

The Clavien Classification of Surgical Complications was used for surgically related complications [12].

Statistical analysis

Relationships between clinicopathological characteristics and response rates were examined using the $\chi 2$ test. Changes in serum creatinine levels were examined using the t-test. Test results were considered significant at $P < 0.05$. All analyses were performed using JMP 10.0.2 (SAS®).

Results

Patients

Cryoablation therapy was performed on a total of 42 patients before December 2014 (Table 1). Their median age was 74 years (range, 31–91). The median tumor diameter was 24.1 mm (range, 10–42 mm).

Percutaneous renal biopsy was performed on 86% of patients (36/42), but was not mandatory. Biopsy data are shown in Table 1. A pathological diagnosis of renal cell cancer (RCC) was reached in 30 out of the 36 patients and benign tumor (AML) in one patient who underwent biopsy. In the other five patients, biopsy specimens were insufficient to make a pathological diagnosis.

Response

Treatment responses were evaluated using mRECIST based on contrast-enhanced CT findings (Table 2). In six patients (14.3%) for whom it was not possible to use contrast medium, plain CT findings were assessed

according to RECIST. After the first course of therapy, 29 (69%) and five (12%) patients achieved complete responses (CR) and partial responses (PR), respectively, while four (10%) and four (10%) patients each had stable disease (SD) and progressive disease (PD). A second course of cryoablation therapy with lipiodol marking was performed on three out of the four patients with PD after the first course of therapy. CR was achieved in two patients and PR in 1. Final treatment responses were evaluated in 42 patients, including three who underwent two courses of cryoablation therapy. CR and PR were achieved in 32 and five patients, respectively. SD and PD were noted in four and one patients, respectively. one patient proved to have AML. The technical success rate was 98%.

Complications

There were 11 episodes (24.4%) of complications during a total of 45 courses of cryoablation therapy regardless of the grade. Grade 3 or higher adverse events were observed in two patients (4.4%). Intra- and postoperative complications included fever, hematoma, hematuria, pleural effusion, hydronephrosis, and ureter perforation in 5, 1, 2, 1, 1, and 1 patient, respectively (Table 3). Grade 3 or higher adverse events were observed in two patients: G3a hydronephrosis and G3a ureteral injury. There were no lipiodol marking-related adverse events.

Renal function after cryoablation

Postoperative renal function was investigated based on serum creatinine levels 3 months after the treatment. Preoperative serum creatinine levels were 0.95 ± 0.4 in patients aged 74 years or younger and 1.19 ± 0.61 in those aged 75 years or older. These values 3 months

Table 1 The characteristics and outcomes of patients underwent cryopablation with or without preoperativeliiodol marking

Preoperative lipiodol marking		(+) (n = 31)	(−) (n = 11)	p value
Mean age (year, range)	74 (31–91)	71.5 (31–86)	71.1 (49–91)	NS
Gender (%)				NS
Male	33 (79%)	27	6	
Female	9 (21%)	5	4	
Laterality (%)				NS
Right	21 (50%)	15	6	
Left	21 (50%)	16	5	
Tumor size (mm)	24.1 (10–42)	27.8 (10–42)	21.3 (15–34)	p < 0.05
Biopsy performed in 36/42 (85.7%)		28	8	NS
RCC	30 (87%)	24	6	
AML	1 (4%)	0	1	
Inappropriate sample	5 (9%)	4	1	
PD (%)	4 (36.4%)	0	4 (36.4%)	p < 0.001
Post ablative hemorrhagic event (%)	2 (18%)	0	2 (18%)	p < 0.05

Table 2 Efficacy of cryoablation. In three of four patients with PD after the first therapy, second cryoablation therapy with lipiodol marking was performed

	No. of cases	CR	PR	SD	PD
mRECIST	36	32 (89%)	3 (8%)	0 (0%)	1 (3%)
RECIST	6	0 (0%)	2 (33%)	4 (67%)	0 (0%)
Total	42	32 (76%)	5 (12%)	4 (10%)	1 (2%)

after surgery were 0.96 ± 0.46 and 1.20 ± 0.55, respectively. The rates of changes were −1 ± 10 and 3 ± 15%, respectively, which were not significantly different ($p = 0.3282$).

We conducted preoperative lipiodol marking before cryoablation therapy on 31 patients with guidance difficulties under plain CT. Baseline patient demographics and operative outcomes are listed in Table 1. No significance differences were observed in mean age (71.5 vs. 71.1), gender (male/female) (27/5 vs. 6/4), or tumor laterality (15/16 vs. 6/5). On the other hand, significant differences were detected in tumor sizes (27.8 mm (10–42) vs. 21.3 (15–34) mm).

A case of cryoablation therapy with preoperative lipiodol marking was shown (Fig. 1). The red circle indicates the primary tumor. (A) The right renal tumor was detected by a preoperative dynamic CT scan. (B) The tumor was easily detected by intraoperative plain CT after lipiodol marking. (C) A postoperative CT scan showed no enhancement in the cryoablated area. CR was achieved by cryoablation according to mRECIST.

Among all 42 patients, relapse was detected in four (36.4%) out of 11 patients for whom lipiodol marking was not conducted and was not observed in any (0%) of the 31 patients for whom lipiodol marking was conducted showed relapse, with a significant difference between with and without marking ($p = 0.01$). Moreover, a significant difference was detected in postoperative hemorrhagic events (18% vs. 0%) ($p < 0.05$) (Table 1).

No deaths occurred within 1 month of cryoablation therapy. Although one patient died during the follow-up period, her death was not related to cryoablation therapy;

she died of primary disease (malignant lymphoma) 20 months after cryoablation therapy.

Patient survival was evaluated at a mean follow-up time of 17 (range, 6–26) months (SD, 6.13 months). One- and 2-year overall survival rates were 100 and 94.4%, respectively.

Discussion

Nephrectomy has been performed as a standard treatment for renal cancer for a long time. However, the detection rate of SRM has increased with recent advances in diagnostic imaging procedures. A paradigm shift in treatment approaches to renal masses is underway, leading the AUA to release guidelines for the management of clinical stage 1 renal masses in 2009 for the first time [1]. Partial nephrectomy or ablative therapy for T1a renal cancer may be useful for preventing nephrectomy-related chronic kidney disease (CKD) [13, 14]. In elderly patients or patients with comorbidities, who are likely have a lower estimated glomerular filtration rate (eGFR), rapid reductions in renal function have been implicated in early death [15]. Therefore, not only partial nephrectomy, but also ablative therapy including cryoablation therapy, which may be performed under local anesthesia without renal ischemia, thereby facilitating the preservation of renal function, may be useful for patients with comorbidities and the elderly. In the present study, the impact of cryoablation therapy on renal function in patients aged 75 years or older was not significant.

Treatment options for SRM include ablation therapy. In our hospital, RFA therapy has been performed as advanced medical care and its usefulness has been reported [16, 17]. However, in Japan, RFA for renal tumors is not yet covered by national health insurance. Therefore, cryoablation therapy, which is covered by national health insurance, is primarily performed in our hospital.

CT- or MRI-guided puncture is optional as a percutaneous approach. Plain semi-real-time CT-guided puncture is performed in our hospital. However, the major limitation of plain CT is the difficulty associated with the localization of the tumor, when the tumor resembles

Table 3 Postoperative complication in 45 sessions of cryoablation according to Clavien-Dindo classification

	<75 yo (n = 21, 23 sessions)		≥75 yo (n = 21, 22 sesseions)		Total	
	All grade	Grade 3≤	All grade	Grade 3≤	All grade	Grade 3≤
	5 (22%)	1 (4%)	6 (27%)	1 (5%)	11 (24%)	2 (4%)
Fever	2 (9%)		3 (14%)		5 (11%)	
Hematoma	1 (4%)		1 (4%)		2 (4%)	
Hematuria	1 (4%)		1 (5%)		1 (2%)	
Pleural effusion			1 (5%)		1 (2%)	
Hydronephrosis	1 (4%)	1 (4%)			1 (2%)	1 (2%)
Ureter perforation			1 (5%)	1 (5%)	1 (2%)	1 (2%)

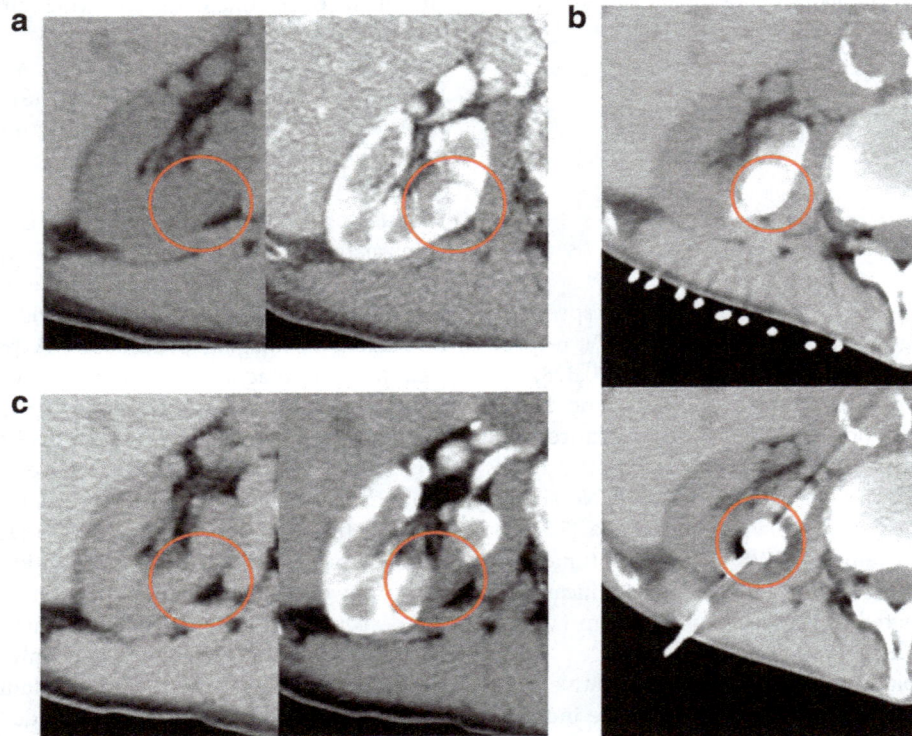

Fig. 1 A case of cryoablation with preoperative lipiodol marking. The red circle indicates the primary tumor. **a** The right renal tumor was detected by a preoperative dynamic computed tomography (CT) scan. **b** The tumor was easily detected by intraoperative plain CT after lipiodol marking. **c** A postoperative CT scan showed no enhancement in the cryoablated area. A complete response was achieved by cryoablation according to the mRECIST criteria

the renal parenchyma, and, importantly, patients indicated for ablative therapy may have renal dysfunctions that are a contraindication for the frequent intraoperative use of a CT contrast agent. In order to overcome these limitations, we evaluated the usefulness of lipiodol marking to identify the tumor center prior to percutaneous cryoablation with plain CT guidance. In the selected patients with submerged tumors or those in whom the tumor margin was difficult to recognize, marking with lipiodol was conducted prior to cryoablation therapy. We previously reported the usefulness of preoperative lipiodol marking prior to the ablation of lung cancer [18]. The use of cryoablation therapy for renal cancer has facilitated accurate evaluations of target tumors, thereby improving the accuracy of the treatment. In contrast, cryoablation therapy may also be performed with the confirmation of tumor contours by administering contrast medium. However, the use of contrast medium needs to be avoided in patients with renal hypofunction. Furthermore, a previous study indicated that embolization prior to cryoablation therapy was useful for reducing the incidence of complications related to cryoablation therapy [19]. Regarding lipiodol marking, lipiodol with a gelatin sponge is transarterially infused. It may be useful for identifying

the tumor location or its margin on CT-guided probe insertion and preventing hemorrhage-associated complications because it reduces intra-tumor blood flow.

When the tumor was adjacent to peripheral organs, such as the intestinal tract, hydrodissection [20], which is useful for avoiding thermal ablation-related intestinal injury, was performed. There were no intestinal injuries in any patients (0%).

In 115 tumors were treated using PCA, technical success rate was achieved in 97% by post-procedure CT (with and without IV contrast or MRI on POD 1). There was no evidence of local recurrence in 80 tumors that were followed for a mean of 13.3 months by CT imaging [21]. Kapoor et al. reported that the maximal and minimal percentages of cancer-specific survival were 100% and 84.3% in follow-ups of 11.4 months (median) and 64 months (mean), respectively, by reviewing a total of 2104 analyzed tumors from 2038 patients in the literature [22].

On the other hand, the timing of follow-ups after cryoablation therapy has not yet been established. One exception was the series by Gill and colleagues; the authors routinely performed biopsies 6 months post-CA. In this series, two out of 56 tumors were positive 6 months post-CA, at a rate of 3.6% [23]. In our hospital, follow-ups are performed using dynamic CT 1, 3, 6, 9, and 12 months after the treatment. In the present study, treatment responses were evaluated after 6 months. The success rate for the treatment was 98%, which was consistent with previous findings. When biopsies revealed no malignancy, follow-up CT was performed 6 and 12 months after the treatment.

Primary complications include hemorrhage. Hemorrhage or significant bleeding requiring blood transfusion has a reported incidence of 1–8% [24].

In the present study, postoperative hemorrhage was observed in two patients (4%) in whom it was impossible to discontinue anticoagulant therapy. However, these patients did not require blood transfusions. There were no cases of hemorrhage requiring blood transfusion (0%). This percentage is lower than that previously reported and may be attributed to the artery-embolizing effects of preoperative marking with lipiodol, which is conducted in our hospital where necessary, thereby decreasing the incidence of postoperative hemorrhage. Transcatheter renal arterial embolization with a mixture of ethanol and lipiodol for unresectable RCC has been reported [24], and this study is the first to demonstrate the efficacy of cryoablation with lipiodol marking. A previous study showed that embolization before cryoablation therapy reduced the rate of complications [25]. In the present study, there were no intestinal injuries. However, based on previous findings, we prepared preventive strategies, such as cryoablation therapy after hydrodissection, for patients for whom the anterior surface of the kidney was suspected to be in contact with the intestinal tract [26].

Regarding complications in the urinary tract, ureteral perforation was noted in one patient. However, the insertion of a Double J stent catheter for 6 months led to improvements. The thermal ablation of renal tumors in close proximity to or abutting the renal pelvis, uretero-pelvic junction (UPJ), or proximal ureter represents a higher risk scenario for ureteral or collecting system injury, with resultant obstruction or renal loss [16]. Cryoablation is more likely to be recommended than RF ablation for the treatment of a renal tumor in proximity to the ureter because the former procedure has been shown to result in fewer urinary tract injuries than the latter, as demonstrated in a porcine model [27].

According to a recent review on treatments for localized renal masses in the United States, nephrectomy still accounts for a high proportion, but its rate has decreased. Partial nephrectomy and thermal ablation, such as cryoablation and RFA, have been indicated for an increasing number of patients [28]. This may also be the case in Japan in the future. Partial nephrectomy is now primarily performed as a renal function-preserving treatment; however, cryoablation therapy may be useful for elderly patients and those with complications. A percutaneous thermal ablation procedure for renal cancer appears to be a useful treatment option for SRM. In the present study, preoperative marking with lipiodol was helpful for achieving successful cryoablation.

There were several limitations in the present study. The total number of cases was too small to reach definite conclusions. In addition, complete preoperative histological information was unavailable, limiting the oncological outcomes. Furthermore, this was a retrospective study. Therefore, controlled randomized trials need to be designed that compare preoperative lipiodol marking followed by cryoablation and cryoablation without lipiodol marking.

Conclusions

The results of the present study suggest that cryoablation with preoperative lipiodol marking improves the safety and success rate of CT-guided cryoablation for SRM. This approach was even shown to be useful for patients with renal dysfunctions, who were likely contraindicated for the intraoperative use of a contrast agent to visualize renal tumors.

Abbreviations
CA: Cryoablation; CKD: Chronic kidney disease; CT: Computed tomography; eGFR: Estimated glomerular filtration rate; HCC: Hepatocellular carcinoma; Lipiodol: Ethiodized oil; mRECIST: Modified Response Evaluation Criteria in Solid Tumors; MRI: Magnetic resonance imaging; PCA: Percutaneous cryoablation; POD 1: Post operative day 1; RCC: Renal cell cancer; SRM: Small renal masses; TACE: Transcatheter arterial chemoembolization; UPJ: Ureteropelvic junction

Acknowledgments
The authors thank Ms. Morioka Y and Ms. Nakamura S for data acquisition and Ms. Katsurai M for organizing the follow-up schedule after the treatment.

Funding
None.

Authors' contributions
FH carried out cryosurgery on patients, collected and analyzed data, and wrote and drafted the manuscript, YY, TU, and YI carried out cryosurgery on patients, YN and KK participated in the acquisition of data, TN and KO participated in the design of the study and performed the statistical analysis, and TM, KY, and OU conceived the study, participated in its design and coordination, and helped to draft the manuscript. All authors read and approved the final manuscript.

Competing interests
The authors declare that they have no competing interests.

Author details
[1]Department of Urology, Kyoto Prefectural University of Medicine, 465 Kajii-cho, Kamigyo-ku, Kyoto 602-8566, Japan. [2]Department of Radiology, Kyoto Prefectural University of Medicine, Kyoto, Japan.

References

1. Campbell SC, Novick AC, Belldegrun A, et al. Guideline for management of the clinical T1 renal mass. J Urol. 2009;182:1271–9.
2. Ljungberg B, Bensalah K, Canfield S, et al. EAU Guidelines on renal cell carcinoma: 2014 update. Eur Urol. 2015;67:913–24. doi:10.1016/j.eururo.2015.01.005. Epub 2015 Jan 21.
3. Fujioka T, Obara W, Committee for Establishment of the Clinical Practice Guidelines for the Management of Renal Cell Carcinoma; Japanese Urological Association. Evidence-based clinical practice guidelines for renal cell carcinoma (Summary–JUA 2007 Edition). Int J Urol. 2009;16:339–53. doi:10.1111/j.1442-2042.2008.02242.x.
4. Uchida M, Imaide Y, Sugimoto K, et al. Percutaneous cryosurgery for renal tumours. Br J Urol. 1995;75:132–6. discussion 136–137.
5. Gill IS, Novick AC, Meraney AM, et al. Laparoscopic renal cryoablation in 32 patients. Urology. 2000;56:748–53. doi.org/10.1016/S0090-4295(00)00752-4.
6. Matsumoto T, Yamagami T, Kato T, et al. The effectiveness of lymphangiography as a treatment method for various chyle leakages. Br J Radiol. 2009;82:286–90.
7. Johnson NP, Farquhar CM, Hadden WE, et al. The FLUSH trial–flushing with lipiodol for unexplained (and endometriosis-related) subfertility by hysterosalpingography: a randomized trial. Hum Reprod. 2004;19:2043–51.
8. Ikeda M, Arai Y, Park SJ, et al. Prospective study of transcatheter arterial chemoembolization for unresectable hepatocellular carcinoma: an Asian cooperative study between Japan and Korea. J Vasc Interv Radiol. 2013;24:490–500.
9. Beksac AT, Rivera-Sanfeliz G, Dufour CA, et al. Impact of tumor histology and grade on treatment success of percutaneous renal cryoablation World J Urol, 2016 Aug 2 [Epub ahead of print]
10. Llovet JM, Decaens T, Raoul JL, et al. Modified RECIST (mRECIST) assessment for hepatocellular carcinoma. Semin Liver Dis. 2010;30:52–60. doi:10.1055/s-0030-1247132. Epub 2010 Feb 19. Review.
11. Lencioni R. New data supporting modified RECIST (mRECIST) for hepatocellular carcinoma. Clin Cancer Res. 2013;19:1312–4. doi:10.1158/1078-0432.CCR-12-3796. Epub 2013 Feb 4.
12. Dindo D, Demartines N, Clavien PA. Classification of surgical complications: a new proposal with evaluation in a cohort of 6336 patients and results of a survey. Ann Surg. 2004;240:205–13.
13. Huang WC, Huang WC, Elkin EB, et al. Partial nephrectomy versus radical nephrectomy in patients with small renal tumors–is there a difference in mortality and cardiovascular outcomes? J Urol. 2009;181:55–61. doi:10.1016/j.juro.2008.09.017. discussion 61–2. Epub 2008 Nov 13.
14. Van Poppel H, Da Pozzo L, Albrecht W, et al. European Organization for Research and Treatment of Cancer (EORTC); National Cancer Institute of Canada Clinical Trials Group (NCIC CTG); Southwest Oncology Group (SWOG); Eastern Cooperative Oncology Group (ECOG) A prospective randomized EORTC intergroup phase 3 study comparing the complications of elective nephron-sparing surgery and radical nephrectomy for low-stage renal cell carcinoma. Eur Urol. 2007;51:1606–15. Epub 2006 Nov 15.
15. Rifkin DE, Shlipak MG, Katz R, et al. Rapid kidney function decline and mortality risk in older adults. Arch Intern Med. 2008;168:2212–8. doi:10.1001/archinte.168.20.2212.
16. Ukimura O, Kawauchi A, Fujito A, et al. Radio-frequency ablation of renal cell carcinoma in patients who were at significant risk. Int J Urol. 2004;11:1051–7.
17. Hiraoka K, Kawauchi A, Nakamura T, et al. Radiofrequency ablation for renal tumors: our experience. Int J Urol. 2009;16:869–73. doi:10.1111/j.1442-2042.2009.02378.x. Epub 2009 Sep 3.
18. Miura H, Yamagami T, Tanaka O, et al. CT findings after lipiodol marking performed before video-assisted thoracoscopic surgery for small pulmonary nodules. Acta Radiol. 2016;57:303–10. doi:10.1177/0284185115576047. Epub 2015 Mar 19.
19. Miller JM, Julien P, Wachsman A, et al. The role of embolization in reducing the complications of cryoablation in renal cell carcinoma. Clin Radiol. 2014;69:1045–9. doi:10.1016/j.crad.2014.05.110. Epub 2014 Jul 16.
20. Bodily KD, Atwell TD, Mandrekar JN, et al. Hydrodisplacement in the percutaneous cryoablation of 50 renal tumors. Am J Roentgenol. 2010;194:779–83.
21. Atwell TD, Farrell MA, Leibovich BC, et al. Percutaneous renal cryoablation: experience treating 115 tumors. J Urol. 2008;179:2136–41.
22. Kapoor A, Touma NJ, Dib RE. Review of the efficacy and safety of cryoablation for the treatment of small renal masses. Can Urol Assoc J. 2013;7:E38–44. doi:10.5489/cuaj.12018.
23. Gill IS, Remer EM, Hasan WA, et al. Renal cryoablation: outcome at 3 years. J Urol. 2005;173:1903–7. http://dx.doi.org/10.1097/01.ju.0000158154.28845.c9.
24. Park JH, Kim SH, Han JK, et al. Transcatheter arterial embolization of unresectable renal cell carcinoma with a mixture of ethanol and iodized oil. Cardiovasc Intervent Radiol. 1994;17:323–7.
25. Finley DS, Beck S, Box G, et al. Percutaneous and laparoscopic cryoablation of small renal masses. J Urol. 2008;180:492–8. discussion 8.
26. Lee SJ, Choyke LT, Locklin JK, et al. Use of hydrodissection to prevent nerve and muscular damage during radiofrequency ablation of kidney tumors. J Vasc Interv Radiol. 2006;17:1967–9.
27. Brashears III JH, Raj GV, Crisci A, et al. Renal cryoablation and radio frequency ablation: an evaluation of worst case scenarios in a porcine model. J Urol. 2005;73:2160–5.
28. Woldrich JM, Palazzi K, Stroup SP, et al. Trends in the surgical management of localized renal masses: thermal ablation, partial and radical nephrectomy in the USA, 1998–2008. BJU Int. 2013;111:1261–8. doi:10.1111/j.1464-410X.2012.11497.x. Epub 2013 Mar 7.

Permissions

The contributors of this book come from diverse backgrounds, making this book a truly international effort. This book will bring forth new frontiers with its revolutionizing research information and detailed analysis of the nascent developments around the world.

We would like to thank all the contributing authors for lending their expertise to make the book truly unique. They have played a crucial role in the development of this book. Without their invaluable contributions this book wouldn't have been possible. They have made vital efforts to compile up to date information on the varied aspects of this subject to make this book a valuable addition to the collection of many professionals and students.

This book was conceptualized with the vision of imparting up-to-date information and advanced data in this field. To ensure the same, a matchless editorial board was set up. Every individual on the board went through rigorous rounds of assessment to prove their worth. After which they invested a large part of their time researching and compiling the most relevant data for our readers.

The editorial board has been involved in producing this book since its inception. They have spent rigorous hours researching and exploring the diverse topics which have resulted in the successful publishing of this book. They have passed on their knowledge of decades through this book. To expedite this challenging task, the publisher supported the team at every step. A small team of assistant editors was also appointed to further simplify the editing procedure and attain best results for the readers.

Apart from the editorial board, the designing team has also invested a significant amount of their time in understanding the subject and creating the most relevant covers. They scrutinized every image to scout for the most suitable representation of the subject and create an appropriate cover for the book.

The publishing team has been an ardent support to the editorial, designing and production team. Their endless efforts to recruit the best for this project, has resulted in the accomplishment of this book. They are a veteran in the field of academics and their pool of knowledge is as vast as their experience in printing. Their expertise and guidance has proved useful at every step. Their uncompromising quality standards have made this book an exceptional effort. Their encouragement from time to time has been an inspiration for everyone.

The publisher and the editorial board hope that this book will prove to be a valuable piece of knowledge for researchers, students, practitioners and scholars across the globe.

List of Contributors

Tushar Patial
Department of General Surgery, Indira Gandhi Medical College & Hospital, Shimla, Himachal Pradesh 171001, India

Girish Sharma
Department of Urology, Indira Gandhi Medical College & Hospital, Shimla, Himachal Pradesh 171001, India

Pamposh Raina
Department of Urology, Indira Gandhi Medical College & Hospital, Shimla, Himachal Pradesh 171001, India

U-Syn Ha, Sung Hoo Hong and Ji Youl Lee
Department of Urology, Seoul St. Mary's Hospital, College of Medicine, The Catholic University of Korea, Seoul, Republic of Korea

Kang Jun Cho
Department of Urology, Bucheon St. Mary's Hospital, College of Medicine, The Catholic University of Korea, Seoul, Republic of Korea

Byung Il Yoon
Department of Urology, Catholic Kwandong University, International St. Mary's Hospital, Incheon, Republic of Korea

Kyu Won Lee
Department of Urology, St. Paul's Hospital, College of Medicine, The Catholic University of Korea, Seoul, Republic of Korea

Jun Sung Koh
Department of Urology, Bucheon St. Mary's Hospital, College of Medicine, The Catholic University of Korea, Seoul, Republic of Korea
Department of Urology, Bucheon St. Mary's Hospital, College of Medicine, The Catholic University of Korea, 327, Sosa-ro, Wonmi-gu, Bucheon-si, Gyeonggi-do 14647, Republic of Korea

Michael A. Liss and Christopher J. Kane
Department of Urology, UC San Diego Health System, San Diego, CA, USA

Tony Chen
University of California, San Diego School of Medicine, La Jolla, CA, USA

Joel Baumgartner
Department of Surgery, UC San Diego Health System, San Diego, CA, USA

Ithaar H. Derweesh
Department of Urology, UC San Diego Health System, San Diego, CA, USA
UC San Diego Moores Cancer Center, 3855 Health Sciences Drive #0987, La Jolla, CA 92093-0987, USA

Satoshi Washino, Masaru Hirai, Yutaka Kobayashi, Kimitoshi Saito and Tomoaki Miyagawa
The Department of Urology, Saitama Medical Center Jichi Medical University, 1-847, Amanuma-cho, Omiya-ku, Saitama city, Saitama, Japan

Dae Ji Kim, Jeong Hwan Son, Seok Heun Jang, Jae Won Lee, Dae Sung Cho and Chae Hong Lim
Department of Urology, Bundang Jesaeng Hospital, 180 Seohyeon-rho Bundang-gu, Seongnam 463-774, Republic of Korea

Hitendra R Patel
Department of Urology, University Hospital North Norway, Sykehusvegen 38, 9038 Tromsø, Norway

Dapo Ilo and Jane Barry
Lilly UK, Basingstoke, UK

Nimish Shah
Addenbrooke's Hospital, Cambridge, UK

Béatrice Cuzin
Department of Urology, Edouard Herriot University Hospital, Lyon, France

David Chadwick
South Tees Hospitals NHS Foundation Trust, Stockton-on-Tees, UK

Robert Andrianne
Centre Hospitalier Universitaire de Liège, Service d'Urologie, Belgium

Carsten Henneges, Katja Hell-Momeni and Hartwig Büttner
Lilly Deutschland GmbH, Bad Homburg, Germany

Julia Branicka
Eli Lilly Polska, Warsaw, Poland

Sabrina Thalita Reis, Kátia R. M. Leite, Nayara Izabel Viana, Roberto Iglesias Lopes, Caio Martins Moura, Renato F. Ivanovic, Marcos Machado, Francisco Tibor Denes, Amilcar Giron, William Carlos Nahas, Miguel Srougi and Carlo C. Passerotti
Urology Department, Laboratory of Medical Investigation (LIM55), University of Sao Paulo Medical School, Av. Dr. Arnaldo 455, 2° floor, room 2145, 01246-903 Sao Paulo, Brazil

Leah Jamnicky
University Health Network, Toronto, Ontario, 200 Elizabeth Street, Toronto, Ontario M5G 2C4, Canada

Daniel Santa Mina
University Health Network, Toronto, Ontario, 200 Elizabeth Street, Toronto, Ontario M5G 2C4, Canada
University of Guelph-Humber, 207 Humber College Boulevard, Toronto, Ontario M9W 5L7, Canada
University of Toronto, 27 King's College Circle, Toronto, Ontario M5S 2W6, Canada

Leslie E. Stefanyk
University Health Network, Toronto, Ontario, 200 Elizabeth Street, Toronto, Ontario M5G 2C4, Canada
University of Guelph-Humber, 207 Humber College Boulevard, Toronto, Ontario M9W 5L7, Canada

Shabbir M. H. Alibhai, Jennifer Jones, Dean Elterman, Neil E. Fleshner, Antonio Finelli, John Trachtenberg and Andrew G. Matthew
University Health Network, Toronto, Ontario, 200 Elizabeth Street, Toronto, Ontario M5G 2C4, Canada
University of Toronto, 27 King's College Circle, Toronto, Ontario M5S 2W6, Canada

Darren Au and William J. Hilton
University Health Network, Toronto, Ontario, 200 Elizabeth Street, Toronto, Ontario M5G 2C4, Canada
University of Guelph, 50 Stone Rd E, Guelph, Ontario N1G 2W1, Canada

Nelly Faghani
Pelvic Health Solutions, 372 Hollandview Trail, Aurora, Ontario L4G 0A5, Canada

Paul Ritvo
York University, 4700 Keele St, Toronto, Ontario M3J 1P3, Canada
Cancer Care Ontario, Toronto, Ontario, Canada

Rajiv K. Singal
University of Toronto, 27 King's College Circle, Toronto, Ontario M5S 2W6, Canada
Toronto East General Hospital, Toronto, Ontario M4C 5T2, Canada

E. Angenete, U. Angerås, J. Ekelund and E. Haglind
Department of Surgery, Institute of Clinical Sciences, Sahlgrenska Academy at University of Gothenburg, SSORG, Sahlgrenska University Hospital/Östra, SE-416 85 Gothenburg, Sweden.

M. Gellerstedt
University West, Trollhättan, Sweden

M. Börjesson
Swedish School of Sport and Health Sciences, Stockholm, Sweden
Department of Cardiology, Karolinska University Hospital, Stockholm, Sweden

T. Thorsteinsdottir
Faculty of Nursing, School of Health Sciences, University of Iceland, Reykjavik, Iceland

G. Steineck
Division of Clinical Cancer Epidemiology, Department of Oncology, Institute of Clinical Sciences, Sahlgrenska Academy at the University of Gothenburg, Gothenburg, Sweden
Department of Oncology and Pathology, Division of Clinical Cancer Epidemiology, Karolinska Institutet, Solna, Sweden

David D. Thiel, Andrew J. Davidiuk and Gregory A. Broderick
Departments of Urology Mayo Clinic, 4500 San Pablo Road, Jacksonville, FL 32224, USA

Michelle Arnold, Nancy Diehl, Andrea Tavlarides, Kaitlynn Custer and Alexander S. Parker
Health Sciences Research at Mayo Clinic, 4500 San Pablo Road, Jacksonville, FL 32224, USA

Pierluigi Bove, Valerio Iacovelli, Francesco Celestino, Francesco De Carlo, Giuseppe Vespasiani and Enrico Finazzi Agrò
Department of Urology, Tor Vergata University of Rome, V.le Oxford 81, 00133 Rome, Italy

Jung Keun Lee, Sangchul Lee, Sung Kyu Hong, Seok-Soo Byun and Sang Eun Lee
Department of Urology, Seoul National University Bundang Hospital, 166, Gumi-ro, Bundang-gu, Seongnam, Gyunggi-do 463-707, South Korea
Department of Urology, College of Medicine, Seoul National University, 103, Daehak-ro, Jongno-gu, Seoul 110-799, South Korea

Masashi Matsushima, Akira Miyajima, Seiya Hattori, Toshikazu Takeda, Ryuichi Mizuno, Eiji Kikuchi and Mototsugu Oya
Department of Urology, Keio University School of Medicine, 35 Shinanomachi, Shinjuku-ku, Tokyo 160-8582, Japan

Ryuta Tanimoto, Yomi Fashola, Kymora B Scotland, Anne E Calvaresi, Leonard G Gomella, Edouard J Trabulsi and Costas D Lallas
Department of Urology, Kimmel Cancer Center, Thomas Jefferson University, 1025 Walnut St. Suite 1112, Philadelphia, PA 19107, USA

Giorgio Franco and Costantino Leonardo
Department Gynaecological-Obstetrical and Urological Sciences, Sapienza University, via del Policlinico n 155 cap, 00161 Rome, Italy

Filomena Scarselli, Valentina Casciani, Pier Francesco Greco, Alessia Greco, Maria Giulia Minasi and Ermanno Greco
Centre for Reproductive Medicine, European Hospital, Rome, Italy

Cosimo De Nunzio
Department Urology, Sant' Andrea Hospital, Sapienza University, Rome, Italy

Donato Dente
Robotic Urology Department, Policlinico Abano Terme, Padova, Italy

Peng Ge, Zi-Cheng Wang, Xi Yu, Jian Lin and Qun He
Department of Urology, Peking University First Hospital and Institute of Urology, Peking University, Beijing 100034, China

National Research Center for Genitourinary Oncology, Beijing 100034, China

Rasa Ruseckaite, Fanny Sampurno and Sue Evans
Department of Epidemiology and Preventive Medicine, School of Public Health and Preventive Medicine, Faculty of Medicine Nursing and Health Sciences, Monash University, Melbourne, Australia

Jeremy Millar
Department of Epidemiology and Preventive Medicine, School of Public Health and Preventive Medicine, Faculty of Medicine Nursing and Health Sciences, Monash University, Melbourne, Australia
Alfred Health Radiation Oncology, Melbourne, Australia

Mark Frydenberg
Department of Surgery, Monash Medical Centre, Melbourne, Australia

Michael Froehner, Ulrike Heberling, Vladimir Novotny, Stefan Zastrow and Manfred P. Wirth
Department of Urology, University Hospital Carl Gustav Carus, Technische Universität Dresden, Fetscherstrasse 74, D-01307 Dresden, Germany

Rainer Koch
Department of Medical Statistics and Biometry, University Hospital Carl Gustav Carus, Technische Universität Dresden, Fetscherstrasse 74, D-01307 Dresden, Germany

Matthias Hübler
Department of Anesthesiology, University Hospital Carl Gustav Carus, Technische Universität Dresden, Fetscherstrasse 74, D-01307 Dresden, Germany

Oliver W. Hakenberg
Department of Urology, University of Rostock, Ernst-Heydemann-Strasse 6, D-18055 Rostock, Germany

Taisheng Liang, Gang Wu, Botao Tang, Xiangdong Luo, Shangguang Lu and Yu Dong
Department of Urology, Ruikang Hospital Affiliated to Guangxi University of Chinese Medicine, Nanning, China

Chenming Zhao and Huan Yang
Department of Urology, Tongji Hospital, Tongji Medical College, Huazhong University of Science and Technology, Wuhan, China

Jundong Zhu, Fan Jiang, Pu Li, Pengfei Shao, Chao Liang, Aiming Xu, Chenkui Miao, Chao Qin, Zengjun Wang and Changjun Yin
Department of Urology, The First Affiliated Hospital of Nanjing Medical University, Nanjing, 300 Guangzhou Road, Nanjing 210029, China

Yoichiro Kato, Renpei Kato, Misato Takayama, Daiki Ikarashi, Mitsutaka Onoda, Tomohiko Matsuura, Mitsugu Kanehira, Ryo Takata, Jun Sugimura, So Omori and Wataru Obara
Department of Urology, Iwate Medical University School of Medicine, 19-1 Uchimaru, Morioka 020-8505, Japan

Shigeaki Baba, Toshimoto Kimura, Koki Otsuka and Akira Sasaki
Department of Surgery, Iwate Medical University School of Medicine, 19-1 Uchimaru, Morioka 020-8505, Japan

Kwaku Addai Arhin Appiah, Roland Azorliade, Kwaku Otu-Boateng, Kofi Baah-Nyamekye, Patrick Opoku Manu Maison, Douglas Arthur, Isaac Opoku Antwi, Benjamin Frimpong-Twumasi, Samuel Kodzo Togbe and George Amoah
Department of Surgery, Komfo Anokye Teaching Hospital, Kumasi, Ghana

Christian Kofi Gyasi-Sarpong and Ken Aboah
Department of Surgery, School of Medical Sciences-KNUST, Kumasi, Ghana

Dennis Odai Laryea
Public Health Unit, Komfo Anokye Teaching Hospital, Kumasi, Ghana

Edwin Mwintiereh Yenli
Department of Surgery, Tamale Teaching Hospital, Tamale, Ghana

Kian Asanad
David Geffen School of Medicine at the University of California Los Angeles, 300 Stein Plaza, Suite 348, Los Angeles, California 90095, USA

Andrew T. Lenis, Nicholas M. Donin and Karim Chamie
David Geffen School of Medicine at the University of California Los Angeles, 300 Stein Plaza, Suite 348, Los Angeles, California 90095, USA
Department of Urology, Health Services Research Group, David Geffen School of Medicine at UCLA, Los Angeles, California, USA

Jonsson Comprehensive Cancer Center, David Geffen School of Medicine at UCLA, Los Angeles, California, USA

Maher Blaibel
Riverside School of Medicine, University of California, Riverside, California, USA

Lucy E. Hackshaw-McGeagh, Richard M. Martin and J. Athene Lane
University of Bristol, NIHR Biomedical Research Centre - Nutrition, Diet and Lifestyle Theme, Level 3, University Hospitals Bristol Education Centre, Upper Maudlin Street, Bristol BS2 8AE, England, UK
University of Bristol, Bristol Medical School: Population Health Sciences, Canynge Hall, 39 Whatley Road, Bristol BS8 2PS, England, UK

Eileen Sutton
University of Bristol, Bristol Medical School: Population Health Sciences, Canynge Hall, 39 Whatley Road, Bristol BS8 2PS, England, UK

Raj Persad and Anthony Koupparis
Bristol Urological Institute, Southmead Hospital Bristol, Southmead Road, Westbury-on-Trym, Bristol BS10 5NB, England, UK

Jonathan Aning
Freeman Hospital, Freeman Road, Newcastle upon Tyne, Tyne and Wear NE7 7DN, England, UK

Amit Bahl
Bristol Haematology & Oncology Centre, Horfield Road, Bristol BS2 8ED, England, UK

Chris Millett
Member of the NIHR Biomedical Research Centre - Nutrition, Diet and Lifestyle Theme Prostate Cancer Patient and Public Involvement Group, Bristol, England, UK

Khaleeq ur Rehman
Department of Urology & Andrology, FMH College of Medicine & Dentistry, Shadman, Lahore, Pakistan

Hafsa Zaneb
Department of Anatomy and Histology, University of Veterinary and Animal Sciences, Lahore, Pakistan

Abdul Basit Qureshi
Department of Surgery, Services Institute of Medical Sciences, Lahore, Pakistan

Ahsan Numan
Department of Neurology, Services Institute of Medical Sciences, Lahore, Pakistan

Muhammad Shahbaz Yousaf, Imtiaz Rabbani and Habib Rehman
Department of Physiology, University of Veterinary and Animal Sciences, Lahore, Pakistan

Yu Mao, Shaoji Chen, Xuejun Wang, Daorui Qin and Yunman Tang
Department of Pediatric Surgery of Children's Medical Center, Sichuan Academy of Medical Sciences & Sichuan Provincial People's Hospital, Chengdu, China

Ru Wang
Department of Burn and Plastic Surgery, West China Hospital of Sichuan University, Chengdu, China

Zhiyuan Shen and Zhongquan Sun
Department of Urology, Huadong Hospital, Fudan University, 221 West Yan'an Road, Shanghai 200040, China

Qiang Cao, Pengchao Li, Xiao Yang, Jian Qian, Qiang Lu and Min Gu
Department of Urology, the First Affiliated Hospital of Nanjing Medical University, 300 Guangzhou Road, Nanjing 210029, China

Yuhki Nakamura, Tsuzumi Konishi and Masashi Ohshima
Department of Urology, Jichi Medical University Saitama Medical Center, 1-847, Amanuma-cho, Omiya-ku, Saitama 330-8503, Japan

Yoshiaki Arai
Department of Urology, Nishi-Omiya Hospital, 1-1173, Mihashi, Omiya-ku, Saitama 330-0856, Japan

Andrew R. Leone, Laura C. Kidd, Gregory J. Diorio, Kamran Zargar-Shoshtari, Pranav Sharma, Wade J. Sexton and Philippe E. Spiess
Department of Genitourinary Oncology, H. Lee Moffitt Cancer Center and Research Institute, 12902 Magnolia Drive Office 12538, Tampa, FL 33612, USA

Wei Chen, Yong Liang, Wei Lin and Guang-Qing Fu
Department of Urology, Zigong No.4 People's Hospital, Sichuan 643000, China

Zhi-Wei Ma
Department of Urology, Sichuan Academy of Medical Sciences & Sichuan Provincial People's Hospital, No.32 West Second Section First Ring Road, Chengdu 641000, Sichuan, China

Fumiya Hongo, Yasuhiro Yamada, Takashi Ueda, Terukazu Nakmura, Yoshio Naya, Kazumi Kamoi, Koji Okihara, Tsuneharu Miki and Osamu Ukimura
Department of Urology, Kyoto Prefectural University of Medicine, 465 Kajii-cho, Kamigyo-ku, Kyoto 602-8566, Japan

Yusuke Ichijo and Kei Yamada
Department of Radiology, Kyoto Prefectural University of Medicine, Kyoto, Japan

Index

A

Adrenal Gland, 207, 211

Adrenalectomy, 133, 137, 206-207, 209-213

Anastomosis, 1-4, 6-7, 12, 18-20, 71-72, 74-75, 78, 82-84

Androgen Deprivation Therapy, 44, 106, 108, 156, 163

Anesthesia, 19, 23, 27, 78, 93, 129, 134, 189, 192, 195, 208, 214-215, 217

Angiogenesis, 42

Azoospermia, 92-93, 98-99

B

Benign Prostate Hyperplasia, 36

Biochemical Recurrence, 72, 75, 85, 88-91, 165

Biopsy, 69, 71, 80, 92-95, 97, 99-105, 115, 147, 173, 175-177, 189, 194-205, 215-216

Bowel Adhesion, 5-9

Brachytherapy, 106, 108

C

Carboxymethylcellulose, 5-6, 8-10

Chemotherapy, 101, 103, 108, 117, 119, 148-149, 153-154, 180-181

Chromophobe, 200-201, 203-205

Chronic Kidney Disease, 202, 205, 217, 219

Circumcision, 1, 138-145

Computed Tomography, 19, 127, 132, 134, 137, 189, 205, 207, 209, 214, 218-219

Cryoablation, 214-220

Cystectomy, 6, 18-21, 100-105, 116, 119-122, 147, 154, 179-181, 183-184, 186-193

Cystoscopy, 22, 27, 80, 147, 153, 173, 175-176, 189

E

Electro Medical Systems, 124, 127

Erectile Dysfunction, 3, 29, 37-38, 52-53, 55, 61, 68, 73

F

Fistula, 3, 71-72, 74, 138-143, 145, 174-175

G

Gene Expression, 40-41

Gleason Score, 54, 65, 69, 71-72, 80-82, 86, 89, 108-110, 113

H

Hematuria, 18-21, 25-26, 72, 80, 100, 126, 129, 147, 149, 194-198, 216-217

Hemophilia A, 18, 20-21

Heterogeneity, 153, 181, 184

Hydronephrosis, 40, 43, 124, 126, 216-217

Hypogonadism, 167, 170

Hypospadias, 138-142, 145, 172-174, 176-178

I

Ileal Conduit, 18-20, 192-193

Ileal Neobladder, 190-192

Immunotherapy, 101, 148

L

Laparoscopic Radical Prostatectomy, 5-6, 9, 55, 61, 69, 76-78, 80-85, 91

Lesion, 147, 153, 195

Lithotripsy, 28, 123-125, 127

Luteinizing Hormone, 93, 98, 173, 177

Lymphadenectomy, 86, 187-190, 192

M

Maturation Arrest, 92, 98

Metastasis, 78, 103, 106, 109, 128-130, 132, 134, 203

Micturition, 52, 77, 79, 83

N

Necrosis, 1-2, 141, 147, 153

Nephrectomy, 63-65, 67, 76, 128-137, 200-205, 214, 217, 219-220

Nephrolithotomy, 123, 127

Nephrostomy, 123-124

O

Octogenarians, 116, 119-122

Ovotesticular Disorder, 172, 177-178

Ovotestis, 172, 174-176

P

Partial Nephrectomy, 63-65, 67, 128-132, 200-205, 214, 217, 219-220

Penile Amputation, 1-4, 138-143

Percutaneous Nephrolithotomy, 123, 127

Polymerase Chain Reaction, 39-40, 42

Postoperative Ileus, 137, 188-189, 192-193

Prognosis, 43, 92, 96-97, 100, 104-105, 113, 131, 172, 203

Prostate Cancer, 6-7, 20-21, 29-31, 34, 36-38, 44-45, 51-56, 61-70, 74-78, 82-83, 85, 90-91, 106-107, 115, 155-158, 162-165, 195, 197, 199

Prostate Specific Antigen, 30, 90, 108, 196-198

R
Radiation Therapy, 44, 67, 86, 91, 106
Radiofrequency Ablation, 132, 202-203, 220
Radiotherapy, 38, 78, 108, 155-159, 163
Renal Artery, 128-132, 135
Renal Cell Carcinoma, 63, 67-68, 132-134, 137, 200, 204-205, 220
Renal Oncocytoma, 200-205
Renal Parenchyma, 42, 129, 218
Retroperitoneal Space, 129

S
Sclerosis, 19, 176
Seminal Vesicle, 86, 189
Sertoli Cell-only Syndrome, 92, 98
Sperm Retrieval, 92-93, 95-99
Stratification, 120, 137, 147-150, 152

T
Tadalafil, 29-38
Thromboplastin, 2-3, 18, 20

T
Transrectal Ultrasound, 195, 198-199
Traumatic Penile Amputation, 1, 3

U
Ultrasonography, 46, 107, 123-124, 126-127, 129, 133, 137, 166-167, 170, 173-174, 178
Ureteral Stent, 20, 22-28
Urethrocutaneous Fistula, 138-143, 145, 175
Urethroplasty, 172-175, 177-178
Urinary Diversion, 18, 20-21, 179, 181, 183-184, 186-189, 193
Urinary Incontinence, 29-38, 44-45, 49, 51-53, 55-56, 61, 72-73, 76-79, 82-83, 155, 159-160
Urinary Tract Symptoms, 23, 25, 28, 36, 38, 147
Urolithiasis, 22-24, 28, 127
Urothelial Carcinoma, 100, 102-105, 147, 153

V
Varicocele Vein, 166-167, 169
Varicocelectomy, 166-167, 169, 171

X
X-linked Recessive Disorder, 18